Evidence-based Therapeutic Massage

For Churchill Livingstone:

Publishing Director, Health Professions: Mary Law
Project Development Manager: Katrina Mather
Project Manager: Morven Dean
Design: Judith Wright
Illustration Manager: Bruce Hogarth

EVIDENCE-BASED THERAPEUTIC MASSAGE

A Practical Guide for Therapists

Elizabeth Holey

Chartered Physiotherapist, Principal Lecturer, University of Teesside, UK

Eileen Cook

Chartered Physiotherapist, North Yorkshire, UK

SECOND EDITION

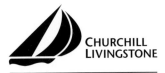
CHURCHILL
LIVINGSTONE

EDINBURGH LONDON NEW YORK OXFORD PHILADELPHIA ST LOUIS SYDNEY TORONTO 2003

CHURCHILL LIVINGSTONE
An imprint of Elsevier Limited

First edition 1997
Second edition 2003
  Reprinted 2004

ISBN 0 443 07230 2   24045675

British Library Cataloguing in Publication Data
A catalogue record for this book is available from the British Library

Library of Congress Cataloging in Publication Data
A catalog record for this book is available from the Library of Congress

Notice
Medical knowledge is constantly changing. Standard safety precautions must be followed, but as new research and clinical experience broaden our knowledge, changes in treatment and drug therapy may become necessary or appropriate. Readers are advised to check the most current product information provided by the manufacturer of each drug to be administered to verify the recommended dose, the method and duration of administration, and contraindications. It is the responsibility of the practitioner, relying on experience and knowledge of the patient, to determine dosages and the best treatment for each individual patient. Neither the Publisher nor the authors assumes any liability for any injury and/or damage to persons or property arising from this publication.

The Publisher

ELSEVIER your source for books, journals and multimedia in the health sciences
www.elsevierhealth.com

The publisher's policy is to use paper manufactured from sustainable forests

Printed in China

Contents

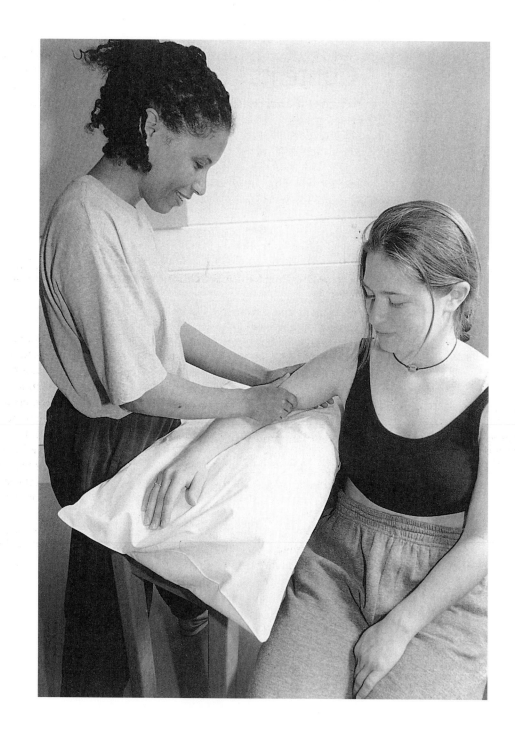

Preface to the Second Edition

Since writing the first edition, there has been much new research into massage. This is variable in quality but, as a whole, offers further evidence of the effectiveness of massage. We have identified and included key research findings and updated clinical approaches within orthodox, integrated and complementary medicine.

Preface to the First Edition

Therapeutic massage is undergoing a regeneration. There is a need for the availability of theoretically based education to enhance the standard of practice both inside and outside orthodox health care. Professionals are progressing toward evidence-based practice to satisfy the requirements for optimum effectiveness. This book has been written to fulfil the need for a massage textbook which presents currently available evidence to guide the therapeutic application of massage. It will assist the student and therapist in extending and justifying the use of massage in health care, whether orthodox or complementary, publicly or privately funded. It encourages the integration of practical massage skills with an understanding of the research-based biological foundation, enabling the application of a problem-oriented approach to therapy.

The anatomy, physiology and pathology included in the text is directly related to massage, so that it informs students of the effects and helps them to appreciate the various massage techniques. There is extensive evaluation of the massage literature to guide and support the student.

Liz Holey
Eileen Cook

Acknowledgements

We are grateful for the assistance of our photographic models, physiotherapy students at the University of Teesside: Alicia Carne, Rosey Foley-Fisher, John Gowland, Wendy Halliburton, Rob MacFadzean, Gavin McAdam, Kendra Smith, Lisa Wood, and to Judy Hume, the photographer.

We acknowledge, with thanks, the help we have received from: Alice Beard, Monica Bono, Belinda Borneo, Emma Bowers, Gill Brent, Nicola Brewin, Pam Crawford, Lisa Fear, Geraldine Forbes, Helen Goldsmith and baby Ellie, Chia Swee Hong, Hilary Illingworth, Jan Kemp, Martyn Jenkins, Shirley Lawrie, Gill Robinson, Martin Watson, Helen Widdowson, Sarah Wood, The University of East Anglia and the photographer, Debbie Besford.

About the Authors

Elizabeth Holey is a Chartered and State Registered physiotherapist. She is Principal Lecturer and head of the physiotherapy subject group at the University of Teesside and is a member of the Chartered Society of Physiotherapists Interested in Massage.

Eileen Cook is a Chartered and State Registered physiotherapist. She is in private practice in North Yorkshire and is a member of the Chartered Society of Physiotherapists Interested in Massage.

Section 1
The Theoretical Basis

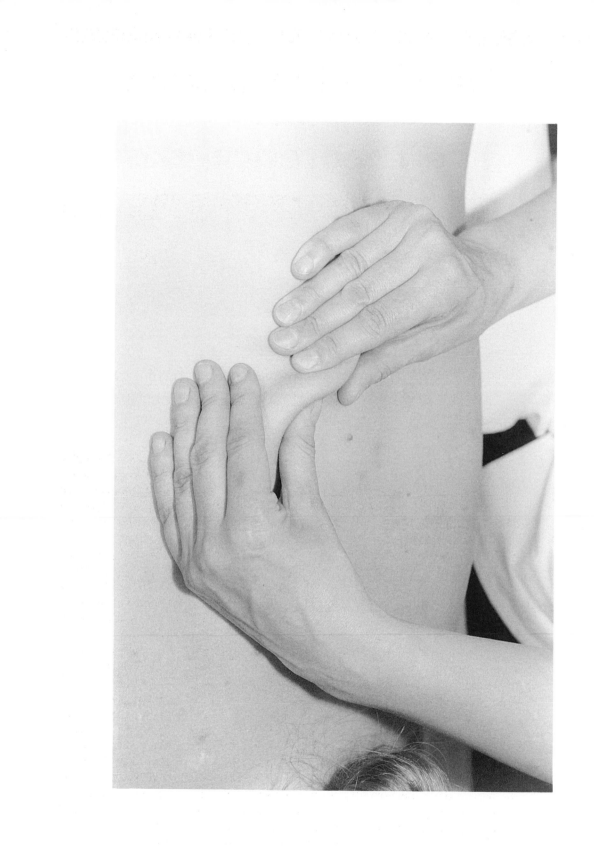

1 Massage in Context

THE PHILOSOPHY OF MASSAGE

A practitioner of massage may choose to be either a technician or a therapist. A technician is competent to administer massage as a manual skill. A therapist, in addition to being competent in the manual techniques, understands human anatomy, physiology, pathology and psychosocial issues, and will apply this knowledge when practising massage. This book is written for those who aspire to be therapists.

The image of massage, as frequently presented in the media, is of a mystical technique which is practised by intuition. Experienced therapists may appear to work intuitively but they are, in reality, applying previously learned and internalized knowledge. It is that vast pool of clinical experience which a proficient therapist draws on during her working day, expanding and modifying her internal memory base as new knowledge is acquired. In its real sense, 'intuition' means immediate unreasoned perception; to state that massage is intuitive is to imply that it can be practised by the use of instinctive actions in the absence of any reasoning.

Instinctual massage is not the way of the professional therapist, whose skills are grounded upon both sound biological and scientific principles and experience gained in clinical practice. This does not invalidate the 'feel-good' factor of massage, which can be as important as the therapeutic effect – massage can both feel good and be of therapeutic value: there is no reason why these two objectives should be mutually exclusive. Of course, these principles need apply only to the professional therapist. Family members, friends and participants in group therapy may have other objectives, such as the giving and receiving of caring touch to promote interaction and feelings of well-being. These aims may also apply to massage with certain client groups, such as people with learning disabilities.

MASSAGE AND HOLISM

Holistic health care practice is an approach to treatment which recognizes the inseparable wholeness of the human organism and views it in the context of its environment, the implication being that every somatic system interacts with every other system and that to isolate one component for therapeutic purposes means that their complex interactions are ignored. Holism is the antithesis of the dualistic Cartesian division of mind and body, which has been integral to the development of Western medicine. Although the concept of holism is not new in global terms, it is only recently that it has been accepted in the West and, in common with other new converts to a cause, we have embraced the idea with enthusiasm without always being aware of the implications. Therapists who work holistically must, by definition, have a detailed knowledge of all the body systems to enable them to coordinate the responses of these systems with a therapeutic intervention. Clearly, this is the opposite of working instinctively and in the absence of a broad knowledge base; massage in those circumstances restricts both the recipient and the therapist to an emotional level only, which is not considered to be holistic.

Properly trained and experienced therapists are able to influence the health of the whole person by using appropriate techniques to achieve the desired effect. For example, they will decide at which interface in the tissues it is necessary to work, light pressure affecting only the epidermis while heavier pressure affects progressively the dermis, fascia, muscle, tendon, ligament, viscera, periosteum of bone and their attendant reflexes. The technique to be utilized will be determined by thorough assessment of the patient, together with the employment of intellectual and clinical skills that are sensitive to both psychosocial and physical needs.

COMPLEMENTARY OR ORTHODOX?

Is massage a complementary or an orthodox therapy? Certainly there is ample evidence that massage has been used, at least since the early twentieth century, as part of mainstream medicine for orthopaedic rehabilitation. In England in 1895 the Society of Trained Masseuses was founded to increase the status of massage and of the professionals who practised the technique under the supervision of medical doctors. In 1907, Araminta Ross, the principal of the Dublin School of Massage, wrote *The Masseuse's Pocket Book*, a small textbook describing the various strokes of massage and how they are to be used for various medical conditions. British trained physiotherapists (physical therapists) have practised massage as a 'core skill' since the inception of physiotherapy as a profession. Despite this history, in many areas of medicine, massage is now regarded as a complementary therapy. In palliative care, for example, it is a therapy which is usually administered by massage/complementary therapists who often train specifically for that purpose (MacDonald 1999). The answer to the question may lie in the definition of complementary therapy: '[it] is diagnosis, treatment and/or prevention which complements mainstream medicine by contributing to a common whole, by satisfying a demand not met by orthodoxy, or by diversifying the conceptual frameworks of medicine' (Ernst et al 1995). This definition has been adopted by the Cochrane Collaboration (Ernst et al 1998). Perhaps it is not the technique or the therapy which is either mainstream or complementary, but the context in which it is used and the perceived status of the therapist using it – in other words, the system of medicine in which it resides and the approach of the individual therapist. Medical systems are embedded in a cultural framework which has an overriding influence on the scientific perspective. For example, there are many similarities between Chinese, Thai and Japanese traditional medicines; therapies which have been regarded as mainstream in the East for centuries are looked upon as complementary in the West because they do not easily or immediately fit into the Western cultural medical framework.

In the USA and some European countries, massage may be used professionally only by those with medical training or those who have undergone massage training and have been licensed to practise, while in other countries anyone may practise, even without training. It would not be in the interest of massage as a dynamic and evolving therapy, or in the interests of society, if massage were to be monopolized by a particular group. If the practice of massage were to be confined to one profession with a relatively narrow interest, its various branches would atrophy and the facility for the exchange of ideas would be lost. This opinion should not, however, be taken as a charter for those who wish to arrive at a quick method of 'practising bodywork'. A good attitude, a caring disposition and a desire to help people are not of themselves qualifications for the practice of massage. The way forward is to acknowledge that by creating factions the path to new discoveries may be obstructed. Adapting to the demands of the time, accepting that the needs of society are changing health care practice and that people require massage for many different reasons is a realistic approach. Being responsive to the views of other groups and professions, but furthering the practice of massage through the scientific method will justify public spending on it and, thus, safeguard its widespread availability. In addition, those who practise massage in a therapeutic context need to be adequately trained.

WHAT IS MASSAGE?

There are many definitions of massage. Reproduced here are a number of published definitions that highlight the variety of opinions which abound:

> Massage is the term used to express certain scientific manipulations which are performed by the hands of the operator upon the body of the patient. It is a means used for creating energy where such has become exhausted, from whatsoever cause, and is a natural method of restoring the part, either locally or generally injured, to its normal condition . . .
> *(Ross 1907)*

> . . . massage may be described as a scientific way of treating some forms of disease, by external manipulations, applied in a variety of ways to the soft tissues of the body. There are many varieties in the technique of massage, but the manipulations in general may be classified as follows . . . [lists *the techniques of Swedish massage*]
> *(Goodall-Copestake 1926)*

> . . . the scientific manipulation of the soft tissues of the body, as apart from mere rubbing . . .
> *(Prosser 1941)*

> . . . the hand motions practised on the surface of the living body with a therapeutic goal.
>
> *(Boigey 1955)*

> . . . manoeuvres performed by the hands of a therapist on the skin of a patient and through the skin on the subcutaneous tissues. Massage manipulations may be stationary or progressive; they may be variable in intensity of pressure exerted, surface area treated and frequency of application.
>
> *(Boni & Walthard 1956)*

> . . . massage is the aware and conscious manipulation of the soft tissues of the body for therapeutic purposes.
>
> *(Westland 1993)*

The authors offer the following definition for *therapeutic* massage:

> Massage is the manipulation of the soft tissues of the body by a trained therapist as a component of a holistic therapeutic intervention.

This is an inclusive definition which embraces the many varieties of manual therapy that are commonly associated with massage, for example Swedish, classical, segmental, connective tissue, aromatherapy and shiatsu; it identifies the integrative nature of the therapy but restricts massage, as a therapeutic intervention, to those who are competent to administer it.

Origins of Massage

Stroking and rubbing of the tissues probably evolved from the instinctive contact that is observed in other mammals. At some time during the course of evolution it is likely that intellectual development led to massage becoming integrated into folk medicine and later into systems of medicine.

The word massage derives from the Arabic *mass*, meaning to press. Many ancient civilizations developed a system of therapeutic massage, notably in China, India, Arabia, Greece, Italy and Egypt. Numerous references survive from these cultures which indicate that massage was used for various medical conditions.

The emergence of therapeutic massage in the West is attributed to French missionaries who, upon returning from China in the early nineteenth century, brought with them *The Cong Fou of the Tao-Tse*, which are Chinese medical writings dating from about 2700 BC. The translation of these writings into French is the reason some massage terminology is still in French to the present day, for example effleurage (from *effleurer*, meaning to skim over), petrissage (from *pétrir*, meaning to knead) and tapotement (from *tapoter*, meaning to pat or tap).

The popularity of massage grew when it was incorporated into a system of medical gymnastics by Per Henrik Ling (1776–1839), who founded a central institute of gymnastics in Stockholm, Sweden, in 1813. Ling's system was published by Augustus Georgii, a pupil of Ling, in 1847 under the title *Kinestherapie*, and the system we now know as Swedish massage began to spread in Europe. Institutes of Swedish massage were founded in London in 1838 and in New York City in 1916.

Massage became a popular treatment in health spas throughout Europe from the mid-nineteenth to early twentieth century. The interest of the medical establishment was aroused by the work of Just Lucas-Championniere

(1843–1913), who used massage in the management of fractures. This period also saw the publication of several notable books on massage, among them *Traité de la Massothérapie* (Weber 1891), *Technik der Massage* (Hoffa 1897) and *Practical Treatise on Massage* (Graham 1884). Hoffa's massage was based upon the now classical techniques of Swedish massage. His system emphasized the treatment of individual muscles or muscle groups, rather than specific body regions or the whole body, which is the more usual approach in other systems.

In the USA the technique of massage was advanced by Mary McMillan, director of physical therapy at Harvard Medical School, and later by Gertrude Beard, director of physical therapy at North-Western University, Evanston, Illinois. In England, in 1895, the Society of Trained Masseuses was founded to increase the status of massage and of the professionals who practised the technique. Further credibility for massage within medicine was established by Dr J. B. Mennell (1890–1957), author of a work entitled *Physical Treatment by Movement, Manipulation and Massage*, first published in 1917.

Interest in massage continued to grow in Germany following new discoveries concerning somatic reflex zones. This led to the publication of Dicke's *Meine Bindegewebsmassage* in 1953 and Gläser and Dalicho's *Segmentmassage: Massage Reflektorischer Zonen* in 1955.

This short summary is the history of massage only in so far as the West is concerned. As with the history of anything, it is confined to information that has been preserved in the form of texts which, in this case, are usually derived from the orthodox medical establishment. There is probably an alternative history of massage in folk medicine. In addition, massage in China did not stop evolving when it was discovered by Westerners, but only in recent years have translations become available of massage techniques that are currently used in China. Typically, a practitioner of massage in China is a doctor with at least 5 years' training in both Western and Traditional Chinese medicine and whose practice is informed by the results of prolific recent research studies. Similarly, Russian medical massage is a well-developed system; however, the authors are unaware of any Russian medical massage texts that have been translated into English.

RECENT TRENDS

The interest in massage within the orthodox medical establishment has been variable throughout the latter part of the twentieth century. Conversely, within the field of alternative and complementary medicine, vigorous enthusiasm for the modality has been awakened via the growth of the human potential movement and a consequent interest in natural therapies. The American Massage Therapy Association was founded in 1943 and has continued to promote massage and training for massage therapists. Although there is no unification of massage training in the UK outside orthodox medicine, there has been a growth of interest in massage as a profession, and practitioners often link it with various Eastern therapies and spiritual, psychological and energetic forms of healing. Massage is increasingly being used by nurses within the health care environment, and many papers on the technique are published in the nursing literature. In the USA there is a thriving National Association of Nurse

Massage Therapists. In the UK the Association of Chartered Physiotherapists Interested in Massage has recognized clinical interest group status within the Chartered Society of Physiotherapy.

Since the 1980s there has been a persistent societal trend demanding the availability of massage, which indicates that the effects of massage are valued by recipients. During the same period, pressures on the health economy have precipitated a move away from the empirical basis of therapy towards evidence-based practice. As a result, although it has the support of popular demand, the scientific foundation of massage as a therapy must continue to expand if it is to survive changes in health care policy.

KEY POINTS

- Therapeutic massage cannot be practised by instinct alone.

- Holism recognizes the inseparable wholeness of the human organism.

- Therapists who practise holistic therapeutic massage need expertise in human sciences and psychosocial skills.

- The practice of massage is embedded within orthodox medicine and has, more recently, become known as a complementary therapy.

- Continuing research is required to maintain massage as an evidence-based therapy.

REFERENCES

Boigey M 1955 Manuel de massage. Cited in: Licht S (ed) 1960 Massage, manipulation and traction. Waverly Press, Baltimore, MD

Boni A, Walthard K 1956 Massage et cinesterapie des rhumatismes abarticulaires. Cited in: Licht S (ed) 1960 Massage, manipulation and traction. Waverly Press, Baltimore, MD

Dicke, E 1953 Meine Bindegewebsmassage. Hippokrates, Stuttgart

Ernst E, Resch K L, Mills S et al 1995 Complementary medicine: a definition [letter]. British Journal of General Practice 45: 506

Ernst E, Rand J, Stevinson C 1998 Complementary therapies for depression: an overview. Archives of General Psychiatry 55(11): 1026–1032

Gläser O, Dalicho A W 1955 Segmentmassage: Massage Reflektorischer Zonen. Georg Thieme, Leipzig

Goodall-Copestake B M 1926 The theory and practice of massage. Lewis, London

Graham D 1884 Practical treatise on massage. Wood, New York

Hoffa A 1897 Technik der Massage. Verlag Von Ferdinand Ernke, Stuttgart

MacDonald G 1999 Medicine hands. Massage therapy for people with cancer. Findhorn Press, Scotland

Mennell J B 1945 Physical treatment by movement, manipulation and massage, 5th edn. Blakiston, Philadelphia, PA

Prosser E M 1941 A manual of Massage and movements, 2nd edn. Faber and Faber, London

Ross A 1907 Masseuse's pocket book. Scientific Press, London

Weber A S 1891 Traité de la massothérapie, Paris

Westland G 1993 Massage as a therapeutic tool. British Journal of Occupational Therapy 56(4): 129–134; 56(5): 177–180

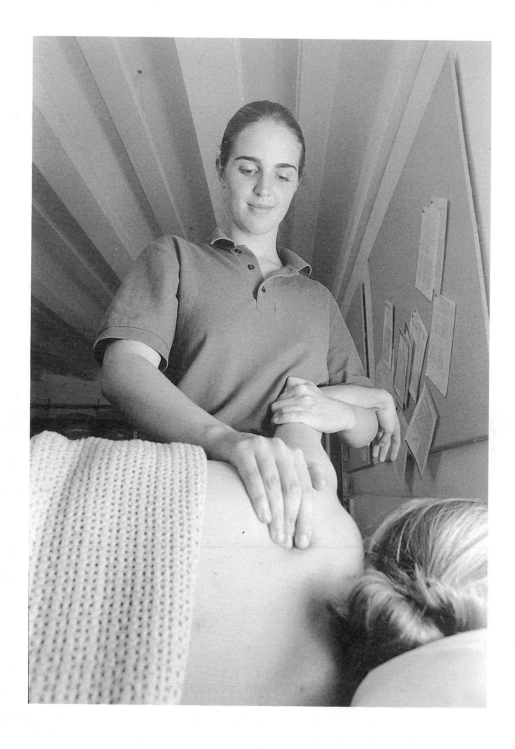

2 A Biological Basis

Touching, stroking and rubbing the skin is an integral part of our lives. Through these actions, we communicate and transmit feelings and emotions to one another. Skin rubbing and caressing can become more formalized and take the form of a massage, to aid relaxation and promote a feeling of well-being. For the massage to progress to a more specific therapeutic outcome it must be directed towards a more specific purpose and be aimed at promoting physical and psychological change. It must therefore be based on sound theoretical principles. The structure, function and dysfunction of the body must be understood so that clinical decisions may be made and appropriate techniques selected to induce desirable change. This chapter discusses a range of anatomical, physiological and pathological issues, providing an essential basis for the therapeutic use of massage. The chapter covers topic areas specific to massage; extrinsic material can be found in greater detail in other texts.

SKIN

The skin is the tough, waterproof, external surface of the body. What makes the skin such a fascinating structure is its ability to combine a protective and insulating function of great physiological significance with an important role in communication. It conveys emotional responses through its vascular changes (flushing with pleasure or embarrassment, blanching with shock or fear, for example); it plays a part in expressing words or emotions through its transmission of the coordinated contractions of the underlying muscles of facial expression and is essential for tactile and sexual communication. By being sensitive to these reactions, the therapist may learn a considerable amount about the patient's psychological and emotional state and can modify massage treatment subtly and appropriately. By using her awareness of these properties, the therapist can communicate attitudes that are essential to obtaining trust and relaxation – friendliness, approachability, concern and understanding – even before touching the skin, thereby enhancing her personal approach.

Skin varies in thickness between 0.5 and 2–3 mm. It is of vital importance for survival: it forms a protective layer for deeper structures and is a richly innervated sensory organ (the largest in the body) to feed information about the environment to the nervous system, thus acting as a warning system and protective mechanism. It regulates temperature due to its neurovascular mechanisms and insulating properties (fat, found in the hypodermis, conducts heat two-thirds less efficiently than other tissues); prevents fluid loss; allows excretion and absorption of substances; and acts as a chemical and bacterial barrier. The rate of blood flow into the vascular plexi associated with the skin varies from 0% to 30% of total cardiac output. It is controlled by the sympathetic response to core or environmental temperature changes, which alters the degree of vasoconstriction of the arterioles and arteriovenous anastomoses feeding into the venous plexi of the skin. This changing of blood flow affects core body temperature as heat is then lost from the body by radiation, a composite of conduction whereby heat is lost into anything the body touches (for example, a chair or bed), and is thus self-limiting, and convection whereby heat is removed as the surrounding air circulates. Heat is consequently lost through evaporation: 0.58 kilocalories of heat are lost for each gram of water that evaporates. It is therefore important to cover any parts of the body not directly involved in the massage or that are awaiting massage, to avoid excessive heat loss during a treatment session.

The first thing to be noticed by the massage student when touching the skin is that it is usually soft and, in most parts of the body, smooth. This top outer layer which can be touched is the *epidermis*, the epithelium of the skin. It consists of keratinized, stratified, squamous epithelium which is arranged in five laminae according to their cell type (Fig. 2.1). It consists of two zones: the deeper is known as the *zona germinativa*, a single layer of columnar cells, and the more superficial zone is the *stratum basale*. Cells are continuously being lost from the surface and replaced from the deeper layer.

This natural process occurs constantly, but certain events will speed it up. Friction on the skin, for example, caused by the clothes when dressing or during massage, results in desquamation. Massage will often remove the top layer, which is readily replaced. This occurs when skin may be seen to 'rub off' or may be left on the treatment plinth following treatment. This is a normal and painless process. It tends to be excessive if the skin is very dry or visibly flaky (following removal of a plaster cast, for example) and can be reduced by the application of an oil-based lubricant. In severe cases, a soap and oil solution is beneficial. The epidermal cells become gradually flatter and more keratinized as they move to the surface. Keratin is important for hydration of the skin. Dry skin has reduced water content and the keratin allows swelling when the skin is wet. This is useful information to have when selecting the appropriate media for massage: the choice of oils, creams or talcs should be based not only on the type and purpose of massage but also on the individual skin quality. Keratin provides protection, and skin that has been soaked and has a

FIGURE 2.1 *Layers of the skin and circulatory plexi. Reproduced, with permission, from 'Layers of the skin with circulatory plexi', Physiotherapy 1995, Vol. 81. Reproduced, with permission, from Schuh (1994).*

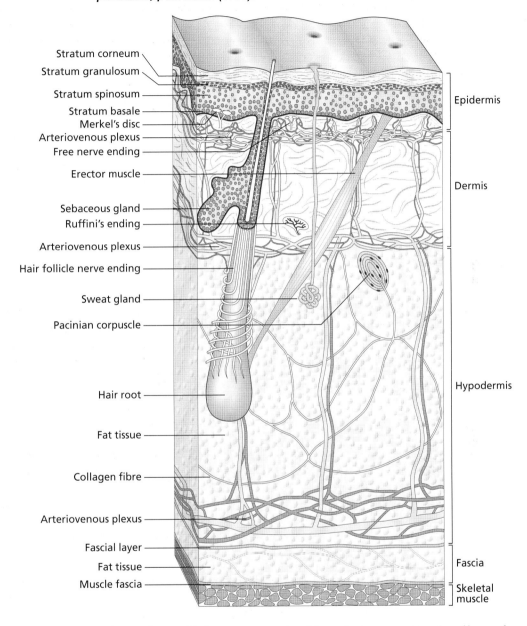

whitened, wrinkled appearance should not be massaged as the effects of treatment on the superficial layer will be difficult to predict and monitor.

The *dermis* lies beneath the epidermis and forms most of the skin thickness. Whereas the epidermis is composed mostly of cells, the dermis contains collagen and elastin fibres, which give the skin its mechanical properties. The dermis is flexible and varies in thickness from the dense layer on the soles of the feet to the thin layer of the eyelids. It is composed of connective tissue (see below) which is arranged in two layers: the papillary layer is superficial to the deeper reticular layer.

The more superficial papillary layer of the dermis connects the epidermis with the dermis. Tiny conical projections, the papillae, project into the under-surface of the epidermis. These are sensitive and vascular, and range from being sparse to lying in dense lines which are seen as ridges on the surface of the skin, for example on the pads of the fingers and toes.

The reticular layer contains mainly thick collagen fibres (for strength) inter-spersed with reticular and elastin fibres (the latter for stretch) which form a tough interwoven layer. The directional lay of the skin in different parts of the body results from some of these fibres lying parallel to the skin surface. Skin is always under tension and the lines along which this tension lies are known as Langer's or Kraissl's lines (Fig. 2.2). They are important because they dictate the natural variation in tension when the skin resists movement and when it heals. If a cut in the skin follows the tension lines, scarring will be minimal – an important principle utilized by surgeons. The fibroblast cells (which secrete the precursor for collagen) and phagocytes, important in immune defence mechanisms, are found in this layer.

The wrinkling in the skin around the nipple and scrotum is caused by the presence of smooth muscle fibres in the dermis. Stretch marks (striae gravi-darum) follow partial rupture of the fibres of the reticular layer. It is com-monly thought that this follows stretching of the skin in pregnancy, or fat

FIGURE 2.2   *Tension lines of the skin. Reproduced, with permission, from Last (1984).*

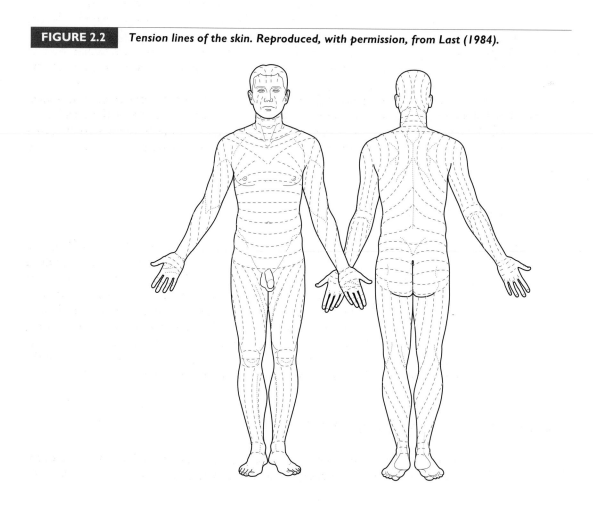

deposition. This does not explain the common occurrence of these marks in thin people or the nulliparous, often on or above the sacrum, which could indicate weakening of the dermis due to the action of hormones or disease. As these marks show some fragility of the tissues, care should be taken when handling them. In particular, this tissue should not be overstretched by manipulation, to avoid possible further rupture of fibres and more extensive marking.

CIRCULATION IN THE SKIN

Blood supply to glabrous (non-hairy) skin is maintained by arteriovenous anastomoses, found in the deeper layers of the dermis. They are surrounded by smooth muscle, the glomera, which maintain blood supply to the skin, despite variations in blood flow due to vascular responses aimed at maintaining body temperature.

Blood vessels within skin are found lying in and running between three flat horizontal plexi. Small arteries pierce the superficial fascia and form a horizontal plexus known as the *rete cutaneum* at the interface between the dermis and superficial fascia. It gives off vessels to supply the adipose tissue, glands and follicles. Some vessels reach the junction between the reticular and papillary layers of the dermis where they form another flat plexus, the *rete subpapillare* or *superficial plexus*. From here, capillaries supply the dermal papillae before travelling back to the venous plexus immediately below the superficial plexus, draining into the flat *intermediate plexus* in the middle of the reticular layer of the dermis which connects to the *deep laminar venous plexus* at the dermis–superficial fascia junction.

As the vessels tend to lie in plexi at the different interfaces of skin, movement in the form of manipulation *between* layers will influence the circulation. Capillaries running *through* the layers will be similarly influenced by gross movements of the tissue as a whole. This is discussed in more detail in Chapter 3.

SUBCUTANEOUS TISSUE

The layer of connective tissue under the dermis is adipose (fat) tissue and may be termed the hypodermis or subcutis. It is a layer of superficial fascia in which fibres from the reticular layer of the dermis extend to lie in bundles between fat lobules, giving it its sometimes characteristic appearance. It varies in density and thickness in individuals; for example, it is generally thicker in women than in men, and varies in different parts of the body. This layer is important in that, apart from its insulating properties, it gives mobility to the skin. One of the effects of massage is that it maintains or restores this mobility, particularly at the tissue interfaces. The sliding of the layers on each other can easily be felt.

INNERVATION OF THE SKIN

Skin has an important sensory function, which gives it a role in communication, reproduction, protection and coordinated movement. Responsibility for this is held by the many nerve endings that are responsive to sensory information. This is transmitted along nerves of the peripheral nervous system to the central nervous system, where it is interpreted and a response is made. The area of innervation of any one nerve fibre varies considerably, with overlap between the receptive fields of two adjacent nerve fibres. In the fingers, for example, each single fibre supplies a small area of skin. This is accompanied by a low sensitivity threshold and a high degree of spatial localization. This means that the nerve is easily triggered by sensory stimuli and the brain can pinpoint the location of the stimulus very precisely. This high degree of sensitivity is particularly marked on the lips and external genitalia. On an area such as the back, however, a single nerve fibre will supply a larger area of skin, the nerve has a higher sensitivity threshold and the brain is less precise in its spatial localization.

These nerves penetrate the superficial fascia and ramify through the dermis. They lie in plexi in the papillary layer of the dermis and around the hair follicles. The nerve endings are predominantly myelinated and non-myelinated 'free' nerve endings which are found in the dermis and lower parts of the epidermis. They monitor temperature and some pain. In addition there are specialized end-organs which include:

- Merkel discs which respond to *shear* forces and *vertical* pressure, which are magnified by hair follicles and structural ridges grouped into Iggo dome receptors, on the underside of the epithelium.
- Meissner's corpuscles, found in the dermal papillae. These are rapidly adapting mechanoreceptors which are responsive to *mechanical deformation*.
- Pacinian corpuscles in the deeper layers of the skin and superficial and deep fascia. They are innervated by a single axon only, and respond to a narrow range of *vibration* frequencies and rapid changes within the tissues.
- Ruffini's corpuscles in the deeper dermis and hypodermis respond to stretch. They have an important tactile function.

The endings show specificity as a result of their differential sensitivities, and interpretation of the modality of sensation is due to the location of their termination in the brain. The endings listed above are those which have most relevance to massage. They are stimulated by mechanical deformation which stretches the membrane, thus opening the channels through which ions pass to depolarize the nerve fibre. The Meissner's corpuscle consists of a central nerve fibre surrounded by terminal nerve filaments within an elongated capsule. The construction of the Pacinian corpuscle consists of a central nerve fibre surrounded by capsular layers (Fig. 2.3). The fibre is distorted in various ways by compression of any part of the capsule. The fluid in the corpuscle immediately redistributes so that the deformation is no longer transmitted to the central fibre until the force is removed. Thus, repetitive forces rather than continuous ones will affect the nervous system more strongly; this demonstrates the importance of the continuous movement in massage.

Sensory stimuli are carried in nerve fibre types II (type A β and γ), III (type A δ) and IV (type C), which are the smaller, slower conducting types. The stimulus enters the spinal cord via the dorsal horn and diverges or converges via neuronal pools. It passes to the brain through either (1) the dorsal column, crossing to the opposite side in the medulla, to the medial lemniscus and the thalamus, or (2) by crossing to the opposite side of the spinal cord, passing

FIGURE 2.3   *Somatic sensory receptors – exteroceptors. Reproduced, with permission, from Thibodeau & Patton (1999).*

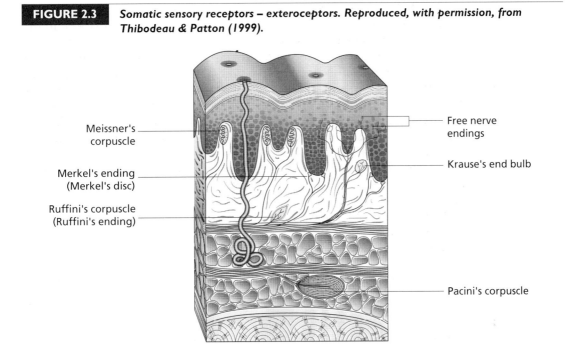

through the anterior and lateral white columns to the brainstem and thalamus. The former is for rapid, sensitive transmission of sensation and the latter for a slightly cruder response. The thalamus relays the sensory information to the cerebral cortex for localization, interpretation and controlled response.

The epidermis and dermis filter mechanical and thermal stimuli, which attenuate in different ways as they are transmitted through the layers. This is probably because different stimuli need to be strongest at specific depths in order to have maximum impact on sensory end-organs.

CONNECTIVE TISSUE

Skin is a type of connective tissue. The connective tissue that lies *under* the skin is important as a base to provide attachment to skin, providing both anchorage and mobility. These tissues are all formed from the embryonic mesoderm (middle layer) and all are basically composed of the same constituents. The presence of specialized cells, or an alteration in the predominance of any constituent in a particular tissue, ensures that the different connective tissues are adapted and well suited to their purpose. Thus, the appearance and properties of the different connective tissues vary significantly. They range from fascia, ligament and tendon to specialized types including cartilage and bone.

The cells of connective tissue lie within a matrix which is formed by fibres lying in ground substance. The fibres are collagen, reticulin and elastin fibres, the first offering resistance to stress while the last allows for stretch. There are more than 10 types of collagen.

Fibrillar collagen types I and III are the most relevant here, being found in tendon, skin, ligament and skin vessels. These types have the greatest stiffness (see below). The ground substance is composed of water and organic molecules, predominantly glycosaminoglycans (GAGs). These molecules have water-binding properties and are responsible for the amount of water present in the tissue. Thus they have a role in the diffusion of molecules through the tissue, notably incoming nutrients and out-going metabolites. They are also important for communication between cells and for their adhesion to collagen. Their structure makes them springy and so able to absorb shock. This mechanism is enhanced by their being held under tension by the surrounding collagen fibres. In a specialized connective tissue such as cartilage, this springiness allows compression when weight-bearing and restoration of shape when the weight is removed. In the superficial tissues, these molecules allow take-up or removal of liquid, which appears to be partly under hormonal control. Skin, therefore, can be 'dry' or well hydrated, terms that refer to the skin itself rather than its surface. This can be palpated as a change in consistency and loss of compliancy of skin and is different from the presence of fluid in the tissue spaces, which gives the skin a 'spongy' feel. Hyaluranon has a role in hydration and enables gliding movement within the tissue (Culav et al 1999).

The cells of connective tissue are:

- Fibroblasts: synthesize collagen and reticulin, important in repair
- Macrophages: phagocytic
- Plasma cells: produce antibodies, present in large numbers in pathological states
- Mast cells: in loose connective tissue, release inflammatory agents of histamine, serotonin, heparin
- Fat cells: mobilization of the contained fat is under nervous, hormonal and chemical control
- Pigment cells (chromatophores): in the corium, contain melanin.

BIOMECHANICS OF CONNECTIVE TISSUE

The main constituent of connective tissue is collagen, the function of which is to resist axial tension and which has been shown to exhibit standard stress–strain behaviour. Collagen is derived from its precursor procollagen, synthesized by the fibroblast. Procollagen becomes tropocollagen, which in turn forms microfibrils. Under the electron microscope, collagen fibres are seen to be arranged in bundles and have a crimped appearance, thought to be due to molecular attachment. There are several types of collagen. Type I collagen (in dermis and fascia) consists of three polypeptide chains, coiled in a left-handed helix; these helical chains are coiled together in a right-handed helix. This type gives resistance to tension and provides filtration and support. The basal lamina of epithelia contains type IV collagen, which synthesizes epithelial cells. Hydrogen cross-links are formed between chains, and also between molecules, giving stability at fibril level and between fibrils, assisting in the formation of collagen fibres. They allow the tissue to function under mechanical stress.

The orientation of fibres depends on the stresses to which the fibre is subjected. Connective tissue needs to be pliable yet very strong. The stress–strain

FIGURE 2.4 *Typical stress–strain curve for connective tissue. Stress = force applied per unit area; strain = proportional elongation; P_{max} = maximum load point.*

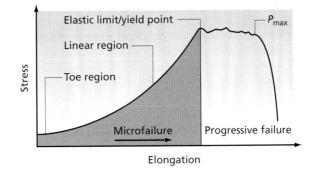

behaviour of biological materials may be demonstrated by a *stress–strain curve* (Fig. 2.4). These have been plotted for various types and constituents of connective tissue, the exact behaviour differing slightly in each:

Stress = force applied per unit area
Strain = proportional elongation

When longitudinal stress is applied, the tissue responds firstly by elongation. This occurs in the *toe region* of the curve and is thought to be due to a straightening out of the crimping in the fibres. It may also be due to some interfibrillar sliding and shear of ground substance which flows between the fibres. Stress and strain are linearly proportional up to the *proportionality limit*. Elongation that occurs in this region will not be permanent. The *elastic limit* is the point to which maximum stress may be applied without permanent deformation. As the loading continues, a greater force is required to increase elongation. This is due to the fact that the tissue becomes stiffer.

The next part of the curve is the *linear region*. Microfailure begins to occur in some of the fibre bundles, but the tissue retains its external appearance of continuity. The end of the linear region is known as the *yield point* of the tissue. Here, elongation (or yielding) can occur without a corresponding increase in load. Once beyond this point, major failure of fibre bundles occurs. The external appearance changes, and the smooth outline is lost; this is termed 'necking'. The same effect is seen, for example, when an elastic band is overstretched or becomes overused and its width changes and appears uneven. It loses strength but still has gross continuity. When the *maximum load point* is reached P_{max}, complete rupture occurs. Its position on the curve designates the rupture strength.

Most changes that occur as a result of massage are in the toe region of the curve. The therapist should take care not to overstretch the tissues, thereby causing damage to the internal structure of connective tissue fibres. Each massage student should learn to be sensitive to the 'end-feel' of the tissues (see Ch. 5). Any permanent deformation is termed *plastic* and occurs with microfailure – breakage of cross-bridges. These are molecular bonds which bind adjacent fibres together. They are broken and then reform further along the fibres, enabling the fibres to reposition themselves in relation to each other, resulting in increased length of the tissue. The undamaged fibres absorb a greater proportion of the load as a new length is established, which reflects the balance between elastic recoil and the resistance of the water and GAGs to compression.

Biological materials also have viscosity, a property of fluids of resistance to flow, and elasticity, a property of solids. They are therefore said to be *visco-elastic*. The response is dependent on how quickly the load is applied or removed (regardless of the size of the strain). The quicker the repetitive loading and unloading occurs, the stiffer the material becomes, as there is less chance for the ground substance to flow between fibres. This continuous loading and unloading causes friction and a rise in temperature, as energy is dissipated as heat when the tissue is returned to its original length. This quality is known as *hysteresis*. Consideration should be given to the speed at which massage is undertaken and the therapist should be sensitive to how stiff the tissues feel. If an increase in tissue mobility is aimed at, the progression of treatment should be partly dictated by this stiffness and the rate at which any lengthening is felt to occur.

If a low constant or repetitive *load* is maintained over a long period, the elongation is by *creep* whereas if the *length* is held constant, elongation occurs by *relaxation*. Excess fluid in the tissues which remains for a long period of time, for example in chronic oedema or lymphoedema, will stretch and produce a creep effect on the surrounding tissues and they will not be restored to their original shape following removal of the fluid. This is important as connective tissue helps to maintain the fluid pressure in the tissue spaces. If the pressure reduces, due to stretching of connective tissue as a result of creep, the pressure within the vessels may be comparatively greater and external pressure must be applied to prevent swelling. For example, pressure stockings or sleeves may be worn to maintain the beneficial effects of oedema massage.

Massage produces low repetitive load over the medium term and may cause a non-permanent creep response. Biomechanical study of connective tissue indicates that the quicker tissue is loaded, the stiffer it becomes owing to its visco-elastic properties. Dry tissue produces more friction, and is known to lose compliance, elongating less readily than when the tissue has good water content. Thus, the rate of massage should be suitable for the type and condition of the tissue.

Goldfarb et al (2001) compared the effects of low-force and high-force rehabilitation on collagen synthesis and extracellular matrix maturation in sutured intrasynovial flexor tendons in dogs. They found that higher force rehabilitation did not accelerate healing, as no changes were seen in the biomechanical composition of the healing tendon over a period of 6 weeks. This suggests that there is no advantage in applying heavy stresses to the tissues in relation to healing speed.

The implications of tissue biomechanics in the different phases of healing are discussed later.

FLUID SYSTEM DYNAMICS

The therapist must be able to recognize subtle changes in the fluid content of the tissues. One of the first things she notices when performing any form of deep massage in the tissues is that the fluid balance between the circulation and the tissue spaces changes, sometimes rapidly. To understand how the squeezing, pulling and stretching manipulations affect the tissue fluid, it is necessary first to examine tissue fluid dynamics.

The fluid of the body serves to transmit nutrients and to bathe structures, ensuring that the correct chemical and electrolyte balance is maintained around the cells. In some instances this is crucial – around the heart, for example, which cannot function correctly without its muscle cells being bathed in a perfect balance of electrolytes. It may appear, simply, that newly oxygenated blood is pumped from the heart and carried in the arteries, arterioles and capillaries (in order of descending size) and, when deoxygenated, returns for replenishment via the capillaries, venules and veins. However, the mechanism by which specific components of the blood flow into and out of the tissues, and maintenance of the delicate balance of fluid inside and outside the tissue spaces, warrant closer examination.

Fluid movement occurs either by diffusion or osmosis along concentration gradients, or by flow along pressure gradients. In diffusion or flow, water flows down the gradient, from an area of high concentration or pressure to one of lower concentration or pressure. However, in osmosis, water flows up the gradient, towards the side of the most concentrated solute. This physiological concept of functional gradient is an attempt by the body to achieve balance and uniformity. So, when two non-uniform areas exist, either in concentration or pressure, fluid will move to try to level them out.

After fluid has been filtered by the capillaries, it returns to the circulation by the venous end of the capillary loop. A small proportion is returned via the lymphatics. There are two key areas involved in maintenance of tissue fluid balance: the capillary loop and its surrounding environment, and the lymphatic vessel. The capillary loop has an arteriolar end and a venule end. This demonstrates that both sections of the blood vessel network are, in fact, continuous and the moment at which blood *coming from* the heart becomes blood *going to* the heart depends on a subtle pressure change.

The important mechanism by which equilibrium of fluid within the blood vessels and tissue spaces is maintained was first described by Starling. It is the mechanism by which the inherent leakiness of the capillaries through their semipermeable membranes is counteracted to maintain the volume of circulating plasma.

To understand these pressure changes, it is necessary to examine the blood, which is composed of plasma (clear liquid containing substances in solution or suspension), red and white cells, and plasma proteins (such as prothrombin and fibrinogen). Nutrients, for example oxygen, enter the tissue spaces from the bloodstream by diffusion, until concentration gradients are equal on both sides of the capillary wall. Plasma proteins are too large to leak out of the tiny pores in the capillary vessel walls and therefore create a pressure (known as osmotic pressure) inside the vessel. If you imagine liquid flowing into an empty vessel, its ease of passage will depend on the relationship between the quantity of liquid and the size of the vessel. If the vessel contains large particles, this effectively reduces the space available for the liquid to occupy and increases the pressure inside the vessel. This is exactly the effect of the plasma proteins. In some situations, they are able to leak out into the tissue spaces when the vessels dilate, which causes the pores in the vessel walls to increase in size. Adipose tissue contains type I capillaries which have uninterrupted membranes

FIGURE 2.5 *Diffusion of fluid and dissolved substances between the capillary and interstitial fluid spaces. Reproduced, with permission, from Guyton (1991), p. 172.*

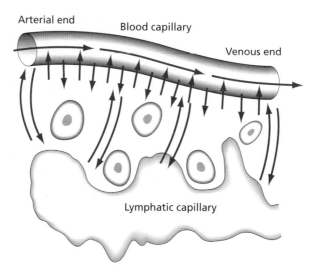

with 'pores' in them. The pressure from the fluid itself is known as the hydrostatic pressure. It is slight outside the vessel, but greater inside owing to the pumping of the heart. This pressure is opposed by the osmotic (or colloid osmotic, or oncotic) pressure, which is a reabsorption pressure resulting from the fluid itself which forces fluid back in the vessel. If the osmotic pressure inside the vessel and the hydrostatic pressure outside the vessel are equal, then fluid flow will not occur. In reality, at the arterial end of the capillary loop, the net result of these different pressures tends to produce an outward force, moving fluid into the tissue spaces. However, at the venous end of the capillary the net pressure tends to move fluid into the capillary, thus maintaining normal balance (Fig. 2.5). The development of oedema and its implications will be discussed subsequently. These pressures can be influenced by compression or movement of the tissue, as in massage, and natural pumping mechanisms can be enhanced mechanically in this way.

THE LYMPHATICS

The pressure in loose subcutaneous tissue is negative, maintained at −3 mmHg as a result of the pumping action of the lymphatics. One-tenth of fluid is removed via the lymphatics rather than the venous end of the capillary. Proteins and other substances of higher molecular size that leak into the interstitial spaces cannot return into the capillaries because of the adverse concentration gradient, and must return via a different route – the lymphatic system. If massage is to enhance this effect and improve this system, it needs to be employed in the correct way; thus an understanding of the lymphatics is necessary for successful massage.

The lymph system mirrors the vascular system in structure. Tiny lymph capillaries have blind endings in the tissue spaces which drain into veins. They form a mesh-like system in the tissue spaces, and are slightly larger than vas-

FIGURE 2.6 *Structure of a typical lymphatic capillary. Reproduced, with permission, from Thibodeau & Patton (1999).*

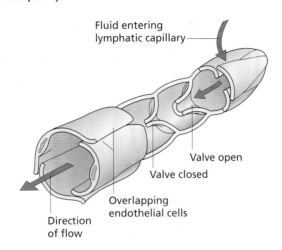

cular capillaries. They are composed of a single layer of endothelial cells, the basement membrane often being absent. The capillaries unite to form larger vessels and have a coating of connective tissue outside the endothelium. The larger collecting trunks resemble small veins structurally, with smooth muscle present in their walls, which is important for the transmission of fluid. Unidirectional flow is maintained by the presence of semilunar, paired, one-way valves, which are found in higher numbers than in veins (Fig. 2.6).

The movement of lymph occurs via the following chain of events. Filtration pressure in the tissue spaces is caused by filtration of fluid from the vascular capillaries. The surrounding muscle pump effect compresses lymph vessels and lymph moves as directed by the valves. Flow is enhanced by respiratory movements, creating a negative pressure in the brachiocephalic veins, the pumping effect of muscle contraction and possibly arterial pulsing. Sympathetic stimulation causes contraction of the smooth muscle in the vessel walls, particularly near the valves. The endothelial cells of the lymphatic capillaries are attached, by anchoring filaments, to the surrounding connective tissue. When fluid enters the tissues they swell and the anchoring filaments pull the capillary open, allowing fluid to flow between the cells. This effect can also result from the mechanical deformation that occurs during massage. The overlapping cells produce a valve-like effect by which fluid can flow in, but not out, as the back-pressure closes the flap. The rate of flow is determined by the interstitial fluid pressure and lymphatic pump activity.

The factors increasing lymphatic flow are:

- increased capillary pressure
- reduced plasma osmotic pressure
- increased interstitial fluid pressure
- increased capillary permeability.

When interstitial fluid pressure reaches a little above atmospheric pressure (0 mmHg), lymph flow fails to continue rising, probably due to fluid compressing the outer surfaces of the larger lymph vessels impeding flow (this is why massage should be directed proximally). The lymphatic capillaries empty into collecting lymphatics. The vessel stretches with increased volume of fluid, and the smooth muscle in the walls of the vessels contracts (Starling's law). This effect is particularly marked immediately proximal to the valves, and so pumps fluid through the proximal valve. Thus, pumping is increased by the compression of the vessel (Guyton 1991). A pumping action is also exerted by actomyosin in the capillary end cells.

The lymph nodes are small oval structures composed of a collagenous capsule and an interior trabecula. Within this framework is a fine reticulum within which many lymphocytes are embedded, with fewer macrophages and reticular cells (littoral cells). Blood vessels and the efferent lymph vessel enter and leave the node at the hilum, while afferent lymph vessels enter it around the periphery. Points at which the reticulum is loose, relatively cell free, and where lymph flows freely are termed lymph sinuses. Within the cortex, collections of cells are termed lymphatic follicles, or nodules, and contain germinal centres.

Lymphatic fluid is transported from the tissue spaces to the nodes where it passes in close proximity to a range of phagocytic cells. The large surface area of the node's interior ensures that numerous cells are available. Microorganisms and foreign bodies are removed from the bloodstream here, to be processed by the lymph glands, and certain cells and proteins are returned via the lymphatics. The lymphatics assist in reducing the threat of toxic spread throughout the bloodstream; however, they also provide a channel for the spread of infection or malignancy.

Fluid eventually returns to the bloodstream via the thoracic duct, which extends from the 12th thoracic vertebra to the root of the neck. It passes through the diaphragm and travels on the posterior mediastinum to the neck, where it drains into the left subclavian and internal jugular veins. At the base of this duct is the cysterna chyli, which extends down to the 1st lumbar vertebra. It receives the right and left lumbar and intestinal lymphatic trunks, which in turn drain the lower limbs, pelvis and abdomen, respectively. In addition, drainage from the intercostal trunks, the left jugular trunk draining head and face, and the left subclavian trunk draining the upper limb, join the thoracic duct. The right lymphatic duct receives drainage from the right jugular trunk, the right subclavian trunk and the right bronchomediastinal trunk. Most drainage from the head and neck enters the deep cervical (superior and inferior) group of nodes, which in turn drain into the jugular trunk. There are also minor groups draining particular areas. Figure 2.7 gives a summary of drainage and shows the position of the nodes.

Lymph drainage from the skin occurs by a system of overlapping skin areas. The tiniest vessels are known as precollectors; they drain from several skin areas into a collector in the hypodermis. The skin area of one collector is a strip of skin – a 'skin zone'. The zones of a single lymph vessel bundle have been termed a territory (Kubik & Manneston 1984). The borders of these territories are known as lymphatic watersheds as there is normally no functional connection across watersheds, although they anastomose with each other.

As lymph drains into a single duct in a proximal direction, it is important that any attempt to increase this drainage mechanically occurs in the same proximal direction. A lymphatic system that is blocked with fluid anywhere on its course will necessitate that extra mechanical drainage occurs in the trunk,

FIGURE 2.7	*Main lymphatic channels and glands. Reproduced, with permission, from Guyton (1991), p. 181.*

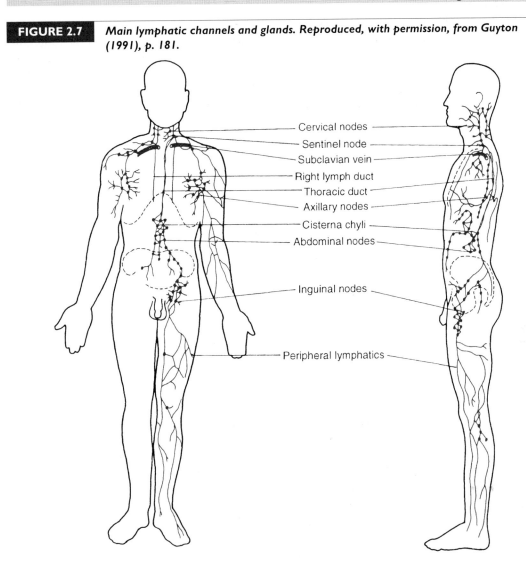

Cervical nodes
Sentinel node
Subclavian vein
Right lymph duct
Thoracic duct
Axillary nodes
Cisterna chyli
Abdominal nodes

Inguinal nodes

Peripheral lymphatics

to clear an area into which the more distal fluid can drain. This is discussed in more depth in Chapter 11.

MUSCLE TONE

Massage can also affect skeletal muscle. A healthy muscle is always in a certain amount of resting tone, which is a response of the muscle fibres to nervous activity; this maintains the muscle in a state of slight, normally imperceptible, contraction. Tone can be increased, especially in postural muscles, by factors such as stress or cold. This is probably, in part, due to the fact that muscle spindles have a sympathetic innervation (Barker & Saito 1981). Tone is dependent on interaction between the muscle spindle (sensitive to length and rate of change in length of muscle) and the central nervous system (CNS). Stretching a muscle will stimulate the spindle and cause reflex muscle contraction, while reflex inhibition of the antagonist occurs. Massage can add an external stimulus to sensory organs and either increase tone by stimulation or reduce it, probably by facilitating an accommodation of the spindle, causing it to 'reset' at a lowered threshold of excitability. The sympathetic supply to muscle spindles means that any influence on the autonomic nervous system (ANS) will affect muscle responses. Massage techniques which have a general relaxation effect, as well as local massage, will therefore change muscle tone.

CONCLUSION

It is important for the massage therapist to understand the effects of massage on the different body systems. The structure and function of the skin, how it is nourished with blood, and the way in which fluid and fibres behave must be understood before the effects of massage can be explored. The mechanisms by which muscle tone is maintained and influenced are pertinent, as are the transmission and interpretation of touch and other types of sensation. Only by a full understanding of these factors can the therapist work autonomously and make effective and informed clinical decisions.

KEY POINTS

- Horizontal arteriovenous plexi lie at the skin interfaces and can be influenced by massage.
- The dermis gives a mobility to the skin which can be maintained or restored by massage.
- Fibres in the tissues can be overstretched beyond their elastic limit, causing damage.
- Failure of fibre bundles occurs beyond their yield point. This can be prevented by not stretching tissue beyond its end-feel.
- Massage principally works within the elastic limit of the stress–strain curve.
- Massage provides a low repetitive load over the medium term and may create a non-permanent creep response by which the tissue is temporarily elongated.
- Massage should not be done too quickly, to avoid a stiffening of connective tissue, as a result of its visco-elastic properties.
- 'Dry' tissue should be massaged more slowly as more friction will be produced between collagen fibres.
- The effectiveness of the venous system can be enhanced, to aid removal of excess tissue fluid, by increasing its pumping effects with massage.
- Lymphatic drainage can be increased by a pumping effect and a pulling on the filaments, which open the gaps between cells in the walls of lymphatic vessels.
- The muscle spindle can be stimulated or caused to accommodate by massage, producing a change in muscle tone.

REFERENCES

Barker D, Saito M 1981 Autonomic innervation of receptors and muscle fibres in cat skeletal muscle. Proceedings of the Royal Society of London B212: 317–332

Culav E M, Clark C H, Merrilees M J 1999 Connective tissues: matrix composition and its relevance to physical therapy. Physical Therapy 79(3): 308–319

Goldfarb C A, Harwood F, Silva M J et al 2001 The effects of variations in applied rehabilitation force on collagen concentration and maturation at the intrasynovial flexor tendon repair site. Journal of Hand Surgery – American 26(5): 841–846

Guyton A C 1991 Textbook of medical physiology. W B Saunders, Philadelphia, PA

Kubik S T, Manneston M 1984 Anatomie der Lymphkapillaren und Präkollektoren der Haut. In: Bonniger A, Partsch H (eds) Initiale Lymphstrombahn, Internat Symp. G Thieme, Zurich, pp. 62–69

Last R J 1984 Anatomy, regional and applied. Churchill Livingstone, Edinburgh

Layers of the skin with circulatory plexi. 1995 Physiotherapy 81(12). Originally published in Schuh 1994 Bindegewebsmassage. Fischer-Verlag, Stuttgart

Thibodeau G A, Patton K T 1999 Anatomy and physiology, 4th edn. Mosby, St Louis

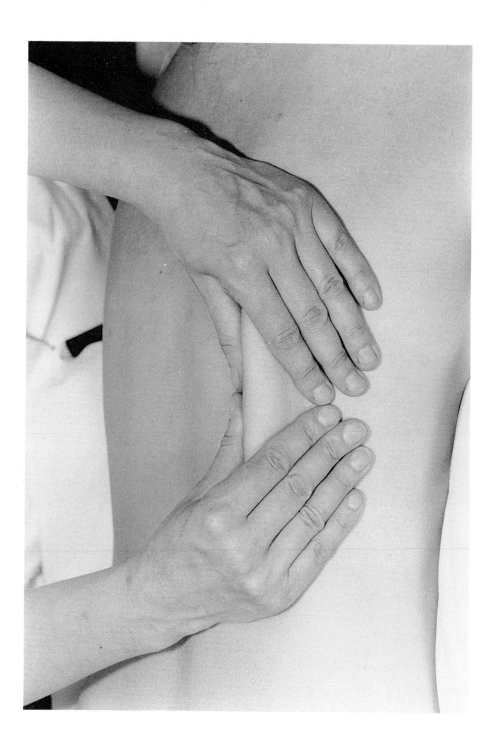

3 Therapeutic and Reflex Effects

It is clear that people like massage. The frequency with which individuals casually touch each other, their children and their pets demonstrates that touch is comforting and is an automatic reaction to another's distress. It is also clear from the increasing willingness of large numbers of people to pay for massage regularly, and their response when receiving it, that it is perceived to be valuable by many individual recipients. Identifying with authority the specific therapeutic effects attributable to massage itself is, however, difficult. There are many postulated effects which are widely believed and documented throughout the massage literature. Unfortunately, not many have been substantiated scientifically.

The aim of this chapter is to discuss the accepted effects, passed on through the oral tradition and literature of physiotherapy and, more latterly, of massage therapy, and examine them in the light of the underlying pathophysiology and available research findings.

An interesting starting point is the widespread popular belief that massage can 'break down' fat tissue and reduce its bulk. Perhaps, as therapeutic massage becomes more popular, this belief is becoming less well promulgated as there is neither convincing evidence nor a plausible theoretical basis for it. Fat is stored as triglycerides in liquid form and held in globules within the cells themselves (Guyton 1991). It is liberated into the bloodstream by enzymatic activity in response to energy demands, to be utilized as a metabolic and biochemical event. A passive mechanical manipulation of the storage area cannot affect the cells in the same way. The fat cells are collected together and compartmentalized by fibrous septa, each compartment having its own blood supply (Williams et al 1989). If the fluid balance within this tissue alters and the collagen fibres become tight, the subcutaneous tissue loses smoothness in outline and takes on a characteristic 'cellulite' appearance. It appears to worsen under the influence of the autonomic nervous system. It may be unevenly distributed, for example where there is nerve root irritation.

Manipulation which alters the fluid balance in this layer and restores mobility and length to the fibrous tissue may change its appearance, but this is in no way due to reduced fat *content*, rather a surface smoothing-out effect. Possibly, toxins are removed as the tissue fluid is replaced with new protein-free fluid fresh from the bloodstream. Clinical experience shows that massage can indeed improve the appearance and mobility of the subcutaneous tissues as the circulation is improved and mobility restored, especially techniques such as manual lymphatic drainage and connective tissue massage. However, clients should not be misled into believing that massage can replace a reducing diet, should they wish to lose weight.

There have been many effects claimed for massage, and examination of massage texts reveals that authors vary somewhat in their opinions, and few rigorously support the claimed effects with research findings. It is necessary, then, to examine which of these effects are likely, in the light of the previous chapter on the pathophysiology underpinning therapeutic massage, in order to progress thinking and debate in this therapeutic area. We start by logically following through the layers of tissue as they are affected by massage, before summarizing the likely effects; these are later compared with research findings.

EVENTS IN THE TISSUES

The first events begin on the surface of the skin, when it is touched. It is now widely accepted that human touch is a prerequisite for the healthy functioning of the individual. At the same time, in the area of health care, prolific technological advances are decreasing our opportunities for physical intervention. In addition, Western culture is largely moving away from physical activity towards intellectual activity, with the result that many are losing the ability to integrate body and mind, suffering consequently from a lack of sensory unity. Touching and being touched is a basic human need but there is little opportunity outside of families to express or receive feelings of care by touching. This situation is magnified for many elderly people and those people who reside in an institutional care environment (Barnett 1972). Massage can offer valid human contact to counterbalance the potentially dehumanizing effects of tactile deprivation.

The anatomy and physiology of touch receptors and their interaction with the central nervous system (CNS) were discussed in Chapter 2. We know and understand a great deal about the mechanisms of touch; what is less clear is how the physical phenomenon of touch affects our moods, emotions, and levels of autonomic, cortical and behavioural arousal. Knowledge of this would enable us to predict the responses that might occur as a result of any tactile intervention.

The sense of touch is one of the earliest senses to develop. The human embryo has been observed to withdraw reflexly from stroking stimuli at 6 weeks after conception (Montagu 1978). Preterm infants have been observed not to tolerate massage but to prefer 'containment', that is, holding or cuddling, which is thought not to stimulate developmentally uninhibited reflexes (Hartelius et al 1992). Containment may be perceived by the infant as a similar stimulus to the pressure exerted by amniotic fluid in the uterus. However, a later study (Field et al 1986) found that not only did preterm infants tolerate massage, but they showed increased weight, alertness and maturity.

Observations on young animals have provided some information about their response to touch, the implications of which may be transferable to humans. Among many mammals tactile rituals occur after birth which serve physiological functions and may promote normal emotional development. There is a relationship between the stroking of young animals by humans and a reduction in the animal's physiological response to stress, demonstrated by a decreased output of adrenocorticotrophic hormone (ACTH) (Seyle 1950) and reduction in blood pressure and heart rate (Lund et al 1999). Young animals that are handled also show greater development of the cortex and subcortex of the brain; they learn faster and have a more advanced stage of neural development than non-handled animals (Ruegammer et al 1954). Resistance to infection later in life may also be influenced beneficially by cutaneous stimulation experienced by the infant animal (Soloman & Moos 1964).

It is thus probable that cutaneous stimulation during critical periods of a human infant's development will promote similar normal organic and behavioural growth. After the age of about 3 months, the infant begins to utilize his/her sense of touch to learn about the immediate environment. Deprivation of this primary learning process may compromise later social and learning responses, and adversely affect the way the adult utilizes tactile information (Frank 1957, Mason 1985).

Touch

Throughout our lives, contact with the environment ensures that our skin receives continual stimulation. We receive tactile messages from, for example, the clothes we wear, the water we wash in, the rubbing of lotions on our skin, and from people and animals we touch or are touched by. Depending on the quality of tactile stimulation perceived, we can feel such emotions as pleasure, pain, fear or revulsion. Similar feelings are engendered by the type of human contact we experience, which is often tempered by integration with other somatic senses. Contrast, for example, the feelings experienced by the touch of a warm hand or a cold one; the sense of smell may influence our response; auditory and visual information may also influence our response to touch. Usually we permit touch when we perceive it as safe or desirable but avoid physical contact with people whom we dislike. The subjective experience of the touch determines our neural and hormonal responses, which in turn influence our integrated response to the touch. As massage necessarily involves touch, the therapist needs to consider not only the mechanical and physiological effects but also the emotional responses that are likely to result. This careful thought will begin before the massage, while taking the client's medical history and during the assessment.

Therapeutic Considerations

The first fact to be established is whether the client has given permission to be touched. A major factor will be how the patient perceives the therapist and the environment. The variables may include the way the therapist presents herself, the degree of privacy involved, and whether the environment is perceived to be safe. Careful attention should be given to differentiating between verbal permission and any non-verbal indicators to the contrary. Some individuals involuntarily interpret touch as threatening, and the sympathetic nervous system may be aroused as a result; these individuals are described as being 'tactually defensive'.

An explanation should be given of the method of massage to be used; a patient who has previously experienced only a pleasant skin rub with essential oils may be unprepared for deep tissue manipulations. The quality of touch which is conveyed to the patient may be predetermined by the therapist's intention and may vary through caring, sensitive and professionally based to cold, hasty and clumsy. Invasion of the body surface by unwelcome types of touch will be perceived as threatening or undesirable, and is likely to produce an unwanted effect. Conversely, the effects of appropriate touch will enhance the rapport between patient and therapist, thus enabling further therapeutic intervention. Constant monitoring of the patient is required throughout treatment to ensure that changes in technique are made when appropriate.

As professional therapists, we are concerned with *all* the effects our massage may produce. When administering a massage the main objective is often to have a mechanical effect with the aim of restoring normal function. However, we should not neglect the fact that there may be other stimuli, extrinsic or intrinsic to the massage, which are capable of producing undesirable effects. Such factors as the environment, the temperature of the environment, the degree of privacy and background noise will all affect the response of the client; similarly, the various sensations provoked by the quality of touch can produce a variety of responses. Our responsibility as therapists is to ensure that all the effects of our treatment are desirable and none detract from our aims. In this respect the therapist should have an understanding of autonomic and emotional arousal.

Stressors

The main centres of autonomic nervous system (ANS) activation are in the spinal cord, brainstem and hypothalamus, with control also being influenced by the limbic cortex. Visceral functions such as arterial pressure, heart rate, gastrointestinal motility and secretion, temperature and sweating are controlled. When the system is working optimally, there is a state of homoeostatic equilibrium. The ANS is also influenced through visceral reflexes, sensory signals that trigger reflex responses of the visceral organs. Change of function can be rapid: the heart rate can increase to twice its normal level in 3–5 seconds, and arterial pressure can double in under 15 seconds (Guyton 1991).

Any agent that provokes sympathetic arousal is termed a 'stressor'. Stressors may be physical, psychological or sociocultural (Seyle 1982). One current theory of stress is that it is cognitively controlled; that is, an individual's response to a stressor is dependent upon that particular individual's previous experience of similar stessors, and his/her present ability to cope with the stressor. While a moderate level of sympathetic arousal is desirable to facilitate most everyday activities – it keeps us mentally and physically alert – prolonged exposure to a stressor that produces a high level of autonomic arousal can have undesirable physiological effects, resulting in, for example, decreased immunity, and increases in hypertension and vascular disorders (Willard 1995).

Current concepts of stress take account of the neuroendocrine changes in the body in response to a stimulus (see Fig. 10.1, which summarizes some of the current concepts of stress responses).

An emotion is an expression of subjective feeling which is accompanied by neural and hormonal activity; emotions are determined by learned, cognitive and biological factors. The systems that control autonomic and emotional activity are interactive, being linked by neural impulses and hormones. A therapist who has a good understanding of the integration between these systems will work holistically with clients, thus ensuring that the whole person benefits from her intervention.

THE TISSUE LAYERS

Changes can actually be seen on the surface of the skin during vigorous massage, when some reddening occurs. The amount depends to some extent on the reactivity of the skin, which is determined by skin type, although vaso-dilatory reactions in the skin are common. Fundamentally, it is as a result of release of histamine from the mast cells. Mast cells are found in connective tissue and contain histamine, heparin and hyaluronic acid and it is known that cells respond to mechanical signals (Banes et al 1995). Cell deformation may activate calcium ion channels and influence calcium transport. Mechanical stress has specifically been found to activate mast cell secretion (Theoharides 1996). It is unclear why this mechanical irritation and its resulting vasodilata-tion should occur, and to what purpose. Further reddening seen in the skin may be due to shear forces acting on the endothelium of blood vessels, causing release of the vasodilator nitric oxide (Noris et al 1995), which is angioprotec-tive. Vasodilatation is accompanied by an increase in capillary permeability and it is likely that the tissue fluid released from these capillaries has a flushing effect on the tissues, both removing irritants and allowing protective chemicals to be brought to the area via the bloodstream. The reddening may increase if the hands glide over the surface of the skin, particularly with speed as this increases friction. Reddening can be reduced by massaging more slowly and by using an oily medium.

When a hand is held over the surface of another person's skin, heat can be felt between the two surfaces. If the hand is placed on skin and held in a sta-tionary position, this heat can be felt to increase. Rubbing over the surface of the skin causes friction and this increases heat even further. Heat is a form of energy and some schools of massage, particularly those grounded in Eastern practices, utilize the energy field which exists around the body. This is some-times referred to as the aura, an electromagnetic radiation around the entire body, which can be identified by Kirlian photography, and is thought to be affected by abnormal states in the body. It is felt as heat and therefore identified by palpation at a small distance from the body. Energy fields are also believed to run through the body, along specific pathways known as meridians, and also to exist more generally. Philosophies concerned with this type of energy have not yet been incorporated in standard biomedical practice or texts but the principle is utilized in orthodox health care systems through acupuncture (mainly used by physiotherapists and doctors), reflex therapy (used by physiotherapists) and therapeutic touch (popular with nurses in the USA). Therapeutic touch, non-contact therapeutic touch and other energetic forms of massage use this principle to varying degrees as they attempt to normalize the energy fields, promoting healing and well-being. Within biomedicine, it is often interpreted as ANS activity, as discussed below.

With a slight increase in pressure, layers of tissue are moved with the hands, rather than the hands gliding lightly over the skin surface. A very light glide necessitates some movement of the epidermis. If there is friction between the therapist's hand and the patient's skin, the epidermis moves with the therapist's hands and is gently stretched. As this layer is so thin, the dermis must move simultaneously because of traction between the dermis and epidermis which results from natural adherence between the layers. The application of slightly more pressure with friction (but note the massage still feels very light) and some traction effect occurs between the dermis and subcutis. Resistance or tension is felt when this traction reaches its limit and all layers are stretched. This is referred to as the *end-feel* of the stroke and at this point, if the hands glide or continue to push into the resistance, the massage is deepened as traction occurs at the next interface down.

So far, we have recognized that massage involves an interaction of energy between the patient and therapist; that it utilizes the effects of touch to induce relaxation, communication and a sense of well-being; and that it produces movement of the tissues in subsequent layers as a result of traction at tissue interfaces. In addition, a complete variety of strokes lifts, pulls, squeezes and twists the skin, connective tissue, tendons, ligaments, muscles, blood vessels and nerves. Sensory and autonomic nerves are stimulated, inducing changes in the nervous and circulatory systems, and movement is effected in abnormal tissue, for example scar tissue or where layers are adherent.

CIRCULATORY EFFECTS

The pressure of the massage itself increases pressure in the tissues. Pressure gradients are created between the tissue spaces and vessels as discussed in Chapter 2. As the hands are moved, so the increased pressure is moved, creating a *fluctuating* pressure difference between one area of tissue and another. Thus fluid moves constantly from tissues to vessels and back again, as it flows from areas of high to low pressure. This can occur in two ways: if pressure is increased only in the tissue space and not in the vessel, fluid will move from the tissue into the vessel. Slightly more pressure, however, also increases the pressure in the vessel, so there may be a tendency for fluid to move out of the vessel into tissue space which is at lower pressure. If the vessel is compressed and this pressure moves longitudinally along its course, as in effleurage, then the fluid is pushed proximally along the vessel, leaving the collapsed vessel behind the hand to fill again rapidly. This refilling or milking effect can push fluid towards the heart. If it occurs in veins, a suction-like effect will take place, aided by the valves which prevent back-flow. In addition, manipulation of the tissues at a careful depth will cause a pull on the filaments, which are connected to the flaps in the walls of lymphatic vessels, allowing larger plasma proteins to be removed from the tissue spaces, thus restoring a normal osmotic pressure to the extracellular fluid.

While there appear to be several ways in which fluid balance in the tissues is influenced, the mechanisms are probably more complex than the theoretical supposition described here. It is not possible for the therapist to know exactly where the smaller vessels lie as their exact positions are subject to individual variation. The deep vessels cannot be palpated if they are normal. The massage manipulations themselves are complex and involve a combination of squeezing, stretching, pulling and traction forces, with movement occurring in different directions and in different tissue planes: for example, kneading consists of circular movements, skin rolling produces transverse movements, stroking and effleurage produce longitudinal forces. Consequently, there are complex repetitive pressure changes occurring in varying directions and at different depths. This is likely to have an effect on fluid *interchange*, whereby fluid is pushed from the tissue spaces into the vessel, towards the lymph nodes and heart, and new fluid is pushed or drawn into the spaces. Generally, it seems less logical to assume that massage will reduce the amount of fluid in the spaces when it is more likely to replenish it.

This flushing effect in the tissues is important. New circulation is brought to the area with fresh nutrition, and the stasis by which inflammatory products, chemical irritants and toxins linger in the tissues is corrected. The local environment is therefore changed for the better. The mechanism by which chemical irritants in the tissues can cause an undesirable plasticity in the spinal cord, lowering the threshold to pain within a whole neuronal pool, is discussed further in Chapter 4. Replenishing tissue fluid and removing inflammatory products will reduce this effect, preventing or reducing some types of chronic pain. Removing metabolites and chemicals such as potassium from muscles by releasing them from muscle cells and 'flushing' the muscle tissue with new circulation will reduce muscle soreness following exercise. This effect will reduce pain in situations where metabolites have built up due to prolonged muscle spasm, increased tone (for example, where there is excessive anxiety or tension) and conditions such as fibromyalgia. Indirectly, massage can promote healing by bringing new circulation to the area. Occasionally, in a chronically swollen limb or when fluid is trapped in a tissue space (as in the hand or around the ankle, for example), or where there is fibrous swelling, massage can soften and release the swelling, facilitating its removal.

A much-cited study into massage and blood flow was carried out by Wakim et al in 1949. This team measured blood flow by plethysmography and spirometry in the forearms and hands and in the lower legs. In a group of 15 asymptomatic subjects they found that arm massage increased blood flow to significant levels in 11 of 12 observations and that leg massage increased it to significant levels in 11 of 14 observations. This increase was maintained 30 minutes after the cessation of the massage. The massage given in this instance was a vigorous type involving deep stroking, deep forceful kneading and friction. After a modified Hoffa type of massage, which included stroking and deep kneading, 16 of 32 readings on the upper limbs showed insignificant results while 10 of 32 showed an increase and six of 32 a decrease in blood flow. Lower limb readings were insignificant in 15 of 24 subjects, with five of 24 showing an increase and four of 24 a decrease. In paralysed limbs, four of six had a significant increase and three of five limbs with spastic paralysis showed an increase. Rheumatoid limbs showed readings fairly evenly distributed across the significant increase, non-significant increase and reduced flow categories. Of further interest is the fact that, following two sessions in two patients with poliomyelopathy, all observations were significant. This research was conducted some time ago and plethysmography has been criticized by Hansen & Kristensen (1973) as a technique which only measures blood flow in the skin. Significance levels were arbitrarily set at 15% and improvement was measured in percentages. There was no statistical analysis, so it is not a statistical significance referred to here. There was no account taken of probability in the calculations; the results are of clinical significance only if the pattern of results occurs more frequently than they would by chance, which is why statistical analysis is important. The stimulating massage that produced better results is unlikely to be carried out frequently in a real clinical situation, and the trauma and irritation of such a massage would be expected to increase blood flow in skin, but with a limited therapeutic value. The results of this study are of interest but should be treated with caution, as little convincing scientific evidence is offered.

A further attempt to measure the effects of massage on blood flow was made by Hansen & Kristensen (1973) by the more sophisticated ^{133}Xe clearance technique. This substance was injected into the calf muscles and measured with scintillation detectors during and after massage. The 'centripetal effleurage' was conducted for 5 minutes in the legs of two women and 10 men, aged 20–32 years. The mean disappearance rate during massage was statistically significant, with the significance reducing 0–2 minutes after the massage. The results show a slight effect, with none in avascular subcutaneous tissues. Unfortunately, little detail was given concerning the massage itself, for example the amount of pressure used. Also, some traditional principles of circulatory massage were not respected, namely, massaging proximal areas before distal ones and using an assortment of techniques. In addition, differences in amounts of massage time were not monitored. This research supports the assertion that massage increases blood flow in muscles but missed the opportunity to increase its impact by informing us more about types of massage and lengths of treatment. The study was, in fact, designed to compare the effects of massage with those of shortwave diathermy and ultrasound (found to be not significant) and therefore did not examine massage in particular detail. As the blood flow effects were short-lived, this would suggest that these effects are as a result of *mechanical* stimulation of blood vessels rather than chemical or reflex responses.

The following year produced a publication which to some extent substantiated these findings (Hovind & Nielsen 1974). Blood flow was measured in the brachioradialis and vastus lateralis muscles of nine volunteers aged 22–32 years, following intramuscular injection of saline and ^{133}Xe. The results showed that, following tapotement, blood flow rose significantly for 10 minutes after cessation of the technique, but petrissage results were inconsistent, short-lasting and not statistically significant. As the tapotement results were similar to those found during active isometric muscle contractions, it is probable that this technique (described by the authors as 'unpleasant to the experimental volunteers') stimulated reflex muscle contractions, which increased the blood flow.

Shoemaker et al (1997) studied the effect of massage to the forearm flexor muscle and the quadriceps on blood flow (mean blood velocity (MBV)). Blood flow was measured by pulsed Doppler ultrasound and vessel diameter by echo Doppler ultrasound. Ten subjects were studied, with readings of MBV taken prior to treatment and at 5, 10, 20 seconds and 5 minutes following the onset of massage. Vessel diameter readings were taken before and after massage. Massage did not significantly increase blood flow in either muscle group, whereas light exercise *did* elevate blood flow from rest. This is a sound study in which the massage was conducted by a registered massage therapist. It is not indicated whether the massage was superficial (with the hands gliding over the skin, using an oily medium) or whether it was deep. It is logical to assume the effects on blood flow of deep and superficial massage would differ and a comparison of different depths would make an interesting study.

In normal limbs, then, there appears to be some increase in blood flow, either in the skin or intramuscularly, during massage, particularly effleurage, although this is not universally substantiated by all studies. Small sample sizes and inconsistent methodologies leave results inconclusive. Increases in circulation occurring during, but not following, massage suggest that it results from the mechanical, rather than the reflex or chemical effects of massage, although it has been asserted for many years (Carrier 1922) that vasodilatation during fairly vigorous massage occurs as a result of stimulating the axon reflex, observed as a reddening of the skin. Massage has, in fact, been shown to increase the effect of a vasodilator substance in the skin following superficial massage and in muscles following deep massage (Severini & Venerando 1967). As physiological compensating mechanisms are extremely efficient in healthy tissues, any alteration in local blood flow will be compensated for by autoregulatory processes; these researchers are perhaps limiting their results by using subjects with normal circulatory systems. Severini & Venerando also found, surprisingly, that deep and superficial massage *decreased* skin temperature. Deep massage demonstrated 'appreciable' increases in blood flow in both the massaged and non-massaged legs; increases in cardiac stroke volume; and decreases in heart rate and systolic and diastolic arterial pressure. Unfortunately, only the abstract is available in English.

Morhenn (2000) found that massaging the cheeks of the face increased skin temperature in seven out of eight human subjects, which plateaued after 40 minutes of massage. It was accompanied by erythema. The effect was blocked by pre-treatment of capsaicin, a chemical which causes release of substance P by peripheral nerve endings which suggests that the raised temperature effect can be partly controlled by substance P. A point of less relevance than interest is that the researchers conclude that social grooming in animals may be necessary because of the survival effect of neurotransmitter release. Zoologists, however, have conducted much research into this subject and their explanations for animal grooming vary from stress reduction, care of the coat/feathers, parasite control, communication and the spread of chemicals (such as pheromones in bees), depending on the species.

In 1988, Flowers compared massage with string wrapping and a combination of the two in 56 upper limb digits in 10 women and four men aged 24–61 years. They used a retrograde 'milking' massage along the whole length of the digit and monitored its effectiveness by measuring the distal interphalangeal joint girth with a tape measure. Using sound statistical tests, they found that neither the string wrap nor the massage alone demonstrated significant results but, when combined, results were significant. Continuous stroking was better than intermittent stroking. This is interesting, as the combined effect would operate at a much deeper level in the tissues than manual lymphatic drainage, which is the current treatment of choice for *protein-rich* oedema. Presumably, the swelling in this study was more acute and was possibly trapped in the tissue spaces, needing mechanical assistance to return back into the bloodstream. The string wrapping maximized the principle of pressure gradient-induced fluid dynamics, and the massage mechanically aided the process. It is illuminating that a combination of these two modalities produced good results. This indicates that the pumping effect of rhythmical effleurage may be important in oedema removal and that the constant pressure produced by the string wrapping ensured the swelling did not return to the tissues through leaky capillaries. This points to the need to combine oedema massage with some form of pressure to maintain its effects between treatments.

While the results of different studies can appear confusing, it seems that general massage, arbitrarily used, can produce erroneous results. When massage is more specific, however, and carried out sensitively, is anatomically correct and applied at a precise depth, specific strokes can indeed achieve a specific purpose. Trubetskoy et al (1997) conducted research which showed that gentle manual massage for 5 minutes increased absorption of subcutaneously injected substances from the tissues into the lymphatics. Effleurage and manual lymphatic drainage can mechanically produce a milking effect or open lymphatic flaps for the removal of proteins. A rhythmical pumping effect can then be achieved. The choice of technique or combination of techniques should therefore be selected carefully, the selection being informed by relevant pathophysiology.

Blood constituent readings following massage can offer further elucidation on the mechanism by which massage works. Arkko et al (1983) conducted research in which vigorous conventional whole body massage, using oil as a lubricant, was carried out for 1 hour in nine healthy male volunteers. Stroking, kneading, friction and shaking were applied by an experienced therapist. Blood samples were taken before, immediately after and at 2, 24 and 48 hours later. A variety of blood and serum constituents were measured and results showed wide individual variation, none reaching statistically significant levels. The results did, however, substantiate the findings of Bork et al (1971) that serum levels of creatine kinase (CK) and lactate dehydrogenase (LDH) were raised. These are enzymes that can be examined for skeletal muscle specificity. Bork and co-workers suggested that LDH was liberated by muscle cells, probably as a result of the mechanical trauma of the massage. This work was not in agreement with the claim by Wood & Becker (1981) that haemoglobin levels and erythrocyte count are raised. Unfortunately, there was no check on the activity levels of the subjects earlier in the day. This group of volunteers was not compared with a control group which did not receive massage. Nine is too small a number to conduct the statistical tests used here with confidence (such as the one-tailed paired *t* test). A larger group may have shown more (or, indeed, less) significant results and, in comparison with controls, would have increased the validity of this study.

Ernst et al (1987) found that a standard 20-minute massage treatment reduced the haematocrit, blood and plasma viscosity. The suggestion here is that the fluid immediately surrounding poorly perfused vessels has low viscosity owing to its lack of cells and that the vasodilatation caused by massage nearby creates a need for these almost dormant vessels to be recruited. This may be useful where it is desirable to increase local circulation, for example to promote healing. It can also be a help to athletes whose performance would benefit from increased recruitment of blood vessels. In addition, the mechanical effect of the massage causes a removal of the low-viscosity tissue fluid into the circulation. The study offers further evidence that massage produces a flushing and mechanical effect on the circulation, as the local effects here were detected within the bloodstream.

Research has shown that massage can reduce the incidence of deep vein thrombosis (DVT). Sabri et al (1971) found that the incidence of DVT was reduced by 82% in the massaged limb when compared with the non-massaged limb. Knight & Dawson (1976) demonstrated that the occurrence of DVT in the leg can be reduced by massage of the arm. Both these studies, however, used pneumatic compression devices which simply squeeze the whole limb in a rhythmical manner. This does not mirror a manual massage; rather it mirrors the effect of rhythmical muscle contraction on the muscle pump, which increases venous return. This does not indicate that the reduced incidence of DVT on these occasions was due to massage causing reduced blood viscosity, nor that pneumatic compression devices are superior to regular muscle-pumping exercises in anyone confined to bed or undergoing surgery. A comparative study would be helpful for clarification.

EFFECTS ON MUSCLE

It is claimed that the circulatory effect of massage can reduce muscle soreness and thus aid conditions that cause muscle soreness, muscle injury or post-exercise recovery. Danneskiold-Samsoe et al published important research in 1982. Thirteen women aged 24–55 years with muscle pain and tension in the shoulder region and back had ten 30–45-minute massages over 4 weeks. The index of fibrositis was taken, based on scores attached to the size of tension areas. Venous blood samples were taken before and at 1, 2, 3, 4, 5 and 6 hours following massage at the first treatment, and then before and at 1 and 2 hours after massage. Levels of myoglobin, a protein found only in muscle tissue and associated with oxygen transport in the blood, were measured. The results were statistically significant. There was a peak value of myoglobin within 3 hours of the massage. Gradually, the level of significance fell between treatments. The fibrositis index scores fell between the fourth and seventh treatments, and there was no difference in either myoglobin levels or index scores between treatments 7 and 10. LDH levels showed no change (giving no support to Arkko and colleagues' (1983) suggestion that this was raised as a result of mechanical trauma of the massage itself) and serum creatine concentration rose slowly during 6 hours to double its normal value. The fact that myoglobin levels gradually declined in the blood samples until there was no difference between treatments 7 and 10 showed that this was not, in this case, due to mechanical damage produced by the massage. These results also offer an indicator to treatment length. There was a significant difference between the group and controls after treatments 1 and 4. According to these findings, treatment programmes for this condition should ideally consist of seven sessions.

Further effects of massage on muscle can be divided into effects on tone and performance, as influenced by discomfort. Muscle tone ensures that skeletal muscles remain in a mild state of contraction. It is maintained by a complex interaction between stimulating impulses from the muscle spindle (stretch receptor) and inhibitory impulses from the Golgi tendon organs (Fig. 3.1).

The anterior horn cells in the cord receive these impulses, and activity in these cord cells is further mediated by descending brain activity. Various factors affect muscle tone in situations where functioning of the CNS is normal. This is little understood, but varies from local spasm in response to injury (for example, near a recently fractured bone) to increased muscular tension around the neck and shoulder area and to myofascial trigger spots.

It seems that spasm occurs in response to pain, in an attempt to prevent movement and further damage. This can be useful in indicating potentially serious underlying damage which warrants further investigation. More frequently, however, the cause is either unknown, has resolved or cannot be alleviated; therefore the spasm or, more likely, the muscle shortening itself becomes the problem and the cause of further pain (Fig. 3.2). It has long been assumed that ultimately, a situation can exist where spasm itself becomes the overriding symptomatic factor. Changes then occur in the muscles as their blood supply becomes compromised, resulting in oedema, adhesions and

| **FIGURE 3.1** | *Sensory receptors in muscle – proprioceptors. Reproduced, with permission, from Thibodeau & Patton (1999).* |

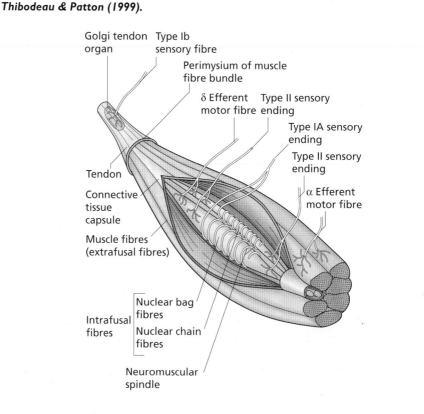

FIGURE 3.2   *Self-perpetuating muscle spasm cycle.*

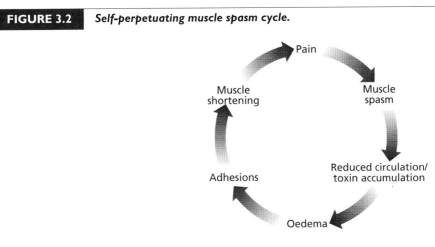

muscle shortening. Massage has long been advocated to relieve this cycle (Jacobs 1960). However, Mense et al (2001) remind us that not all painful muscles which feel tense are in spasm and may sometimes show no electromyographical activity, and that not all muscle spasm is painful.

Where this situation exists, however, massage is also said to reduce tone in muscles that are tense or in spasm, and to reduce the soreness and tenderness of tense or over-exercised muscles. Certainly, muscles can be felt to 'soften' during massage, an effect which is followed by a reduction in pain. Further investigation of the pathophysiology is clearly indicated. Massage can also prepare muscle for exercise and is also sometimes used to reduce hypertonus in spastic muscles.

It is thought that muscles which maintain excess tone or static contraction for prolonged periods of time work beyond their oxidative capacity and an algesic substance, possibly potassium, is released (Jones & Round 1990). Discomfort reduces as its cause is removed by circulating blood. A cycle may be produced of excess (for example, postural or occupational) tone causing release of algesic substances producing pain, which increases tone, causing further toxin release and an increase in pain. This probably explains the discomfort experienced around the neck and shoulder girdle region in tense individuals or those with poor posture. Posture can also be influenced by emotions or body language, hence the typical clinical picture of a very controlled individual who is 'cool in a crisis', holding her/his emotional tension in the muscles of the upper back and neck. Massage appears to soften the tissues, reducing tone, liberating fluid from the muscle tissue and flushing out the algesic substance as new circulation is brought to the area. Often the muscles of the back, particularly paraspinal muscles, are felt to be 'ropey', that is, they feel as if they have rolled tissue, like thin ropes, in them. This is thought to be due to spasm of muscular fascicles as a result of increased sensitivity in the spindles which control them (Yates 1990).

Exercise that works the muscles eccentrically, or which generates high forces in muscle, produces delayed-onset soreness and a feeling of stiffness. It is thought that this is due to swelling in the muscle and inflammation of the connective tissue which sensitizes mechanoreceptors (Jones & Round 1990). Once the initial tenderness has passed, or before it develops, massage can help to limit the painful episode. It is also claimed that massage can help to prevent subsequent post-exercise pain, in a similar way to increased training. Sports physiotherapists describe regularly massaged muscles as being more pliable and less hard. It is possible that the stretching manipulations increase extensibility and strength in the connective tissue. It may also reduce oedema in the muscle tissue and produce a flushing effect, removing algesic substances.

The work of Danneskiold-Samsoe et al (1982), discussed above, substantiates the assertion that massage can reduce muscle discomfort. They assumed that, because myoglobin levels in plasma correlated with a reduction in pain (indicated by the fibrositis index), the regional pain and tension in fibrositis is associated with muscle, rather than connective tissue, damage. They also measured levels of CK and LDH, which are muscle enzymes, and found that CK rose twofold during the 6 hours following massage, with no significant increase in LDH. Pain has been found to occur on activity in muscles if the metabolic demands of the muscle cannot be met. This is thought to be due to the release of algesic substances (for example, potassium). Delayed-onset pain is experienced after the exercise has stopped and is caused mainly by exercising with the muscles in a lengthened position or by eccentric (isotonic lengthening) muscle work. The muscles also feel stiff, tight and tender, and may be oedematous. This type of pain is thought to be due to connective tissue inflammation rather than muscle damage, which may explain why it occurs when the muscle is exercised in a lengthened position. Massage may assist the performance of muscle by increasing pliability in the connective tissue around the muscle fasciculi. It will maintain mobility between the interfaces within the muscle and will flush this relatively avascular tissue. It will also stretch any fibrous adhesions or scarring in the tissue, which may be particularly troublesome when they occur between the connective and muscle tissue, binding them together.

Muscle tension can sometimes produce symptoms elsewhere. A well-known example is that of tension headache. Puustjarvi et al (1990) studied the effects of 10 sessions of deep-tissue upper body massage in 21 women suffering from chronic tension headaches. It was found that the range of neck movements (measured with a Myrin goniometer), surface electromyographic (EMG) activity on the frontalis muscle, pain scores on the visual analogue scale (severity) and scores on the Finnish Pain Questionnaire all improved significantly, together with the incidence of neck pain, at 2 weeks, 3 and 6 months of follow-up. Beck Depression Inventory scores also improved but surface EMG recordings from the trapezius muscle were not significantly changed. The authors suggest that the headaches reduced as a result of a relief of 'cephalic spasm' (Poznick-Patewitz 1976) and endorphin release.

Recent research, based on a series of cadaveric dissections, has found a fascial connection between the rectus capitis posterior minor muscle and the posterior atlanto-occipital membrane which is attached to the dura mater layer of the spinal meninges (Hack et al 1995). The researchers postulate that contraction of the muscle exerts tension on the dura through the fascia and atlanto-occipital membrane. The dura is known to be richly innervated with sensory nerve endings and the authors suggest that this is a common mechanism for tension headaches. Massage techniques along and below the occipital ridge, which reduce tone in this muscle, should therefore reduce the pain of headache. Any underlying cause should of course be investigated and treated to prevent reccurrence. If the cause is muscular tension arising from stress, then massage and relaxation techniques as part of a stress management programme should benefit the patient considerably.

Interest has been shown in the effects of massage on the H (Hoffman) reflex, which indicates the excitability in α-motoneurons, or anterior horn cells. Goldberg et al (1992) investigated the effectiveness of two different depths of massage on depression of spinal motoneurone excitability. The subjects were 20 neurologically healthy volunteers, 10 women and 10 men, aged less than 40 years. They were controlled for activity, caffeine and alcohol intake. One-handed petrissage was performed at both deep and superficial levels. The decision regarding what constituted deep and superficial was subjective but the therapist was trained to standardize massage to the agreed depth. The massage was interspersed between control periods and the order of deep or superficial was allocated randomly. Deep massage showed a 49% reduction in H reflex activity and the light massage a 39% reduction. The order of massage or gender of the subjects produced no differences in result, indicating that gender-based placebo effects did not influence the results. It was concluded that influencing cutaneous mechanoreceptors and pressure receptors reduces H reflex activity. Comparable results were found when the study was repeated on patients with spinal cord injury (Goldberg et al 1994).

In a study conducted by Sullivan and co-workers (1991), 16 subjects (eight women and eight men aged 21.9 ± 1.3 years) received effleurage over triceps surae and the hamstring muscles at a standardized rate of 0.5 Hz. Recordings of peak-to-peak H reflex activity demonstrated stability during control periods and significant falls in activity during periods of massage. This was a well-controlled study which utilized sound statistical tests and demonstrated a reduction in α-motoneurone excitability of the massaged muscles. This substantiated the work of Morelli et al (1990), who conducted a similar study in the triceps surae muscles of two men and seven women. The H reflex peak-to-peak amplitude was measured at 10-second intervals during two pre-treatment control periods, a massage period and two post-treatment control periods. The massage was found to produce a significant reduction in spinal motoneurone excitability during, but not after, massage. Morelli et al did further work in 1998 to determine whether the H reflex, diminished in amplitude by massage, is really due to decreased motoneuronal excitability or whether it is due to another cause. This study showed that motoneuronal excitability is reduced as peak-to-peak mean amplitude of the gastrocnemius muscle H reflex was reduced when the soleus muscle was massaged for 3 minutes. As this close synergic muscle was also affected, this suggests that the effect must be due to reduced α-motoneuronal excitability.

These findings disagreed with the work of Newham & Lederman (1997). In their study, 5 minutes of massage to the quadriceps muscle was found not to affect the quadriceps reflex peak-to-peak amplitude in 20 healthy volunteers (age range 18–64 years).

Similarly, Dishman & Bulbulian (2001) found that massage did not reduce the amplitude of the tibial nerve H reflex when the massage was done locally or paraspinally. Spinal manipulation, however, produced a transient reduction in amplitude.

The suggestion (Goldberg et al 1992) that the effects of massage on H reflex excitability may be due to its influence on cutaneous mechanoreceptors has been tested by Morelli et al (1999). Massage was conducted both with and without the application of a topical anaesthetic and no difference was found between the two groups, but there was significant difference in result between the two experimental groups and the control group. The authors concluded that deep, rather than superficial mechanoreceptors were likely to be influenced by massage.

The positive reports of massage reducing α-motoneurone excitability have involved measurements taken *during* the massage. The studies reporting negative findings, however, took measurements *after* the massage. This area of research would suggest that massage reduces H reflex amplitude during massage, but there is no sustained effect after the cessation of massage.

Nordschow & Bierman (1962), in an earlier, less sophisticated, study of 25 healthy subjects (22 women and three men aged 20–35 years), found that, following Swedish massage to the back and Hoffa massage to the back and leg, fingertip-to-floor measurements with a tape measure increased in all subjects, with a mean increase of 1.35 inches. Tests for statistical significance were not carried out but results showed a trend towards greater increased flexibility after massage than after rest.

EFFECTS ON PAIN AND SENSATION

Many of the effects discussed above would contribute to a reduction in pain and have already been examined in relation to muscle soreness. Pain can be reduced by massage as a primary intervention or as a secondary effect if massage removes the cause of the pain. Ueda et al (1993) demonstrated that massage has a sensory effect. They compared two groups of 16 patients who had had minor obstetric or gynaecological surgery under a lidocaine (lignocaine) epidural block. One group received 30 minutes of gentle massage of the epigastric area, and the proximal extent of the sensory analgesia was monitored before the massage and at 0 and 30 minutes after massage (i.e. every 30 minutes). The analgesic boundary changed in the controls from T9 (before massage) to T10 (at 0 minutes) and T10 (at 30 minutes), whereas that in the massage group progressed by two segments every 30 minutes: T9 (before), T11 (at 0 minutes) and L1 (at 30 minutes). This study suggests that mild sensory stimulation can facilitate regression of sensory analgesia, with possible implications for sensory recovery in other situations.

The effects of massage on levels of pain perception have been studied by Carreck (1994). She compared a minimum of 20 subjects who had painful stimulation (by transcutaneous nerve stimulation) before and 15 minutes after Swedish massage of the leg. The massage was substituted by rest in the control group. Pain threshold was raised to significantly higher levels in the massage group, although individuality of response was seen. Massage can therefore be used to manage pain or reduce treatment soreness, but care should be taken if other modalities are also used in which pain levels are an important guide.

Massage has been shown to contribute to a reduction in pain in various situations. Massage and unspecified physiotherapy decreased post-thoracotomy pain as measured by a visual analogue scale in a study of 116 patients (Marin et al 1991). Less clear was the work of Weinrich & Weinrich (1990), who studied cancer pain in 28 patients who were randomly assigned to either a control or a massage group. Patients in the massage group received a 10-minute back massage, while the others received a visit for the same amount of time, to take into account the effect of one-to-one contact and attention. Pain levels in men decreased significantly immediately following the massage. This measure was not significant in women; neither were reductions of pain levels significant for either group 1 or 2 hours after massage. The age range of these patients was 36–78 years, which is wide for a relatively small study. Also, the levels of pain were actually higher in the experimental group than in the control patients. This study could have been more elucidating had the authors compared homogeneous groups and identified particular patients who may have benefited from massage. The difference in the sex-specific responses contradicted the findings of Goldberg et al (1992), which demonstrated no sex differences in the effect of massage, although this may reflect a difference in the way patients and healthy volunteers respond.

Massage causes traction to occur at tissue interfaces. Horizontal plexi lie at interfaces in the tissues, and gentle pulling on these vessels may stimulate the accompanying sympathetics which supply the mechanoreceptors. These receptors are distorted by the manipulation and there is therefore a dual effect in which mechanoreceptor sensitivity might be lowered, reducing pain and tenderness. If delayed-onset pain in muscle is caused more by connective tissue inflammation than by metabolic build-up in the muscle, as previously supposed, the flushing effect in the surrounding fluids, removing inflammatory mediators, may increase the speed at which the inflammation resolves. Substance P, for example, is known to play a role in chronic inflammation and pain (Harrison & Geppetti 2001). Promoting the flushing of the tissues through massage will inevitably reduce such irritants and therefore contribute to an alleviation of pain.

EFFECTS ON CONNECTIVE TISSUE

It is necessary to examine the purely mechanical effects of massage on the non-contractile or vascular tissues. Connective tissue is primarily composed of collagen fibres held together by fibrous cross-bridges. Following injury or disease processes, inflammation causes increased vascular permeability, which allows fluid to seep into the tissues in the form of oedema. This oedema contains plasma proteins, in particular fibrin-secreting fibrinogen, responsible for fibrous tissue. Adhesions thus form within the tissues, binding tissue interfaces or individual fibres together. These adhesions appear to increase the cross-bridge effect between pairs of fibres, preventing normal glide of fibres upon each other and also reducing the ability of the fibres to spread apart.

It has been asserted that massage will stretch tissues that have become short, tight or adhered. Some authors (Wood & Becker 1981, Ylinen & Cash 1988) describe the 'breaking down' of adhesions, which suggests a vigorous, destructive response. The adhesions, however, become part of the tissue; such a violent effect would be destructive to the surrounding tissue as the technique cannot differentiate between adjacent structures and the normal, more vascular and sensitive, surrounding tissue, which may also yield. This would cause further inflammation and pain, and would precipitate more extensive fibrin deposition.

In speculating about what does actually happen, we know that petrissage manipulations stretch and pull the tissues in various directions, thus mobilizing adjacent connective tissue fibres. The molecular cross-bridges between fibrils will be influenced and plastic changes may occur, and their length maintained or increased due to elongation or 'creep' (see Ch. 2). Mobility will be increased biomechanically at the fibrous cross-bridges, between fibres and where there are adhesions, by stretching connections between the fibres. This will promote width, spread and glide at tissue interfaces, and longitudinal elongation which will increase flexibility. These effects can be observed and palpated readily in scar tissue. Following surgery or accidental laceration, scars can become bound down to the underlying tissue, and massage will mobilize and soften by means of increased fluid exchange, elongation and creep.

Collagen fibres align themselves along the lines of stress; thus they are not found to lie in parallel formation in many muscles and tendons, as the directional forces on the intramuscular septum or ligament vary with changing range of motion. Techniques that stretch the fibres and adhesions in different directions will eventually restore their mobility, promoting remodelling along the lines of their normal stresses. The stretching and pulling may ensure that the connective tissue maintains its pliability and length, and could account for the subjective observations of sports therapists that regularly massaged muscles feel softer and more pliable, despite intensive training. Local flexibility contributes to general flexibility, and structures that regain their full length after injury are less likely to be reinjured during sudden stretching movements. Massage may be important, therefore, in optimizing the functional recovery of a structure and preventing reinjury, by ensuring mobility at interfaces both inside and outside the structure. It cannot replace accurate, controlled, longitudinal stretching exercises but the two complement each other well.

There is currently much interest in the way components of the body are interconnected through the connective tissue levels. Elements of the cytoskeleton connect, across the cell surface membrane, with the extracellular matrix. Theories are being developed which are based on the belief that effects on one part of this system can spread throughout (Oschman 2000). As connective tissue is influenced, the effects can occur on both the micro and the macro level and can be generalized throughout the body. Connective tissue may, therefore, contribute to the quality of movement, mood and general well-being. Some bodyworkers believe it is the 'underlying determinant' of these functions (Schultz & Feitis 1996). One explanation for how widespread influence can be achieved by localized manipulation of connective tissue is the piezo-electrical effect. Some molecules operate as liquid crystals. Stretch or compression creates an electrical field and sets up pulsations and oscillations in the crystal. This represents the movement created in the tissue and the information is transmitted through the tissue electrically and electronically. This mechanism forms the basis of realignment of structure and is the way in which weight-bearing stimulates bone remodelling (Oschman 2000). Connective tissue can be visualized as being a continuous fascial network supported by struts. This allows tensegrity whereby the body can absorb impacts, which functions more efficiently if the network is flexible and balanced. Mechanical energy, whether in the form of manual therapy or harsher physical impacts (such as in sport or falls), will be more readily transmitted through a mechanically healthy network as information rather than damage (Lederman 1997).

FIGURE 3.5   *The parasympathetic nervous system. Reproduced, with permission, from Guyton (1991), p. 669.*

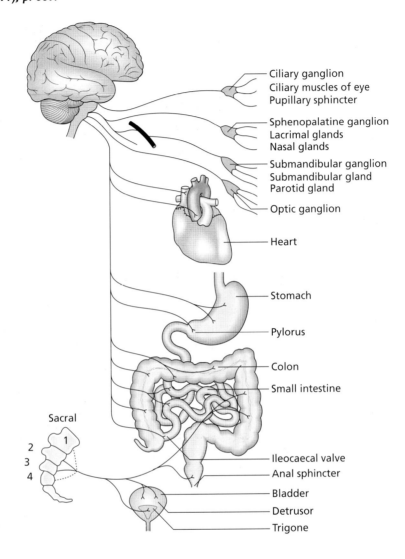

are discussed in some detail by Sato (1975), Koizumi & Brooks (1972) and Sato et al (1997). In addition, Kurosawa et al (1995) found that stroking the abdomen of a rat lowered blood pressure.

It has been shown experimentally that strong autonomic reflexes exist segmentally and that there are suprasegmental reflexes which are weaker. The segmental reflexes produce a sympathetic response when skin of the same spinal segment is stimulated. This reflex reaction is integrated in the spinal cord. In the suprasegmental type, responses are elicited in segments distant from the point of cutaneous stimulation, the organization occurring primarily in the medulla (Sato & Schmidt 1971). Type II and III fibres of cutaneous, visceral and motor nerves contribute to supraspinal reflexes that are integrated at medullary and supramedullary levels, whereas fibre types IV contribute to segmental and suprasegmental reflexes, reaching only as far as the medulla (Sato et al 1969, Sato & Schmidt 1971).

Thus, certain types of skin stimulation can have an autonomic effect. It has also been found that, following somatic afferent stimulation, a silent period in the sympathetic reflex occurs which appears to result from a descending inhibition from the medulla. Polosa (1967) found that repetitive stimuli produce a longer silent period and Koizumi & Sato (1972) demonstrated that a repetitive rate of 10 per second produced a dominant inhibitory effect. There is also an autonomic influence on the receptor mechanism. Merkel's discs are the exteroreceptors that detect shear force in tissue. They are supplied directly by the sympathetic nervous system (Barker & Saito 1981), so sympathetic tone will influence their sensitivity. Sympathetic stimuli and directly applied adrenaline (epinephrine) has been found to modulate the action of cutaneous mechanoreceptors of frog skin *in vitro* (Loewenstein 1956, Loewenstein & Altamirano-Orrego 1956).

There is, then, a connection between skin stimulation and autonomic function, whereby activity in the ANS can be modified by skin stimulation; there is also a converse connection operating in the opposite direction between autonomic output and the structure and functioning of the skin. To summarize, the sympathetic nervous system controls smooth muscle in blood vessel walls. If sympathetic activity increases, the muscles will constrict, causing, among other things, vasoconstriction and altering fluid balance. Sympathetic activity may also alter the threshold of mechanoreceptors causing them to be stimulated more readily, or even to be stimulated by the sympathetic nervous system itself, as in sympathetically maintained pain (Roberts 1986), which occurs in complex regional pain syndrome (reflex sympathetic dystrophy). The concept of autonomic reflexes involving the skin is well accepted but relatively little is known and its relevance to manual therapy is, at present, only postulated. A helpful conceptual model is that of Korr's facilitated segment (Korr 1979).

THE FACILITATED SEGMENT

A spinal cord segment is an anatomical and functional unit which includes a spinal nerve, its root and the section of spinal cord to which it is attached (Bogduk 1989). The spinal nerves form parts of mixed peripheral nerves which contain sensory, motor and autonomic fibres. Sensory stimulation enters the spinal cord via the dorsal horn and motor output leaves via the ventral horn. Convergence of sensory, motor and autonomic impulses occurs in lamina V of the dorsal horn at the wide dynamic range neurones. The segment therefore receives afferent stimuli from sensory fibres, provides electrical supply to muscles via motor nerves, and innervates tissues and viscera via autonomic nerves (Fig. 3.6). Each segment connects to neighbouring ones and to other parts of the CNS via longitudinal connections in the fibre tracts of the spinal cord.

According to Korr's theory, all neuronal components within a single vertebral segment may become 'facilitated' by abnormal activity or irritation in any of the individual components. Facilitation in this context refers to synapses that are easily triggered, probably due to loss of inhibitory factors. In other words, it is 'more easily activated by a stimulus than is necessary in order to

FIGURE 3.6 *The facilitated segment.*

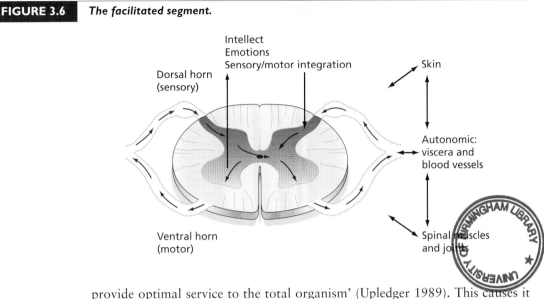

provide optimal service to the total organism' (Upledger 1989). This causes it to fire off a more rapid volley of nervous activity than is warranted by the strength of the incoming stimulus and these are able to pass more easily across the synapses. With reference to pain impulses, for example, the 'gate' is opened. It is thought that, eventually, this facilitation spreads to all nervous tissue throughout the segment, and possibly to neighbouring segments, through neuronal pools. Changes will be seen and felt by the therapist and experienced by the patient in skin, muscle, circulation and viscera. So, the therapist may feel tight, dry or sweaty skin, thickened connective tissue, reduced circulation and increased muscle tone, whereas the patient may feel tightness and soreness between the shoulder blades with visceral symptoms such as an irritated stomach or gallbladder, depending on the spinal segments involved. Normal stimuli can trigger discomfort in an irritated structure and a minor strain, for example in a muscle, will trigger symptoms in a segmentally associated organ.

Eventually, the whole segment can be irritated and abnormal responses of the microcirculation can result. It should be understood that the effects may be extremely subtle, the tissue changes being detectable only by a therapist with very sensitively trained hands. The visceral discomfort may be a slight discomfort, rather than pain. It is believed that it is possible to desensitize the segment by applying altered neuronal programming, by changing the local chemical environment, improving circulation, reducing the muscle spasm, removing the focus of irritation (by stretching a scar, for example, or manipulating a joint), or modifying the diet to 'rest' an inflamed gallbladder.

Clearly, it is preferable to remove the cause of the facilitation but sometimes this is not possible if the problem is a chronically degenerated joint or an ongoing stress response such as a stomach ulcer. Once a state of facilitation exists, it can be 'damped' by treating any part of the segment, to have a reflex reprogramming effect. Massaging the skin, changing the circulation and local fluid balance, reducing muscle spasm and stretching tightened connective tissue will affect sensory, autonomic and motor nerves, and should eventually have an effect through the whole segment. In chronic states, when the facilitation itself has outlived the initial primary problem, this sort of treatment may reduce and prevent symptoms altogether (Upledger 1989).

So, theoretically, stimulus of muscle, skin and viscera can produce responses in the other structures supplied by the same segment; the effect can be positive (if used therapeutically) or negative (if this results in hyperactivity and irritation). This situation should dictate whether intervention should be stimulatory or sedative. A muscle problem may require massage but, if it occurs in association with an area of autonomic tissue change or facilitation, the intervention should ultimately be sedatory and care should be taken not to over-treat.

Reflex effects can also be utilized more specifically through reflex points in the skin and superficial tissues. Myofascial trigger points are not included in this discussion as they fit into this category only loosely, and so are considered elsewhere. The examples chosen for inclusion here are connective tissue zones, Chapman's neurolymphatic reflexes and Bennet's neurovascular points. The therapy associated with the first, Bindegewebsmassage (BGM), or connective tissue manipulation (CTM), has its origins in European physiotherapy (it was developed in Germany), whereas the latter are grounded in osteopathy.

Connective tissue zones (Fig. 3.7) are found on the surface of the body, in the skin and connective tissue (Holey 1995a). They exist in anatomical areas which have a clear, identifiable segmental relationship, occurring in the dermatome which shares the sympathetic supply of the corresponding visceral organ (stomach, for example) or function (such as venous circulation to the

---

FIGURE 3.7   *Connective tissue zones. After Ebner (1962).*

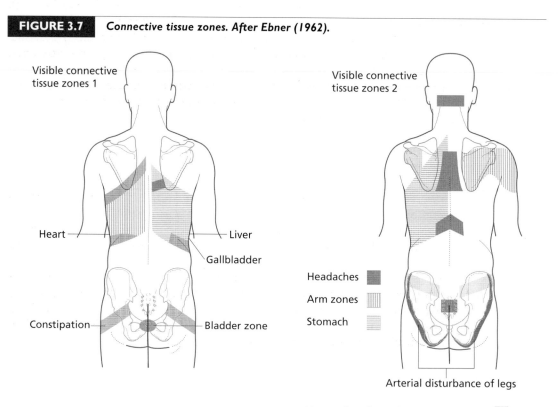

legs). They are found between the dermis and hypodermis when acute, and between the hypodermis and fascia when chronic. Zones appear as tight indrawn areas, often with oedema around their edges. On palpation, the tissues feel dry, adherent, with increased tension and/or thickenings, or can be very oedematous (Dicke et al 1978, Ebner 1980). Stretching the tissue interface to produce a cutting sensation normalizes the tension in the tissue, reflexly increases the circulation throughout the area that corresponds to the zone, and improves visceral function. Working on the sacral and buttock areas, for example, can reduce local pain, increase peripheral circulation and improve bowel and bladder function. CTM may also promote balance within the ANS in patients who present as being sympathetically or parasympathetically dominant (Holey 1995b).

Chapman's reflexes are described as being specific points in deep fascia, palpable as thickenings smaller than the size of a large bean. They assist diagnosis and, when manipulated, alter local fluid drainage and stimulate somatovisceral reflexes. Bennet's neurovascular points are palpated as contraction or induration of the tissues. They are relieved by slight pressure, which is most effective when applied with a fingertip in between two adjacent fingertips, which exert a slight stretch to the skin by drawing away from each other. Bennet believed that this stretch may be followed by a palpable arteriolar pulsing (Chaitow 1987).

Unless the therapist is using a general massage technique such as classical massage, or is following a particular approach such as shiatsu or segmentmassage, she is faced with a bewildering array of reflex points and their postulated effects. Chaitow's solution is to use neuromuscular technique (NMT), in which all the tissues are systematically palpated and treated by specific stroking movements of the finger or thumb tips. These are applied at two depths: the first is a superficial stroke aimed at palpating and identifying a problem area; this is then treated by a deeper stroke which is often sufficient to alleviate the problem. The palpable areas are treated as they are encountered and Chaitow advocates the use of NMT in combination with any other technique necessary, such as stretch and pressure (Chaitow 1987).

CONCLUSION

Several claims have been made for massage. Some have been demonstrated scientifically but, unfortunately, many of the studies are flawed, some in the light of more recent knowledge and some owing to poor research design (Ernst & Fialka 1994). Massage remains both under-researched and difficult to research. Many of the suggested effects for massage can be explained and understood in the context of sound scientific principles, but it is desirable that these beliefs are supported by research evidence. Claims should be regarded sceptically, at least until a convincing explanation has been given, and the therapist should be clear about which parts of our understanding are based on biological explanations rather than scientific validation.

KEY POINTS

- The fat content of tissues cannot be reduced by massage.

- Touching can provoke various responses.

- Massage can influence fluid exchange in tissues without necessarily changing the volume of fluid present.

- Massage can reduce swelling; this effect is considerably enhanced by the use of continuous pressure between sets of strokes and treatment sessions.

- Increased fluid exchange can 'flush' the tissues, clearing the area of chemical irritants and toxins.

- Massage has been shown to increase circulation in immobile limbs.

- The circulation is not increased beyond muscle pump effects in healthy volunteers.

- Vasodilatation caused by massage possibly creates a need for dormant vessels to be recruited.

- Massage has been found to reduce the discomfort of fibrositis, with seven treatments being the optimum number.

- Massage can reduce spasm in muscle fascicles, thought to be due to increased sensitivity in muscle spindles.

- Massage reduces muscle tone, increasing the range of joint movement and reducing associated pain.

- Massage reduces the H reflex, the deep effect being greater than superficial effect.

- Massage increases general flexibility.

- Sensory recovery can occur more quickly with massage.

- Remodelling of connective tissue during the healing process can be facilitated by massage.

- Autonomic reflexes are stimulated by massage; these are the axon and cutaneovisceral reflexes.

- The spinal neuronal segment is said to be facilitated when all its components are hyperactive and the whole is triggered by any one component.

- Reflex points on a patient's skin may be connective tissue zones, Chapman's neurolymphatic reflexes or Bennet's neurovascular points.

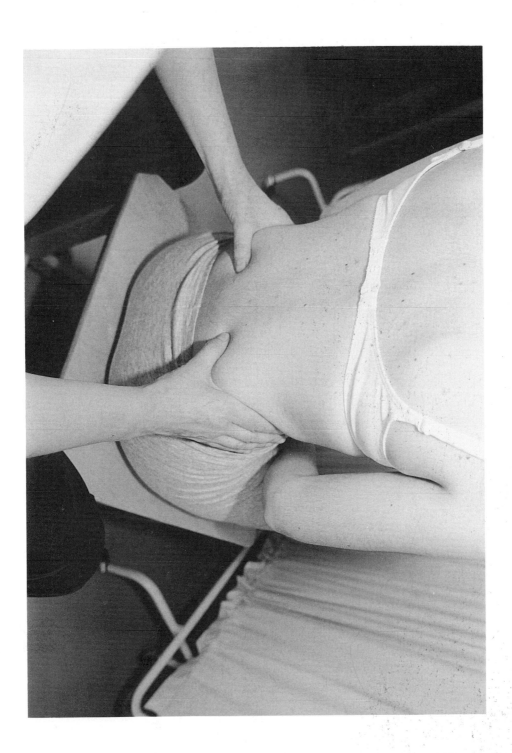

REFERENCES

Arkko P J, Pakarinen A J, Kari-Koskinen O 1983 Effects of whole body massage on serum protein, electrolyte and hormone concentrations, enzyme activities and haematological parameters. International Journal of Sports Medicine 4: 265–267

Banes A J, Tsuzaki M, Yamamoto J et al 1995 Mechanoreception at the cellular level: the detection, interpretation and diversity of responses to mechanical signals. Biochemistry and Cell Biology 73(7–8): 349–365

Barker D, Saito M 1981 Autonomic innervation of receptors and muscle fibres in cat skeletal muscle. Proceedings of the Royal Society of London B212: 317–332

Barnett K 1972 A theoretical construct of the concepts of touch as they relate to nursing. Nursing Research 21(2): 102–110

Bogduk N 1989 The nervous system. In: Palastanga N, Field D, Soames R Anatomy and human movement. Oxford, Butterworth-Heinemann, pp. 800–870

Bork K, Korting G W, Faust G 1971 Serum enzyme levels after a whole body massage. Archiv für Dermatologische Forschung 240: 342–348

Carreck A 1994 The effect of massage on pain perception threshold. Manipulative Physiotherapist 26(2): 10–16

Carrier E B 1922 Studies on the physiology of capillaries: reaction of human skin capillaries to drugs and other stimuli. American Journal of Physiology 11: 528–547

Chaitow L 1987 Soft tissue manipulation. Thorsons, Wellingborough

Chamberlain G J 1982 Cyriax's friction massage: a review. Journal of Orthopaedic and Sports Physical Therapy 4(1): 16–22

Cyriax J 1984 Textbook of orthopaedic medicine. Ballière Tindall, London, vol. 2, pp. 19–25

Danneskiold-Samsoe B, Christiansen E, Lund B, Anderson R B 1982 Regional muscle tension and pain ('fibrositis'): effect of massage on myoglobin in plasma. Scandinavian Journal of Rehabilitation Medicine 15: 17–20

De Bruijn R 1984 Deep transverse friction; its analgesic effect. International Journal of Sports Medicine 5: 35–36

Dicke E, Schliack H, Wolff A 1978 A manual of reflexive therapy of connective tissue. Simon, Scarsdale

Dishman J D, Bulbulian R 2001 Comparison of effects of spinal manipulation and massage on motoneuron excitability. Electromyography and Clinical Neurophysiology 41(2): 97–106

Ebner M 1962 Connective tissue massage. Krieger, Florida

Ebner M 1980 Connective tissue manipulations. Krieger, Huntington, New York

Ernst E, Fialka V 1994 The clinical effectiveness of massage therapy – a critical review. Forsch Komplementarmed 1(5): 226–232

Ernst E, Matrai A, Imagyarosy I et al 1987 Massages cause changes in blood fluidity. Physiotherapy 73(1): 43–45

Field T M, Schanberg S M, Scafidi F et al 1986 Tactile/kinesthetic stimulation effects on preterm neonates. Pediatrics 77(5): 654–658

Flowers K R 1988 String wrapping versus massage for reducing digital volume. Physical Therapy 68(1): 57–59

Frank L K 1957 Tactile communication. Genetic Psychology Monographs 211–251

Gershon M 1981 The enteric nervous system. Annual Reviews of Neuroscience 4: 227–272

Goldberg J, Sullivan S J, Seaborne D E 1992 The effect of two intensities of massage on H-reflex amplitude. Physical Therapy 72(6): 449–457

Goldberg J, Seaborne D E, Sullivan S J, Leduc B E 1994 The effect of therapeutic massage on H-reflex amplitude in persons with a spinal cord injury. Physical Therapy 74: 728–737

Guyton A C 1991 Textbook of medical physiology. W B Saunders, Philadelphia, PA

Hack G D, Robinson W L, Koritzer R T 1995 Previously undescribed relation between muscle and dura. Proceedings of the Congress of Neurological Surgeons, Phoenix, Arizona, February 14–18

Hansen T I, Kristensen J H 1973 Effect of massage, shortwave diathermy and ultrasound upon Xe disappearance rate from muscle and subcutaneous tissue in the human calf. Scandinavian Journal of Rehabilitation Medicine 5: 179–182

Harrison S, Geppetti P 2001 Substance P. International Journal of Biochemistry and Cell Biology 33(6): 555–576

Hartelius I, Ramussen L, Sygehus O 1992 How little you are? Neonatal Network 11(8): 33–37

Holey L A 1995a Connective tissue zones: an introduction. Physiotherapy 81(7): 366–368

Holey L A 1995b Connective tissue manipulation towards a scientific rationale. Physiotherapy 81(12): 730–739

Hovind H, Nielsen S L 1974 Effect of massage on blood flow in skeletal muscle. Scandinavian Journal of Rehabilitation Medicine 6: 74–77

Jacobs M 1960 Massage for the relief of pain: anatomical and physiological considerations. Physical Therapy Review 40(2): 93–98

Jones D A, Round J M 1990 Skeletal muscle in health and disease. Manchester University Press, Manchester

Knight M T N, Dawson R 1976 Effect of intermittent compression of the arms on deep vein thrombosis of the legs. Lancet ii: 1265–1267

Koizumi K, Brooks C McM 1972 The integration of autonomic system reactions. In: Adrian R H et al (eds) Reviews of physiology. Springer-Verlag, New York, pp. 1–71

Koizumi K, Sato A 1972 Reflex activity of single sympathetic fibres to skeletal muscle produced by electrical stimulation of somatic and vaso-depressor afferent nerves in the cat. Pflugers Archiv 332: 283–301

Korr I 1979 The collected papers of Irwin M. Korr. American Academy of Osteopathy, Newark, OH

Kurosawa M, Lundeberg T, Agren G et al 1995 Massage-like stroking of the abdomen lowers blood pressure in anesthetised rats: influence of oxytocin. Journal of the Autonomic Nervous System 56(1–2): 26–30

Lederman E 1997 Fundamentals of manual therapy. Churchill Livingstone, Edinburgh

Loewenstein W R 1956 Modulation of cutaneous mechano-receptors by sympathetic stimulation. Journal of Physiology 132: 40–60

Loewenstein W R, Altamirano-Orrego R 1956 Enhancement of activity in a pacinian corpuscle by sympathomimetic agents. Nature 178: 1292–1293

Lund I, Lundeberg T, Kurosawa M, Uvnas-Moberg K 1999 Sensory stimulation (massage) reduces blood pressure in unanaesthetised rats. Journal of the Autonomic Nervous System 78(1): 30–37

Marin I, Lepresle C, Mechet M A, Debesse B 1991 Postoperative pain after thoracotomy: a study of 116 patients. Revue des Maladies Respiratoires 8(2): 213–218

Mason A 1985 Something to do with touch. Physiotherapy 71(4): 167–169

Mense S, Simons D G, Russell I J 2001 Muscle pain: understanding its nature, diagnosis and treatment. Lippincott Williams and Wilkins, Philadelphia

Montagu A 1978 Touching. Harper and Row, New York

Morelli M, Seaborne D E, Sullivan S J 1990 Changes in H-reflex amplitude during massage of triceps surae in healthy subjects. Journal of Orthopaedic and Sports Physical Therapy 12(2): 55–59

Morelli M, Sullivan S J, Chapman C E 1998 Inhibitory influence of soleus massage onto the medial gastrocnemius H-reflex. Electromyography and Clinical Neurophysiology 38(2): 87–93

Morelli M, Sullivan S J, Chapman C E 1999 Do cutaneous receptors contribute to the changes in the amplitude of the H-reflex during massage? Electromyography and Clinical Neurophysiology 39(7): 441–447

Morhenn V B 2000 Firm stroking of human skin leads to vasodilatation possibly due to the release of substance P. Journal of Dermatological Science 22(2): 138–144

Mosby 1998 Medical, nursing and allied health dictionary, 5th edn. Mosby, St Louis

Newham D J, Lederman E 1997 Effect of manual therapy techniques on the stretch reflex in normal human quadriceps. Disability and Rehabilitation 19(8): 326–331

Nordschow M, Bierman W 1962 The influence of manual massage on muscle relaxation: effect on trunk flexion. Journal of the American Physical Therapy Association 42(10): 653–657

Noris M, Marigi M, Danadelli R et al 1995 Nitric oxide synthesis by cultured endothelial cells is modulated by flow conditions. Circulation Research 76(4): 536–543

Ombregt L, Bisschop P, ter Veer H J, Van de Velde T 1995 A system of orthopaedic medicine. W B Saunders, London

Oschman J L 2000 Energy medicine – the new paradigm. In: Charman R A (ed) Complementary therapies for physiotherapists. Butterworth-Heinemann, Oxford

Pellechia G L, Hamel H, Behnke P 1994 Treatment of infrapatellar tendinitis: a combination of modalities and transverse friction massage versus iontophoresis. Journal of Sport Rehabilitation 3: 135–145

Polosa C 1967 Silent period of sympathetic preganglionic neurons. Canadian Journal of Physiology and Pharmacology 46: 887–897

Poznick-Patewitz E 1976 Cephalic spasm of head and neck muscles. Headache 15: 261–266

Puustjarvi K, Airaksinen O, Pontinen P J 1990 The effect of massage in patients with chronic tension headache. International Journal of Acupuncture and Electrotherapeutics Research 15: 159–162

Roberts W 1986 A hypothesis of the physiological basis for causalgia and related pains. Pain 24: 297–311

Ruegammer W R, Bernstein L, Benjamin J D 1954 Growth food utilization and thyroid activity in the albino rat as a function of extra handling. Science 120: 134

Sabri S, Roberts V C, Cotton L T 1971 Prevention of early deep vein thrombosis by intermittent compression of the leg during surgery. British Medical Journal 4: 394

Sato A 1975 The somatosympathetic reflexes: their physiological and clinical significance. In: Goldstein M (ed) Research status of spinal manipulative therapy. NINCDS Monograph 15. DHEW Publications, Maryland, pp. 163–171

Sato A, Kaufman A, Koizumi K, Brooks C M 1969 Afferent nerve groups and sympathetic reflex pathways. Brain Research 14: 575–587

Sato A, Sato Y, Schmidt R F 1997 The impact of somatosensory input on autonomic function. Reviews of Physiology, Biochemistry and Pharmacology. Springer, Berlin

Sato A, Schmidt R 1971 Somato-sympathetic reflexes: afferent fibres, central pathways, discharge characteristics. Physiology Reviews 54: 916–947

Schultz R L, Feitis R 1996 The endless web: fascial anatomy and physical reality. North Atlantic Books, Berkeley, CA

Severini V, Venerando A 1967 Effect of massage on peripheral circulation and physiological effects of massage. Europa Medicophysica 3: 165–183

Seyle H 1950 The physiology and pathology of exposure to stress. Acta, Montreal

Seyle H 1982 History and present status of the stress concept. In: Goldberger L, Breznitz S (eds) Handbook of stress: theoretical and clinical aspects. Macmillan, New York

Shoemaker J K, Tiidus P M, Mader R 1997 Failure of manual massage to alter blood flow: measured by Doppler ultrasound.
Medicine in Science and Sport and Exercise 29(5): 610–614

Solomon G F, Moos R H 1964 Emotions, immunity and disease. Archives of General Psychiatry 2: 657–674

Sullivan S J, Seguin S, Seaborne D et al 1993 Reduction of H-reflex amplitude during the application of effleurage to the triceps surae in neurologically healthy subjects. Physiotherapy Theory and Practice 9: 25–31

Theoharides T C 1996 The mast cell: a neuroimmunoendocrine master player. International Journal of Tissue Reactions 18(1): 1–21

Thibodeau G A, Patton K T 1999 Anatomy and physiology, 4th edn. Mosby, St Louis

Troisier O 1991 Les tendinites epicondyliennes. La Revue du Praticien 41(18): 1651–1655

Trubetskoy V S, Whiteman K R, Torchilin V P, Wolf G L 1997 Massage-induced release of subcutaneously injected liposome-encapsulated drugs to the blood. Journal of Controlled Release 50: 13–19

Ueda W, Katatoka Y, Sagara Y 1993 Effect of gentle massage on regression of sensory analgesia during epidural block. Anesthesia and Analgesia 76(4): 783–785

Upledger J E 1989 The facilitated segment. Massage Therapy Journal 31: 22–26

Wakim K G, Martin G M, Terrier J C et al 1949 Effects of massage on the circulation in normal and paralyzed extremities. Archives of Physical Medicine 30: 135–144

Walker J M 1984 Deep transverse frictions in ligament healing. Journal of Orthopaedic and Sports Physical Therapy 62: 89–94

Weinrich S P, Weinrich M C 1990 The effect of massage on pain in cancer patients. Applied Nursing Research 3(4): 140–145

Willard F H 1995 Neuroendocrine–immune network, nociceptive stress and the general adaptive response. In: Everett T, Dennis M, Ricketts E (eds) Physiotherapy in mental health. Butterworth-Heinemann, London, pp. 102–126

Williams P L, Warwick R, Dyson M, Bannister L H (eds) 1989 Gray's anatomy, 37th edn. Churchill Livingstone, Edinburgh

Wood E C, Becker P D 1981 Beard's massage. W B Saunders, Philadelphia, PA

Yates J 1990 A physician's guide to massage therapy: its physiological effects and their application to treatment. Massage Therapists Association, British Columbia, Canada

Ylinen J, Cash M 1988 Sports massage. Stanley Paul, London

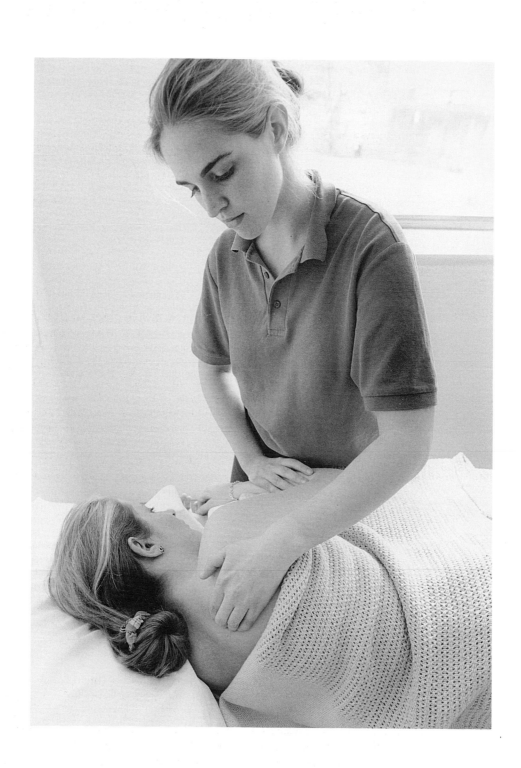

4 Pathological Principles

When massage is applied therapeutically for specific physical problems, the therapist should be guided by knowledge of not only the underlying pathological process but also the stage of healing. Almost all diseases or traumatic states involve a process of inflammation and repair, and the stages in this process must inform decision-making in the planning, progression and modification of treatment. In addition, massage should be applied in the context of the patient's well-being as a whole: the influence of massage on other physical problems must be clearly thought through *before* treatment begins as they may indicate modification of, or even contraindicate, the preferred treatment. Psychological and emotional factors must also be considered carefully to ensure that the psychological effects will be positive and that the massage is appropriate to the patient.

PHYSICAL CONSIDERATIONS

Pathological factors to consider are both local and general.

Local Factors

Inflammation (Fig. 4.1)

Inflammation may have an acute and a chronic stage. Acute inflammation is the response of the tissues to injury. It is a common process which occurs following mechanical or chemical trauma, infection, extremes of temperature, ischaemia, bacterial invasion and faulty immune reactions. It is a necessary and positive event, being an important defensive mechanism which is essential for adequate healing to occur. It can, however, be induced or maintained inappropriately, in which case it may cause severe tissue damage, pain, deformity and loss of function in the affected parts.

FIGURE 4.1   *Inflammation: a comparison of normal capillary exchange and inflammatory response. Reproduced, with permission, from Gould (1997).*

Inflammation

1. Injury

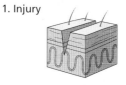

2. Cells release chemical mediators

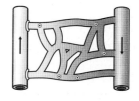

Normal
1. Blood flow

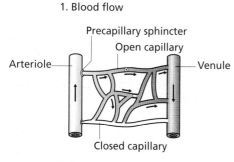

Precapillary sphincter
Open capillary
Arteriole
Venule
Closed capillary

3. Vasodilation - increased blood flow

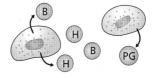

2. Normal fluid shift

Protein remains in blood

F

A

A   G

Water, electrolytes,
glucose to tissue cells

4. Increased capillary permeability

Protein and water leave
capillary - form exudate

Water   F
F

A

A   G

Water,
electrolytes   G

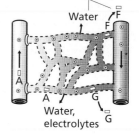

3. Cells remain in blood

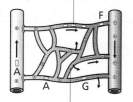

5. Leucocytes move to site of injury

Leucocyte

Chemotaxis

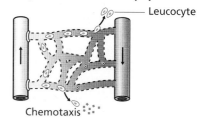

⊙	Cell	B	Bradykinin
A	Albumin	H	Histamine
G	Globulin		
F	Fibrinogen	PG	Prostaglandin

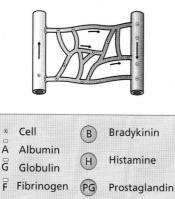

6. Phagocytosis - preparation for healing

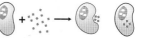

Macrophage Debris   Phagocytosis

Immediately after injury to the tissues, damaged blood vessels constrict under the influence of noradrenaline (norepinephrine) to slow blood loss should that be occurring. During acute inflammation the tissues then undergo sequential change, which begins with arteriolar dilatation, induced by local chemical mediators, causing relaxation of the smooth muscle in the vessel walls. There is a consequent increase in blood flow. This means that the capillaries become dilated with the increased volume of blood entering them from the arterioles, which is seen and felt as a reddening of the skin in the affected area.

There follows an increase in capillary permeability, which allows leakage of plasma into the tissue spaces. The intercellular gaps in the endothelium increase in size due to contraction of the endothelial cells, which contain contractile filaments. Fluid is forced out of the capillary into the extravascular tissue spaces by an increase in hydrostatic pressure within the vessel, created by the extra blood which has flowed into the area. Proteins are also lost from the vessel, as they can escape through the enlarged intercellular gaps; this causes decreased intravessel osmotic pressure and increased osmotic pressure in the tissues. The fluid is seen and felt as a swelling, or oedema, in the affected and surrounding tissues. It is thought that oedema dilutes any toxins that may be present in the tissues and carries important substances which assist in phagocytosis. The fluid is known as inflammatory exudate and the process by which it moves into the tissues is termed transudation.

Stages of acute inflammation

- *Transient phase*: mild injury, caused by histamine, lasts approximately 15 minutes.
- *Delayed persistent phase*: delayed response in which swelling may take up to 24 hours to reach a maximum because of endothelial cell damage.
- *Immediate persistent response*: may last for several days until damaged endothelial cells are replaced.

Note that massage is contraindicated over an area of acute inflammation.

White cells line and adhere to the venule walls (margination) immediately the inflammatory process begins. Once fluid and proteins have leaked into the tissues, blood flow diminishes and blood viscosity increases, with red cells undertaking rouleaux formation in which they are stacked together.

Outside the vessels, white phagocytic cells, mainly neutrophils, migrate to the area. They are attracted by chemotaxis and leave the blood vessels by pushing between the endothelial cells, forcing through their pseudopodia. They are followed by large numbers of macrophages. The exudate is now a cellular aggregate and is viscous in consistency and appearance. Phagocytosis then removes unwanted material from the damaged area. The target cells are coated with protein – antibodies or complement – in the process of opsonization, which allows them to be engulfed by the phagocyte. The material is then ingested, requiring much lysosomal activity.

Once the causative factor has been dealt with and inflammation has slowed, the tissues must return to normal by resolution. The inflammatory debris (including fibrinogen) is removed by macrophages, plasmin and lysosomal enzymes. The exudate and its proteins are removed by the lymphatics. If, however, any exudate persists it must undergo the process of organization. Macrophages, fibroblasts and new capillaries invade the area. The macrophages remove the remains of the exudate while the fibroblasts secrete fibrin, which eventually results in collagen formation (a process that is expanded upon later in this chapter). The new capillaries withdraw and the collagenous tissue shortens, forming a *scar*. If tissue has been lost and the damaged cells are able to reproduce, regeneration next occurs.

The subacute phase lasts from 2 to 4 weeks after injury and is the period when resolution becomes complete and symptoms gradually subside (Kloth et al 1990).

Chronic Inflammation

Inflammation that persists for months or more is termed chronic. It results from a breakdown in the normal process of acute inflammation, caused, for example, by a persistent irritant, inadequate circulation or a failure of exudate, pus or bacterial removal. It may also be caused by an autoimmune response. The presence of increased numbers of macrophages in the tissues will attract collagen-producing fibroblasts, which aim to encapsulate the affected site to prevent the spread of pathogens. Thus, prolonged inflammation will produce excess scar tissue, which can have significant functional consequences.

Inflammation occurs in all damaged tissues; recognition and assessment of the presence and severity of the symptoms will inform accurate clinical decision-making concerning massage.

Symptoms of inflammation
■ Redness
■ Swelling
■ Heat
■ Pain

The symptoms of inflammation (see box) are known as the four cardinal signs. *Redness* is caused by the capillary vasodilatation and increased blood flow; *swelling* is caused by the inflammatory exudate in the tissues, enhanced by a reduction in lymphatic drainage in the area due to fibrinogen clots; *heat* is due to increased blood flow; and *pain* results from the former events, particularly the distension of tissues, pressure exerted by the oedema in limited tissue space and chemical irritation from inflammatory mediators.

Healing (Fig. 4.2)

The next process to consider is that of wound healing. The process is essentially the same in soft tissues whether the wound is caused by a scalpel, a crush or blow, a tear, or non-mechanical trauma. Inflammation is an inherent part of healing as the initial inflammatory process serves to contain the damage, preventing bacterial spread, for example. The other phases of healing must also be considered as they should dictate the type and timing of different massage manipulations. During this process, the tissues show a diversity of the various

| FIGURE 4.2 | *The healing process. Reproduced, with permission, from Gould (1997).* |

A. Healing of incised wound
   by first intention

B. Healing by second intention

1. Injury and inflammation
   - Scab
   - Suture holds edges together
   - Blood clot
   - Neutrophils
   - Inflammation

1. Injury and inflammation
   - Scab
   - Blood clot
   - Inflammation

2. Granulation tissue and epithelial growth
   - Epithelial regeneration
   - Inflammation
   - Macrophage
   - Fibroblast
   - Granulation tissue begins to form
   - New capillaries

2. Granulation tissue and epithelial growth
   - Epithelial regeneration
   - Inflammation
   - Macrophage
   - Granulation tissue
   - New capillary

3. Small scar remains
   - Scar

3. Large scar remains
   - Fibrous tissue contracts
   - Scar

stages of healing. Ongoing inflammation occurs alongside other healing processes and possibly pathologies, for example inflammatory exudate, scar tissue and tissue necrosis.

There are two types of healing, the distinction being whether there is, or is not, tissue loss. If the wound is a neat incision (a cut with a knife, for example) there is no tissue loss, whereas in the case of a skin graze, or a blow leaving crushed muscle fibres which die, tissue loss leaves a gap. Wounds without tissue loss heal by 'first intention' and those with tissue loss heal with 'second intention' (Fig. 4.2).

In either case, granulation tissue is formed, this process beginning 38–72 hours after injury. The area contains large numbers of macrophages and fibroblasts, surrounding capillaries 'bud' into the area, forming new growth to provide nutrition. Collagen, hyaluronic acid and fibronectin (a glycoprotein which enhances cellular adhesion and migration) surround these new leaky capillaries and newly formed lymphatics. This tissue is termed granulation tissue, as its new capillaries give it a red granular appearance.

Meanwhile, a few hours after injury, epidermal cells begin to migrate. The surrounding epidermal cells break their desmosomal attachment with neighbouring cells and produce actin filaments at the edges of their cytoplasm which give them the capacity to move more easily by reaching out with pseudopodia. The cells either roll over the top of each other in a continuous line until the gap is filled, or slide along in a chain until the lead cell reaches the other side of the wound. The surrounding epithelial cells also reproduce, until a thin covering of cells seals the wound surface, and the wound is then closed from the edges inwards, growing progressively smaller in diameter. It is thought that these events can occur because the natural inhibitors of tissue growth – chalones – are absent from the area of tissue loss and are therefore unable to prevent cell division, and because epidermal growth factor is present.

At this stage the connections between the cells are fragile and delicate, and manipulation may damage them, causing breakdown of the new tissue which delays healing. However, good nutrition via the bloodstream is essential for successful tissue repair and careful massage of the surrounding area may be beneficial, particularly where the circulation is poor.

The next visible occurrence is wound contraction. This begins before substantial collagen synthesis in the first 2 weeks after injury; it is thought to be due to the contractile abilities in the actin-containing fibroblast, the myofibroblast. These cells extend pseudopodia, attach to the collagen fibrous network and retract, reducing the surface area of the wound if the conditions are favourable, and if the number of cells is appropriate for the size of collagenous matrix.

Once cell migration is complete, a collagenous basement membrane is laid down and the cells form connections. In scar formation, the fibroblasts form collagen, and polypeptide chains aggregate into a triple helix to become procollagen, at which stage it is released from the fibroblast. Parts of the molecule are lost leaving tropocollagen, and intramolecular and intermolecular crossbridges are formed to give tensile strength to what is not yet a structural fibril. At this point, the collagen resembles type III collagen, which is eventually replaced by type I collagen in response to mechanical stress. This stage is a major part of skin healing, as dermis contains predominantly connective tissue.

Mechanical stress is important at this stage for the remodelling of collagen (replacement of type III with type I collagen) and also for alignment along the lines of stress. This alignment is due to the piezo-electrical effect whereby electrical streaming potentials result from mechanical stress and dictate the remodelling process. This stress is usually produced internally by normal functional activity, for example when muscle contraction exerts a pull on a tendon or when joint movement applies forces to ligaments. The effect may be enhanced with artificial stress, applied externally by manipulation of the tissues. Massage, therefore, will promote remodelling and thereby increase the tensile strength of the tissues. This effect is particularly important where immobility, either local or general, has been enforced. The lack of movement will have resulted in reduced stress being exerted on the tissues which has a weakening effect, even in normal tissues, as demonstrated by research (Akeson et al 1973).

The remodelling occurs during the *maturation phase* of scar formation. The bonding within the intercollagenous molecules strengthens, converting from the weaker hydrogen type to the stronger covalent type of bond. Hydrogen bonding permits stretching in response to gentle stress, whereas mature collagen is more resistant. This is important, as at this stage stress that is correctly applied and not excessive will ensure that the wound or scar heals at optimum length; any shortening is difficult to correct once healing is complete, owing to the stronger covalent bonding in mature collagen.

Occasionally, this remodelling mechanism fails and the balance between collagen removal (or lysis) and deposition (or synthesis) is lost. If excess collagen deposition occurs within the boundaries of a skin wound, a *hypertrophic scar* results. If it extends beyond the wound, and encroaches on normal tissue, then a *keloid scar* results. Keloid scarring is prone to occur in burned skin and the use of pressure garments is common in treatment of the burned patient. These exert a continuous pressure (they must be worn for 24 hours a day), creating a piezo-electrical streaming potential to maximize connective tissue remodelling. They have been found to be extremely successful in reducing hypertrophic and keloid scarring.

Friction massage has been found not to influence the vascularity, pliability or height of hypertrophic scarring (as assessed by the Vancouver Burn Scar Assessment Scale) when it was given to 30 children for 10 minutes daily over a 3-month period (Patino et al 1999). The choice of frictions as a massage technique in this study can be questioned. It places a high level of dynamic mechanical stimulation in tissues in which, in the case of hypertrophic scarring, the balance between the lysis and synthesis of collagen has been lost. It is perhaps unsurprising that this study yielded negative results when there is evidence that continuous pressure is effective in reducing the effects of hypertrophic scarring.

This account of the physiological events that occur during the inflammatory and healing processes may serve to inform our intervention during or following these events. Massage should be employed to:

- enhance natural healing processes
- increase surrounding circulation, thereby increasing local blood flow
- increase venous and lymphatic drainage from the area, enhancing the removal of waste products and proteins
- promote remodelling of collagen
- soften scarring
- mobilize tissue bound in scar formation.

First, it may be appropriate to increase circulation to the area. Blood flow may be compromised as a result of the patient's circumstances – confined to bed, for example, or immobilized for some other reason. The reduced mobility may be general if the patient is unable to function normally, or may be local if only the affected limb, or even joints above and/or below the injured area, is immobilized. Immobility may be of a more subtle nature, for example if pain, or a dressing, prevents normal gait or muscle action. This situation reduces muscle pump activity and consequently venous return, resulting in a reduction of general circulation and a gravitational pooling in the lower limb. Slight puffiness around distal joints, especially the ankles, in the absence of other possible factors (such as heart or kidney failure), indicates reduced muscle pump.

The circulation locally around the wound may need to be increased. If inflammation has reached a chronic stage and healing has been delayed for any reason, then the wound margins may be adherent and congested. Wound contraction may be compromised due to excess adherence of the margins to underlying tissue. Gentle circular kneadings around the edges, taking care not to touch any healing surfaces, may bring nutrition to the area, mobilize the margins from adjacent layers of tissue and speed up wound contraction, and therefore healing.

As the wound heals beyond the cell adherence stage, gentle stress will facilitate remodelling of collagen and therefore maturation of the scar. At this stage, adherence and excessive contracture must be avoided. Massage can help to loosen the scar from underlying tissue, preventing or reducing adherence in a more chronic stage of healing. It can reduce contracture of the scar by repetitive stretching, facilitating a final optimum length of the collagen fibres.

At all times, the stage of healing must be considered – this guides the effectiveness and safety of the techniques. The timetable of healing is now well established and the summary in Figure 4.3 provides a good basis for clinical decision-making and treatment planning.

We will return to the implications of the stages of the healing process in the clinical sections of this book, but from the preceding descriptions it is clear that in the early stages of healing, when the cell connections and collagen fibrils are delicate, manipulation should be avoided. The surrounding area can be massaged gently to increase circulation, an effect that may be enhanced by proximal massage. During the early stages of remodelling, *gentle* mechanical

FIGURE 4.3   *Phases of wound healing. Adapted from Boscheinen-Morrin et al (1992), p. 2.*

Phases of Wound Healing

Phase	Onset	Peak	Duration	Pathophysiology	Wound Strength	Management
Traumatic inflammation	0	12 hours	24–48 hours	Vascular response: bleeding, oedema Cellular (phagocytosis) response: leucocytes, macrophages	Negligible	Rest Elevation Ice
Proliferation of fibroblasts	12 hours	2–5 days	10 days	Fibroblasts proliferate, migrate and bridge wound edges by 5 days	Some	Rest Elevation
Collagen (fibroplasia)	5 days	3 months	6 months	Collagen fibrils: initially weak random fibrils, later strong flexible fibres depending on the stress placed upon them	Rapid rise	Splintage of the repaired tissue Exercise
Remodelling	1 month	→	2 years or more	Collagenase removes excess collagen, fibroblasts contract, and there is vascular and wound shrinkage	Continued gradual rise	Exercise and return of function

Adapted from The Hand Fundamentals of Therapy, p. 2, by Boscheinen-Morrin *et al.* (1992). Butterworth-Heinemann, Oxford.

stress will facilitate healing at the optimum collagenous length and strength. As this period moves into consolidated healing, a stronger stress will correct any shortening and further strengthen the tissue.

Wound contracture is an essential part of the healing process, particularly where there is extensive tissue loss, and over time the scars tend to become smaller and paler in colour. However, occasionally this shrinkage occurs beyond a desirable level. This sometimes happens as healing occurs, but remodelling, stimulated by normal movement of the body part and stretching of the affected tissues, gradually stretches the tissue to a more functional length. If local or general immobility reduces this normal process, or if pathological factors such as infection increase fibrous tissue formation, it may be appropriate to assist in the establishment of tissue length; reduction in tissue extensibility, even temporarily, compromises joint movement and function causing possible joint complications such as stiffness and loss of accessory movements, which may alter the biomechanics of the joint and reduce its range of movement. Complications such as this produce the difficulties experienced by a patient as *functional loss*. This may be considerable, for example if the damage has occurred in the hand, with potentially serious psychological, social and financial effects. Eventually, if left, the tissue may remodel in its newly shortened length and contracture may be permanent. Manipulations that stretch the tissue in all directions are important here.

The effects of excess tissue contracture will be exacerbated if adherence of the scar to underlying tissue has occurred. This will result in loss of excursion, not only of the superficial layers but of the deeper layers also, resulting in increased functional loss. Each time a normal movement places the tissue on a stretch, rather than yielding normally, a pull will be exerted at the point of adherence (and the tissue interface), causing pain. The patient will tend to stop the movement short of that point, to avoid further pain. Remodelling of the tissue will therefore occur in response to non-functional stimuli, resulting in shortened, and initially weaker, collagen because of the reduction in stress. If muscle tissue is involved, shortening and muscle imbalance could result. Where movement is less well controlled, there will be pull exerted at the end-point of mobility, creating an inflammatory reaction at the adherent interfaces. This will result in the formation of further fibrin and collagen, causing thickening and excess scarring. The result will be a permanent adherence and loss of function.

At this chronic stage, massage should be vigorous, focusing on prolonged stretching manipulations.

It is likely that the circulation will be compromised, as chronic inflammation may result in its attendant problems, and there may be involvement of nerve endings, resulting in neural tension in the skin.

Oedema

Oedema is present in many of the patients who consult or are referred for physical therapy. It must be controlled immediately it occurs, as chronic oedema can cause fibrosis, adhesions, resultant loss of joint movement and pain. The excess fluid itself causes pain as pressure is exerted on nociceptors; it further prevents cells from being bathed in fresh, newly nourished tissue fluid, and thus reduces normal cellular metabolism. Metabolic circulation may be reduced together with metabolites, and protein remains in the tissues. Prevention, containment and removal of swelling is the essential hierarchy of care for the tissues, regardless of cause, and massage can be a cornerstone of effective treatment, with skilful application of manual lymphatic drainage (MLD) being essential in the treatment of lymphoedema.

Oedema is a significant feature of the massage therapist's professional life. It is present in many of our patients' tissues for a variety of reasons and hence occurs in many forms. It is essential that we are able to recognize it and identify its type so that we can establish its causative factors. This will enable us to decide whether massage can assist its removal, which type of massage will be most effective, whether an alternative intervention is required, or whether massage should be avoided altogether. Excess tissue fluid is present in many people, from the 'puffy ankles' of the shop assistant on a hot day or the holiday-maker at the end of a long flight, to more long-standing intractable oedema, as in lymphoedema. Normal fluid balance in the tissues is dependent on many factors, any of which, if operating suboptimally, can result in excess tissue fluid.

Fluid Balance in the Body

To maintain a perfect balance of fluid between the circulatory system and the tissues, the circulation must be operating normally, both in the structure of the carrying vessels and the constituents of the blood itself. The heart pumps arterial blood into the periphery of the body, through the arterial system, so the veins must operate an efficient system of return. They must be sufficiently pliable to be squeezed by contracting muscles, to pump the blood from the superficial veins into the deep veins and then upwards along the venous system, against gravity. Valves stop the back-flow of blood when the muscles relax, thus contributing to the pumping effect. A strong dynamic muscle pump will make this system extremely efficient, and weakened muscles or immobility will decrease its effectiveness. The volume being returned to the heart must match the volume being pumped by the heart, and a system of fluid balance maintenance must operate successfully at the arteriovenous capillary loop, through pressure equalization between the tissues and vessels (see Ch. 2). Adequate tissue pressure around the muscles created by the fascial layers will give the muscles a firm covering to contract against, ensuring that good squeezing of the veins occurs.

Causes of Oedema

There are several components to the circulatory system, and oedema can occur when any component operates at less than optimum efficiency:

- Inflammation, as in an acute injury or an allergic response in the skin, causes increased permeability of the capillaries, and excess fluid will leave the circulation for the tissues.
- If pressure is placed on any part of the circulatory system, as in pregnancy, varicosity or thrombosis in the veins, the increased hydrostatic pressure within the vessels will be in excess of that in the tissues, resulting in oedema.
- Pressure can be increased in the circulatory system by heart malfunction. Cor pulmonale results from pulmonary conditions in which the pressure in

the pulmonary artery is increased, exerting a back pressure on the right ventricle, resulting in hypertrophy and reduced output by the insufficient musculature. The back pressure causes congestion in the veins of the periphery, raising the hydrostatic pressure in the venous blood with inevitable oedema.

- Insufficiency of the lymphatic system, for example congenital absence or damage to the lymph glands by radiotherapy or surgery, means that proteinous fluid accumulates in the tissues.

- Other medical conditions can create oedema in the tissues. Heart failure, which lowers cardiac output, leads to a lowered capillary pressure, which affects perfusion in the kidneys. Sodium and water are retained by the body, some of the fluid being pushed into the tissues. Primary renal disease invariably leads to a reduced filtration rate with excess retention of salts and fluid (Woolf 1988).

- If the veins lose their compliance and the valves become incompetent, then venular distension occurs due to an increased volume of blood. The resulting increased hydrostatic pressure in the veins will produce oedema in the tissues. Primary varicose veins can be severe enough to allow blood from the deep veins to flow back across the saphenofemoral junction down the long saphenous vein. The veins will be very distended after standing and often reduce in size quite drastically after lying down. Secondary varicosity often follows an undetected deep vein thrombosis, which may exist without producing symptoms of its own, for example after surgery or childbirth (Hurst 1987).

- In situations where oedema has been long standing, the fascia may become stretched and the muscle pump becomes less efficient, so the problem becomes self-perpetuating.

- Ascites is the name given to the accumulation of fluid in the peritoneal cavity and is seen where the hepatic venous outflow is restricted in liver disease or malignancy. It also occurs in nutritional oedema resulting from prolonged starvation (particularly kwashiorkor, the name given to protein undernutrition in children).

Tissue fluid is also determined by sympathetic control of the capillary bed. The amount of arteriolar constriction is dependent on sympathetic stimulus and occurs in response to local metabolic need, chemical and mechanical irritants, temperature, activity elsewhere in the body (redistribution effect) and psychological factors such as stress. Normal tissue fluid balance is maintained by a balance between the hydrostatic pressure (outwards force) and colloid osmotic pressure (inwards force) in the vessel and the hydrostatic and colloid osmotic pressure in the tissues.

Factors disturbing any of these pressures will disrupt the balance and result in oedema. Dilatation increases the size of the gaps between cells in the capillary walls, allowing more fluid to escape from the bloodstream. This typically occurs in an acute injury as an essential part of the healing process. It is thought that the fluid flushes the area of damaging substances and chemical irritants. Plasma proteins are released into the tissues and must then be removed by an efficient lymphatic pump as they are too large to re-enter the bloodstream any other way. If fluid is formed more rapidly than it can be removed, the balance is lost and oedema accumulates. As one of the plasma proteins is fibrinogen, fibrin is secreted in an attempt to 'wall off' destructive agents and stop them spreading through the tissues. Eventually, fibrous tissue is laid down and this may trap the swelling, preventing its removal, or it may form adhesions between adjacent structures (for example between tendon and sheath, or between fibres within a ligament, or between a nerve and the connective tissue of a surrounding muscle). Once formed, it has a tendency to collect in pockets behind the malleoli or between the metacarpals or metatarsals (for example following local injury), or to become trapped around scars, or more extensively in dependent parts – the lower leg and ankle. It was speculated in 1952 by Ladd and co-workers that metabolic circulation is reduced by oedema as the circulation is separated from the cells and massage was suggested as being important in assisting in its removal.

The Need for Caution

Massage can indeed help in the removal of excess tissue fluid but there are also situations in which it is ineffective or could even exacerbate the swelling:

- Where the fluid is due to organic disease such as heart or kidney problems or nutritional factors.
- Swelling due to an acute injury. In the first 24 hours after a soft tissue injury, massage may increase the inflammation and swelling and disrupt the healing process. A system of:
  - Rest – with controlled movement
  - Ice
  - Compression
  - Elevation
    is the treatment of choice here.
- In the presence of a deep vein thrombosis or phlebitis. Venous problems can lead to skin ulceration and the veins can become inflamed and thrombosed (superficial thrombophlebitis). Massage could possibly dislodge a thrombus, precipitating its movement throughout the bloodstream. This could result in it causing blockage of a smaller vessel and could be fatal should this occur in the lungs. The signs to look for are increased pain, swelling and local erythema occurring in an area of venous varicosity which could indicate phlebitis; in this case a medical opinion and subsequent treatment should be sought. Pain and swelling in the calf, often fairly severe, could indicate a deep vein thrombosis. Homans' test (Fig. 4.4) should be carried out and, if positive, the patient should be referred to a medical practitioner.

Massage for Hydrostatic Oedema

Aims

To force blood mechanically along the vessel, to reduce the internal hydrostatic pressure to less than the hydrostatic pressure in the tissues, and to push fluid from the tissues into the vessel by increasing tissue pressure beyond that of the vessels.

Position

The limb should be elevated on pillows or a covered wedge, to utilize the effects of gravity. Care should be taken to ensure that the distal part of the

FIGURE 4.4 *Homans' test for deep vein thrombophlebitis.*

Hold the knee
straight

Passively dorsiflex
the ankle

If this increases
the exact pain,
the test is positive

A thrombus can
sometimes be
palpated between
the heads of
gastrocnemius

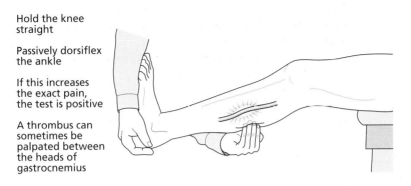

limb is slightly higher than the proximal part but not raised so high the axillary tissues are stretched in the case of an arm, or the lymph nodes are not compressed in the groin in the case of a lower limb. An elevation of approximately 45 degrees is suitable (Hollis 1987).

Media

The skin should be carefully inspected, as it is often dry and fragile, particularly if the oedema has been long standing; oil may be the medium of choice to protect and improve the skin.

Principles

The limb should be divided into sections and proximal areas should be worked before distal ones. As much of the procedure involves pushing the fluid mechanically towards the lymph glands, it is important that the way through is clear; therefore, the proximal sections must be drained to make room for fluid that has collected distally. Milking and pressure techniques will push blood along a vessel and push fluid from the tissues into the vessels. Effleurage may be done to coincide with static muscle contraction to increase the pressure on the vessels, or deep breaths to utilize this suction effect.

Progression of treatment involves modifying the strokes as the tissues begin to feel different, increasing the size of each movement, for example. This will occur automatically as the tissues soften if they are worked to their end-feel. When the oedema has resolved, a general massage should be given to stretch and mobilize the tissue layers fully. In more acute injuries and in fibrous areas such as the soles of the feet, little soft pockets can be felt which seem to 'pop' and disappear when gentle pressure is put on them.

Self-care

The use of limb elevation, support stockings or bandages, breathing and circulatory exercises, and skin care as appropriate should be understood by the patient.

Strokes

Whole Limb:

- Effleurage (done slowly, as tissue fluid can be viscous) the whole limb

In Section:

- Vibrations if the oedema is soft; omit if consolidated
- Deep kneading in box formation (hands on opposite aspects of limb)
- Effleurage
- Squeeze kneading for deeper tissues
- Effleurage

Whole Limb:

- Effleurage
Repeat for each section.

In addition, when a joint is reached, finger and thumb kneading should be carried out around the joint line and ligaments specifically to mobilize these structures.

Tissue spaces – between the metacarpals and metatarsals, the dorsum of the foot and around the malleoli – should be effleuraged with the thumb, interspersed with finger kneading to release the fluid.

Massage for Venous Ulcers

If the massage is prescribed for an area of circulatory insufficiency, a venous ulcer may be present. This requires specific treatment which can be aided by massage. Hygiene is of the utmost importance and, if the ulcer is open, the therapist should wear medical gloves to prevent cross-infection. Latex gloves must not be worn if the patient has a latex allergy. If the massage causes discomfort or the ulcer haemorrhages, massage should be discontinued around this area (Whittaker 1987).

Aims

To increase the circulation to the surrounding tissues and mobilize the edges of the ulcer, promoting healing. As the ulcer heals and becomes smaller in diameter, massage aims to free the healed skin from the underlying layers and promote remodelling, thus increasing the tensile strength of the new skin.

Principles

The edges of the scar should be stretched and moved on underlying layers. Any open surface should not be touched. The treatment should complement, not undermine, the dressing regimen and should preferably take place when a new dressing is due, so coordination with the nursing staff responsible may be essential. Extra changes of dressing which may disturb the healing process and introduce infection should be avoided.

Strokes

Around the Edges of the Wound:

- Finger kneading
- Thumb kneading
- Skin rolling

Friction should be avoided where the circulation is poor. A record can be kept of the progress of healing, to monitor the rate at which the wound shrinks in size. A tracing of the wound can be taken on a double layer of sterile cellophane (the top layer, which is not in contact with the wound, is retained). This can remain as a purely visual record, or the wound area can be calculated after dividing the tracing into measured squares. Alternatively, an estimation can be made from a scale comprised of concentric circles (Fig. 4.5).

Around the ulcer, where there is superficial oedema, the skin feels very soft and spongy. Where the ulcer is long standing, the skin will feel more solid and occasionally hard. The tissues may feel thickened and indurated. As the fluid reduces and circulation improves, solid areas and fibrous bands can often be felt which require treating in the usual way with deep circular finger kneading and friction techniques.

Self-care

The therapist should ensure that the patient understands good hygiene, skin care, support bandages, limb elevation, and breathing and circulatory exercises.

FIGURE 4.5   *Concentric circle grid for measuring wound diameter.*

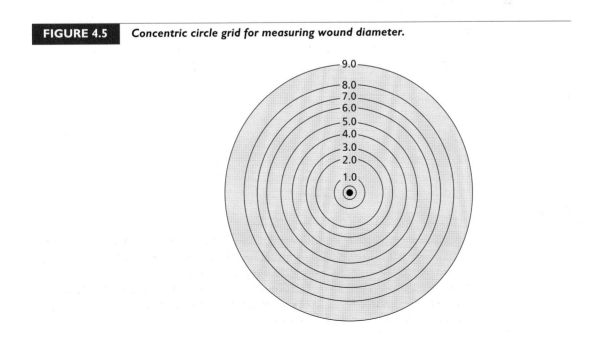

Massage should NOT be undertaken to the area around a decubitus ulcer (pressure sore). These are often found in tissues which are de-nutritioned due to poor circulation and/or generalized ill health where nutrient intake or absorption is reduced. There is often an infective element. Skin rubbing has long been advocated as part of nursing care, to improve circulation, although massage around decubitus ulcers has not been part of the tradition of physiotherapy because of the risk of damaging poor quality tissues (Pritchard & Mallett 1993). A temporary drop in skin temperature may occur after massage (Tyler et al 1990) which may be clinically significant in this group of patients.

General Factors

Adverse Neural Dynamics

This situation can occur in nervous tissue. Fibrous adhesions will produce tension at any interface – intraneurally or extraneurally. It is important that nervous tissue can glide in relation to the surrounding tissues, particularly when movement places a stretch on the nerve fibre. If not, stretch will increase the tension at the point of adherence, producing irritation. In severe cases, the nerve may be compressed by the adhesions. Injury involving the nervous tissue will produce this effect, but adjacent injury that produces inflammation and swelling may lead to compromise of the neural tissue (known as a subclinical entrapment) (Butler 1991).

Neural tension can lead to:

- altered mechanics of the nerve and increased friction
- changes in the interior of the neurone which increases the irritability of the nerve
- abnormal chemosensitivity
- minor demyelination as a result of entrapment
- increased autonomic sensitivity producing trophic changes (Gunn 1989).

If the nerve is irritated, a 'double crush' scenario may exist in which pathology in one part of the neurone (nerve roots, for example) may produce distal symptoms. Conversely a 'double crush' may occur in which the pathology is distal and symptoms proximal. According to Lundborg (1988), this is caused by reduced retrograde transport.

PAIN

Most pathological changes result in varying degrees of pain. It has been found that, under normal conditions, pain is elicited by thermal, mechanical or chemical trauma. Furthermore, damage to the tissues causes chemical release which in turn may cause pain and damage the tissues even further. Substances such as potassium and bradykinin cause pain. In addition, there are various substances that are believed to have an indirect effect in producing pain. Acetylcholine, 5-hydroxytryptamine (5-HT), enzymes and prostaglandins can all have algogenic properties. There are situations in which chronic pain itself becomes the condition suffered by the patient, because it is disproportionate to the

Complications of Healing that may be Helped by Massage

Contracture

This occurs when the tissue has healed in a shortened position. Sometimes this is necessary to prevent traction on the wound edges (for example, following tendon or nerve suture). Once healing is complete, passive and active stretching is necessary. The passive form can be applied longitudinally or transversely by massage.

Adherence

Healed tissue is often bound to the underlying layers of tissue by fibrous tissue. This must be freed by the loosening of the fibrous adhesions by vigorous massage. Adhesions can also occur between adjacent fibres in the same strata of tissue and will prevent the sideways spread necessary during contraction in a muscle or tension in a ligament. They can be loosened by a transverse friction technique.

Neural Tension

The fibrous tissue produced in healing will inevitably involve any structures in the vicinity. Nerve endings may become involved in scars. This can affect the nerve by interfering with the conductivity, causing hypersensitivity. Where this occurs in autonomic nerves, it is believed that widespread effects can result throughout the autonomic nervous system (ANS). Thus, attempts to minimize the extent or effects of scarring may help to prevent neural tension occurring. Promotion of normal fluid balance, both intraneurally and extraneurally, will help to minimize fibrin formation. Mobilizing the tissues will prevent intraneural and extraneural contracture of fibrous tissue.

cause, or because it persists after the causative factor has been resolved. To explore how massage might be used to alleviate pain, pain mechanisms must first be described.

Pain Mechanisms and the Relief of Pain

In the Tissues

Any individual can identify two types of pain: fast and slow. The fast pain is experienced as sharp or pricking pain and typically occurs when one is pricked by a pin. The impulse travels so quickly that the reflex motor response by which the hand is sharply drawn away from the pin is already occurring as the pain becomes registered by the conscious mind. The slower type is of a more aching, throbbing variety. This phenomenon is accounted for by the different fibres in which the pain impulses are transmitted (Fig. 4.6). The painful stimulus is detected via nociceptors (pain receptors) and is transmitted along the large-diameter myelinated A-delta fibres at 15 ms (or 35 miles per hour).

FIGURE 4.6   *Physiological classifications and functions of nerve fibres. Reproduced, with permission, from Guyton (1991), p. 500.*

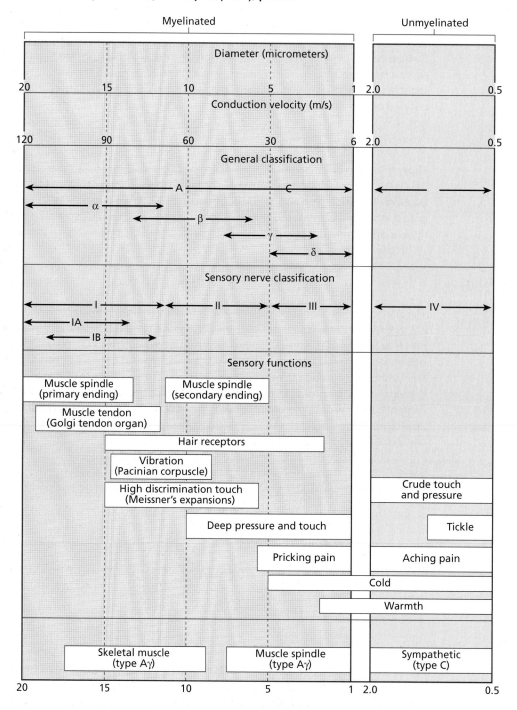

Alternatively, it is picked up by the free nerve endings of polymodal C fibres which also detect chemical, thermal and mechanical stimuli. These use substance P as their neurotransmitter and, being unmyelinated and of small diameter, conduct impulses more slowly at 1.5 ms (or 2.25 miles per hour) (Bowsher

1991). The impulse travels along the sensory nerve to enter the spinal cord at the dorsal horn.

Sensory nerve endings are also able to 'taste' the chemical environment in the tissues. These chemicals, which change following tissue damage, are transmitted antidromically through the axoplasm of the nerve fibre to the cell body. If chemical change persists, the presence of these chemicals within the nerve cell induces plastic changes in the neurone; for example, the cell becomes more sensitive, operating at a lower threshold. This is caused by the development of a subthreshold excitatory postsynaptic potential whereby the synapse becomes more likely to fire but a single stimulus is not sufficient to cause firing – several are needed. Normally, there is a balance between the excitatory postsynaptic potential and the descending inhibitatory influences. The long-term effect of a *subthreshold* excitatory postsynaptic potential increases the level of excitability and converts acute into chronic pain. In chronic states, this effect can spill over throughout a neuronal pool. This is probably why tenderness of the tissues occurs and why this area of tenderness extends over a wider area if a painful state lasts for any length of time. It is commonly experienced by patients suffering from chronic pain. Repetitive stimulus of C fibres lowers their threshold, which may be another source of tenderness. Prolonged excitation of nociceptors may be responsible for hypersensitivity and reflex responses. It is also known that bradykinin, for example, sensitizes muscle nociceptors to mechanical stimuli such as weak local pressure. A recurring cycle can be produced in chronic pain states whereby algogenic substances cause altered local circulation. This increase of capillary permeability creates further biochemical disturbance which sensitizes the cell bodies (for a review see Iggo et al 1984). This should be taken into account when massaging: tissues in this state should be massaged very gently. In chronic pain, the wide dynamic range (WDR) neurones in lamina V of the dorsal horn, at which convergence of sensory, motor and visceral impulses occurs, can become sensitized, causing abnormal responses to normal sensory stimuli throughout the segment.

In the periphery, massage can alleviate pain by removing waste products and chemical sensitizers from the tissues via the venous and lymphatic systems and by increasing blood flow, bringing fresh blood and plasma to the area. By stretching fibrous tissue and altering the pressures in the vessels and tissue spaces, massage releases fluid trapped in the tissue spaces and promotes transfer of fluid between the circulation and tissues. Thus, the local chemical environment can be altered and pain reduced. Removal of excess fluid from the tissues will lower pressure on nerves that may be causing pain. As fibrous tissue is stretched, this will relieve the pain-producing tension on nerve endings, including autonomic endings.

In the Spinal Cord

On arrival in the spinal cord, the A-delta and C fibres synapse. The point at which this occurs depends on the neuronal tract each fibre travels in to reach its final destination. Initially, the pain fibres ascend or descend several segments in Lissauer's tract before synapsing. Afferent A-delta fibres synapse in lamina I and lamina V, whereas C fibres mostly synapse in the substantia gelatinosa (lamina II), releasing excitatory chemicals, amino acids such as glutamate for fast transmission or neuropeptides (for example substance P, or vasoactive intestinal polypeptide) for a slower or modulating effect. Some fibres synapse in the ventral horn via interneurones and produce reflex motor activity, for example the flexor withdrawal response whereby a burned hand is rapidly withdrawn from the source of damage. They are also responsible for increased muscle tone in less acute pain states. If prolonged this can lead to muscle spasm, a type of *reactive pain*. From the dorsal horn, the fast (A-delta) impulses are transmitted in the neospinothalamic tract of the opposite side after crossing in the spinal cord, to travel in the anterolateral fibre columns to the brain. Most of these fibres terminate in the thalamus but connect with the periaqueductal grey area prior to this (Fig. 4.7). The A-beta impulses reach the cuneate and gracile nuclei of the same side without synapsing. The slower, chronic types of pain impulses are transmitted across a synapse in the substantia gelatinosa (lamina II) in the dorsal column before crossing to the opposite side to travel in the paleospinothalamic tract, eventually reaching the thala-

FIGURE 4.7 *Scheme of large- and small-fibre afferent systems and the ascending–descending inhibitory loop. Reproduced, with permission, from Hertling & Kessler (1990), p. 49.*

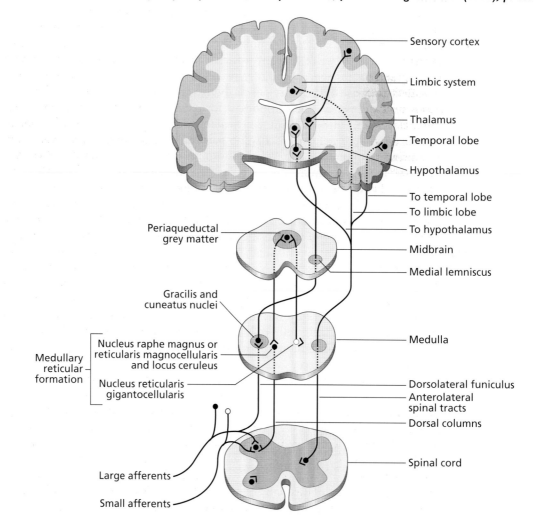

mus, and connecting with the reticular formation of the medulla. The reticular formation exerts an arousal response, the thalamus crudely interprets the stimulus as pain and has a localization function, and the cerebral cortex, the final destination, is important for fine interpretation of the quality of pain and detailed spatial localization. Communication occurs with the limbic system for emotional response to the pain. This is a highly significant factor as the emotional interpretation we place on a stimulus helps us to recognize it as unpleasant and damaging. The connections within the brain are more complex than described here and it is important to appreciate that reactions to pain are also complex. It is known that the hypothalamus is an important integrative area for various types of stimulus.

In addition to the ways in which massage may help to reduce pain by its effects in the tissues, as discussed earlier in this chapter, it is postulated here that massage may be able to interfere with the pain mechanism at the spinal cord level. A-beta fibres are mechanoreceptors which have a low threshold and therefore register mechanical stimuli very readily. As these fibres move from the dorsal horn, *en route* to the brain, they send a small collateral to the terminal of the C and A-delta fibres, partially exciting these terminals when they are transmitting impulses. If the dorsal horn is bombarded with A-beta fibre impulses, the stimulus in the collateral will block the C fibre synapse (by causing the terminal to be in a refractory state), ensuring that it cannot transmit further impulses. Thus, a repetitive mechanical stimulus may prevent pain impulses reaching the brain. It has been found that vibratory stimuli reduce pain (Lundeberg 1983); therefore massage techniques that have a vibratory effect in the tissues and probably other techniques that operate at the same frequency will have the same effect. This is the 'closed pain gate' of Melzack & Wall (1965). As it occurs before the synapse it is termed *presynaptic inhibition*.

Postsynaptic inhibition can occur by a descending mechanism. When the pain stimulus arrives in the raphe nucleus, the reticular formation and the periaqueductal grey area of the brain, it causes the release of endogenous opiates (endorphins, enkephalins) at these sites and in the substantia gelatinosa of the dorsal horn. These are substances released naturally by the body which act like morphine on opiate receptors (on the nerve cell membrane), causing relief of pain and a feeling of euphoria and well-being. Stimuli that travel in the A-delta fibres, such as those from acupuncture, produce this effect. It is possible that a mechanical stimulus which occurs at the same frequency (two or three times a second) will have a similar effect. Massage may also produce postsynaptic inhibition because of the positive effects it has on the limbic system and cerebral cortex. Massage can produce relaxation and positive psychological effects, as discussed in Chapter 10. The patient may feel calmer, less anxious or stressed, may feel relaxed and cared for, and more in control of physical and emotional states. A *tonic* downflow of neural activity has been described in response to cultural, experiential and personality factors. A *phasic* downflow is more transient and is due to factors such as attention, anxiety and expectation. It is suggested that this influences the way each person responds to events and other forms of stimuli, emotional or physiological. As the experience of pain is a combined emotional and physiological event, these factors must influence the response to pain as it occurs in individuals and also as it occurs in each unique set of circumstances. Thus, any change in the client's emotions, as induced by massage, may alter this phasic downflow, helping him/her to cope with any pain that is occurring. In addition, this altered activity within the cortex and limbic system may cause release of endorphins, which could explain the feeling of well-being that patients often report following massage.

In summary, massage is thought to assist in relieving pain both in the periphery and in the central nervous system (CNS) in three ways:

1. The fluid exchange and increased circulation it causes will improve the local chemical environment.
2. It may produce presynaptic inhibition by closing the 'pain gate' in the dorsal horn of the spinal cord.
3. It may cause postsynaptic inhibition through its effect on the limbic system and cerebral cortex.

CONTRAINDICATIONS

Finally, consideration of pathological factors must include discussion of contraindications to massage. Knowledge of what these are, understanding their relevance, and the ability to recognize their existence are what makes massage safe, and safety is the baseline of competence.

Some of the contraindications derive from theoretical understanding or common sense; some are speculative and unproven; and some are suggested as a result of recently reported occurrences. They can be divided into three types. The first type are absolute contraindications for all situations. The second type may not be absolute, and certain techniques in some of these circumstances may be safe. The third type require care and are more accurately regarded as dangers rather than contraindications in the true sense of the word.

To understand the contraindications, it is helpful first to explore the potential dangers of massage. The known effects of massage will prove to be a danger in any situation where those effects are deemed to be undesirable.

Dangers of Massage

- Massage is thought to increase blood flow. However, increasing blood flow could be dangerous if a thrombus is attached to a vessel wall. Mechanical stimulation of the vessel and increased blood flow may cause the thrombus, or a small portion of it, to detach from the vessel wall to become an embolus. This can become lodged in the heart, lungs or brain to cause serious – potentially fatal – damage.
- It is possible that massage can disturb implants in the body such as silicone implants or pacemakers. Kerr (1997) reported an incident which occurred in the accident and emergency department of a hospital. A ureteral double J stent being used to treat ureteral stenosis and calculi was displaced by a session of Rolfing (manipulation of the fascial tissues). The patient was alerted to the problem by left flank pain during treatment. The resulting pain and incontinence resolved when the stent was repositioned.
- Massage increases lymphatic flow. Increased lymphatic flow may increase the rate at which bacteria or metastases are carried around the body.

    Massage creates compression and shear forces within the tissues. Mechanical manipulation over a foreign body or sharp bony fragment will cause damage to the surrounding soft tissues.

- Manipulation of the tissues involves manipulation of blood vessels. Damaged, leaking blood vessels will be further damaged, and bleeding will increase if they are manipulated. For example, bruising will increase in recent muscle tears (in the first 24–48 hours after injury) or fragile blood vessels will be disrupted by massage. Excess bleeding may occur in haemophilia if deep vigorous techniques are used.
- Manipulation of the tissues too early in the healing process will damage the delicate cellular and fibrinous network, delaying healing and even causing excess fibrous tissue to be produced.
- Massage stretches connective tissue and scar tissue. Internal infection can be spread if the fibrous tissue, which is produced in an attempt to encapsulate infective material, is damaged. Bacterial and fungal skin infections can be spread to non-infected areas through touch. Likewise, infection can be spread between patient and therapist, or between patients if a poor standard of hygiene is maintained.
- Infection can be introduced into an open wound if the surface is touched by a non-sterile object.
- Massage media can cause allergies or irritations. Schaller & Korting (1995) reported the case of a patient suffering from relapsing eczema which was resistant to therapy. Its distribution was generalized but occurred mostly on the scalp, neck and hands. Patch-testing revealed allergic airborne contact dermatitis from the use of oils in aromalamps. Despite previous exposure to lavender, jasmine and rosewood, laurel, eucalyptus and pomerance tested positive. Allergic contact dermatitis has occurred as a reaction to tea-tree oil (Khanna et al 2000) and lavender (Sugiura et al 2000). (See Ch. 7 for further discussion.)
- Any excess activity in the tissues (for example, malignant growth, calcification) can be exacerbated by mechanical stimulation, which may speed up local metabolism.

Absolute Contraindications to Massage

- Massage over an open wound surface.
- In the presence of inadequate circulation, thrombophlebitis or fragile blood vessels – look for petechiae or haemophilia.
- When haemorrhage is occurring.
- During the early stages of healing.
- When there is active bacterial or fungal infection (skin infections such as cellulitis, impetigo, ringworm or athlete's foot, abscesses, septicaemia).
- In febrile conditions (very high temperature, childhood diseases, influenza).
- Over areas of acute inflammation.
- Over active bone growth – a healing fracture site, in myositis ossificans or periostitis, such as Osgood–Schlatter disease.
- Directly over skin affected by conditions such as psoriasis.
- Undiagnosed cancer.
- In situations where increased blood or lymphatic flow is undesirable such as active malignancy, in the region of a tumour or deep venous thrombosis.
- Over a foreign body or bony fragment.

Potential Contraindications Where Caution Must Be Applied

- *Malignant disease*: Manual lymphatic drainage or deep manipulations which stimulate the circulation or metabolic rate should be avoided over areas of active disease or in the vicinity of tumours.
- *Fragile skin*: Light pressure only should be used, with a suitable medium to reduce friction, or this type of skin may tear.
- *Collagenous weakening*: For example, in long-term steroid use or diabetes or advanced rheumatoid arthritis.
- *Patients with heart problems*: The anterior chest or neck must not be massaged and care should be taken between the shoulder blades, because of potential reflex effects. Grimes (1988) and Searle (1987) conducted research which showed that 10 minutes of effleurage (as a nursing back rub) in subjects who had undergone coronary artery bypass surgery produced an immediate rise in systolic and diastolic blood pressure, followed by a steady decrease in blood pressure. While the gradual drop in blood pressure may be of benefit to some cardiac patients, such as those who are post myocardial infarction, the initial blood pressure rise suggests that massage may be contraindicated in others. Patients unable to adapt to the initial rise, such as patients in the first 48 hours post surgery, should not be massaged (Labyak et al 1997).
- *Dermatomyositis*: It has been suggested by Bork et al (1971) that massage should be avoided in this condition as whole body massage has been shown to increase serum levels of gonadotrophin, creatinphosphokinase, lactate dehydrogenase and myokinase in a patient with this condition. As high levels of these enzymes indicate the severity of dermatomyositis, it should not be treated by massage.

When Caution Should Be Applied

Stationary Pressure Techniques

If using shiatsu or acupressure techniques, for example, excess pressure should be avoided and the underlying anatomy should be clearly understood. Herskovitz and co-workers (1992) described a situation in which degeneration of the recurrent thenar motor branch of the median nerve occurred as a result of direct pressure exerted during a shiatsu session. Although pressure was applied for only 30 seconds, it resulted in weakness of the abductor pollicis brevis muscle. A point of interest in this report is that the pressure caused 'notable transient discomfort'. This could have indicated to the therapist that she was compressing a nerve fibre; this emphasizes the fact that massage therapists should be aware of the effects any treatment is having on a patient, and that patients should be encouraged to describe any discomfort as it occurs. The therapist should act on this information immediately, modifying the technique to suit the individual. It is surprising in this particular case that a shiatsu pressure was sufficient to produce neuropraxia, as focal pressure on the tissues occurs as part of many daily activities. It may be that this particular massage was, as the authors suggest, 'overzealous' or there could possibly have been an underlying problem. The muscle did, however, recover fully. A similar case was reported by Giese & Hentz (1988) in which a neuropraxia of the posterior interosseous nerve was caused by deep tissue massage of the forearm, with static pressure. The patient presented with extensor paralysis of the metacarpophalangeal joints and an inability to abduct the thumb. Again, the massage was kept within the patient's pain threshold.

In the Vicinity of Endocrine Glands

A case of destructive thyrotoxicosis which occurred following massage of the head and neck was reported by Tachi and colleagues (1990). The patient was diagnosed as having autoimmune thyroiditis (Hashimoto's disease) 12 years previously, and severe symptoms of destructive thyrotoxicosis were found when the patient attended the doctor's clinic 10 days after the massage. The authors suggest that the mechanical manipulation of the massage techniques injured the thyroid follicles, resulting in antigen release and antibody production. It seems surprising that massage could damage a gland as these structures are usually protected by a fibrous outer layer, although the malfunctioning thyroid is particularly susceptible to mechanical manipulation. Tachi et al based the suggestion on a study by Carney et al (1975), which found palpation thyroiditis to have occurred in 91% of a sample of 32 patients with thyroid disease. The massage therapist must know the patient's past medical history and massage should proceed with caution in the vicinity of active or remitting disease. A positive suggestion raised in Tachi et al's paper is that massage of the thyroid gland (Fig. 4.8) may promote altered hormonal secretion in a way that could be clinically significant.

Cancer

The early writers on massage placed little emphasis on cancer as a contraindication. It was not listed by Goodall-Copestake (1926) or Tidy (1932), although this omission could indicate the scant attention the disease received generally at that time. Hollis (1987) gives tumour as a contraindication and Tappan (1988) lists melanoma, as this type of cancer metastasizes easily through lymphatic and blood vessels. Massage therapists with non-medical training are meeting this condition more frequently and the use of massage in

---

FIGURE 4.8 *Surface position of the thyroid gland.*

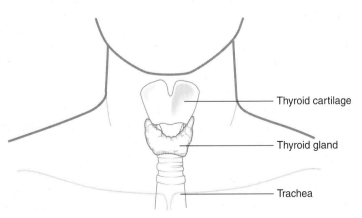

Thyroid cartilage

Thyroid gland

Trachea

people suffering from cancer has become a controversial point. In its traditional use, within orthodox medical care, massage has been regarded as being contraindicated for patients with active malignant disease. Physiotherapists, by taking a detailed medical history and having access to patients' medical records, have avoided techniques that may increase local metabolic rate or blood flow in the vicinity of active disease. This statement needs some clarification, as massage has been used to reduce local symptoms, or to aid relaxation in the patient at the later stages of the condition, when emphasis is being laid on comfort rather than cure. It has also proved useful, for example, in spinal cancer which has produced uncomfortable sensory changes such as hyperaesthesia. This can be sufficiently severe to make touch uncomfortable to the point where washing becomes distressing. Gentle rhythmical stroking can prove useful to desensitize the skin, and the use of warm water to massage the skin gently (via gentle movements in a hydrotherapy pool, for example) may be helpful. Heavier stroking can be used as a counterirritant, acting through the pain gate to reduce pain. Further discussion of the use of massage in patients with cancer can be found in Chapter 11. Traditionally, massage has been taboo in the earlier active stages of the disease but acceptable at the later (including terminal) stages. After radical mastectomy, for example, patients have been given and taught oedema massage for the arm following removal of the lymph glands. Effleurage was the main treatment of choice; this has now largely been superseded by the more superficially applied manual lymphatic drainage.

Of course, patients with cancer have the right to treatment of other injuries and physical problems unrelated to the cancer. They also have the right to support for symptoms of stress, and help with coping mechanisms. Thus, as long as the tissues are not actively manipulated over any active disease site, increase in lymphatic and venous flow is avoided in patients with melanoma or Hodgkin's disease, and the lymph nodes are not directly stimulated mechanically, then massage can be a useful adjunct to other therapies. Stationary and pressure techniques are probably the safest (holding, therapeutic touch, acupressure, shiatsu, for example); the more superficial techniques as used in gentle stroking, whole body sedative massage or through an oily medium would be the next treatment of choice from a safety viewpoint. It is unlikely that these techniques would be physiologically more stimulatory than the everyday activities of walking or housework. In relation to drug therapy, it has been suggested that massage may increase the rate at which chemotherapeutic agents flow around the body when administered into the bloodstream, that it increases the rate at which drugs enter the bloodstream when administered by other means, and that the dosage should be reduced accordingly (McNamara 1994). However, this has not yet been substantiated experimentally. Also, it has been suggested that massage increases the rate at which chemotherapy and its toxins will be lost from the body, although it should be recognized that we have insufficient experimental evidence to support these suppositions and the disease should always be treated with respect. Of course, as in all conditions, techniques and approaches should be modified to match the stage of disease.

A pertinent study was undertaken by McNamara (1994). She sent out questionnaires to 24 volunteer massage practitioners and asked for their views and knowledge on the use of massage for people with cancer. The main findings in relation to dangers and contraindications were that practitioners had often been taught or read that massage was contraindicated in the earlier stages of the disease but not in the terminal stages. There was obviously some concern about the lack of research evidence to support or refute this suggestion, but massage was generally being offered to people with cancer.

An *absolute contraindication* for massage is undiagnosed cancer. It is important that the massage therapist is alert to the possibility and that any patient experiencing symptoms which may relate to a serious condition should be urged to seek advice from a doctor immediately. Look for:

- intractable pain – no relief on rest, significantly disturbed sleep (this may indicate inflammatory or malignant disease)
- feeling of being generally unwell
- change in temperature
- inflammation and heat in the absence of trauma
- unexplained weight change
- any lump bigger than 5 cm, especially if it is a recurrence of a previous lump or is deeper than fascia or is increasing in size (Grimer & Dalloway 1995).

SUMMARY

This chapter has reiterated the message, relayed throughout this book, that the therapist must take responsibility for her treatment decisions and that these should be based on sound theoretical knowledge. Decisions should be justified from a theoretical perspective, based on evaluation of research findings. If the therapist is unable to do this in any situation, then treatment of the condition must depend on the referral and advice of a medical practitioner. At all times, it is wise to err on the side of caution: patients rely on us not to make mistakes.

KEY POINTS

- Local areas of acute inflammation should not be massaged.

- Massage can help to reduce swelling, prevent adhesions and promote remodelling of fibrous tissue in chronic pathophysiological states.

- Massage used in the early stages of healing can disrupt delicate tissue but can assist healing in the later stages by improving circulation and tissue mobility.

- Massage can be used to improve general circulation at any stage.

- Massage can promote remodelling of connective tissue and can mobilize shortened, adherent scar tissue.

- Oedema can occur as a result of inflammation, pressure on part of the circulatory system (for example in pregnancy), heart malfunction, lymphatic insufficiency, venous problems or other medical conditions.

- Excess tissue fluid can reduce nutrition to the cells.

- Oedema leads to adhesions in the tissues.

- Massage should not be used when oedema is due to organic disease, acute injury or thrombosis.

- Swedish massage should be used for hydrostatic oedema; selected techniques applied around the edges of an ulcer or wound; and manual lymphatic drainage used for lymphoedema.

- The effects of massage in oedema are considerably enhanced if the patient wears a pressure garment or bandage between treatment sessions.

- Massage can reduce pain by flushing the tissues with new circulation, facilitating the removal of chemical irritants which can lead to chronic pain changes in the spinal cord.

- Massage can have a counterirritant effect.

- Stimulation of mechanoreceptors may close the pain gate.

- Absolute contraindications must always be followed.

- The therapist should understand the dangers of massage and be aware of cautions.

REFERENCES

Akeson W H, Woo S L-Y, Amiel D et al 1973 The connective tissue response to immobilisation: biomechanical changes in periarticular connective tissue of the rabbit knee. Clinical Orthopaedics 93: 356–362

Bork K, Korting G W, Faust G 1971 Serum enzyme levels after a whole body massage. Archiv für Dermatologische Forschung 240: 342–348

Boscheinen-Morrin J, Davey V, Conolly W B 1992 The hand fundamentals of therapy. Butterworth-Heinemann, Oxford

Bowsher D 1991 Nociceptors and peripheral nerve fibres. In: Wells P, Frampton V, Bowsher D (eds) Pain management and control in physiotherapy. Butterworth-Heinemann, Oxford

Butler D 1991 Mobilisation of the nervous system. Churchill Livingstone, Edinburgh

Carney J A, Moore S B, Northcult L C et al 1975 Palpation thyroiditis (multifocal grannulomatous folliculitis). Annals of the Journals of Clinical Pathology 64: 630–647

Giese S, Hentz V R 1998 Posterior interosseus syndrome resulting from deep tissue massage [letter]. Plastic and Reconstructive Surgery 102(5): 1778–1779

Goodall-Copestake B M 1926 The theory and practice of massage. Lewis, London

Gould B E 1997 Pathophysiology for the health-related professions. Saunders, Philadelphia, PA

Grimes D L 1988 The effects of effleurage back massage on psychophysiological parameters of relaxation in coronary artery bypass patients. Unpublished Master's thesis, University of Michigan, Ann Arbor. Cited in: Labyak S E Metzger B L 1997 The effects of effleurage backrub on the physiological components of relaxation: a meta-analysis. Nursing Research 46(1): 59–62

Gunn C C 1989 Treating myofascial pain: intramuscular stimulation for myofascial pain syndromes of neuropathic origin. University of Washington, Seattle

Guyton A C 1991 Textbook of medical physiology. W B Saunders, Philadelphia, PA

Herskovitz S, Strauch B, Gordon M J V 1992 Shiatsu-induced injury of the median recurrent motor branch [letter]. Muscle and Nerve October: 1215

Hertling D, Kessler R 1990 Common musculoskeletal disorders, 2nd edn. J B Lippincott, Philadelphia, PA

Hollis M 1987 Massage for therapists. Blackwell, Oxford

Hurst P A E 1987 Venous and lymphatic disease – assessment and treatment. In: Downie P A (ed) Cash's Textbook of chest heart and vascular disorders for physiotherapists. Faber and Faber, London, pp. 654–665

Iggo A, Guillbaud G, Tegner R 1984 Sensory mechanisms in arthritic rat joints. In: Kruger L, Kind J (eds) Advances in pain and therapy. Rowan Press, New York, vol 6, pp. 83–93

Kerr H D 1997 Ureteral stent displacement associated with deep massage. WMJ: official publication of the State Medical Society of Wisconsin 96(12): 57–58

Khanna M, Qasam K, Sasseville D 2000 Allergic contact dermatitis to tea-tree oil with erythema multiform-like id reaction. American Journal of Contact Dermatitis 11(4): 238–242

Kloth L C, McCullough J M, Feedar J A 1990 Wound healing: alternatives in management. F A Davis, Philadelphia, PA

Labyak S E, Metzger B L 1997 The effects of effleurage backrub on the physiological components of relaxation: a meta-analysis. Nursing Research 46(1): 59–62

Ladd M P, Kottke F J, Blanchard R S 1952 Studies of the effect of massage on the flow of lymph from the foreleg of the dog. Archives of Physical Medicine 33(10): 604–612

Lundborg G 1988 Nerve injury and repair. Churchill Livingstone, Edinburgh

Lundeberg T C M 1983 Vibratory stimulation for the alleviation of chronic pain. Acta Physiologica Scandinavica 523(Suppl.): 1–51

McNamara P 1994 Massage for people with cancer. Wandsworth Cancer Support Centre, London

Melzack R, Wall P D 1965 Pain mechanisms: a new theory. Science 150: 971–979

Patino O, Novick C, Merlo A, Benaim F 1999 Massage in hypertrophic scars. Journal of Burn Care and Rehabilitation 20(3): 268–271

Pritchard A P, Mallett J 1993 Wound management. In: Pritchard A P, Mallett J (eds) Royal Marsden Hospital manual of clinical nursing procedures. Blackwell Science, Oxford, p. 525

Schaller M, Korting H C 1995 Allergic airborne contact dermatitis from essential oils used in aromatherapy. Clinical and Experimental Dermatology 20(2): 143–145

Searle P M 1987 Psychophysiological effects from an effleurage back massage in adults with acute myocardial infarction: a replication and extension. Unpublished Master's thesis, University of Michigan, Ann Arbor. Cited in: Labyak S E, Metzger B L 1997 The effects of effleurage backrub on the physiological components of relaxation: a meta-analysis. Nursing Research 46(1): 59–62

Sugiura M, Hayakawa R, Kato Y et al 2000 Results of patch testing with lavender oil in Japan. Contact Dermatitis 43(3): 157–160

Tachi J, Amino N, Miyai K 1990 Massage therapy on the neck: a contributing factor for destructive thyrotoxicosis? Thyroidology 2: 25–27

Tappan F M 1988 Healing massage techniques. Appleton and Lange, Norwalk, CT

Tidy N M 1932 Massage and remedial exercises. John Wright, London

Tyler D O, Winslow E H, Clark A P, White K M 1990 Effects of a one minute back rub on mixed venous saturation and heart rate in critically ill patients. Heart and Lung 19(5): 562–565

Whittaker R 1987 Peripheral vascular disease – the place of physiotherapy. In: Downie P A Cash's Textbook of chest heart and vascular disorders. Faber and Faber, London, pp. 666–684

Woolf N 1988 Cell tissue and disease: the basis of pathology. Ballière Tindall, London

Section 2
Practical Application of Massage

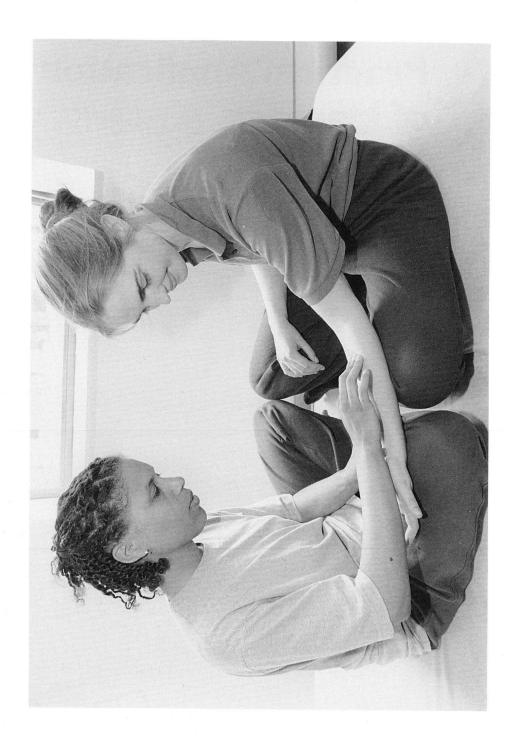

5 Palpation

One of the main keys to success with massage lies in the sensitivity of the therapist's hands. A well-developed manual sensitivity is important for:

- examining and assessing tissues
- recognizing the end-feel of the tissue, which influences the effectiveness and comfort of the massage
- modifying techniques to different tissues and tissue layers
- adapting techniques to suit an individual's tissues
- adapting techniques so that they are appropriate to various pathological states and stages of healing.

EXERCISES TO DEVELOP PALPATION SKILLS

The student therapist may increase her sensory awareness by practising on inanimate objects as well as the human body. To begin, it is helpful to find a friend who is willing to model; it is easier to develop palpatory skills when you do not have to concentrate on giving a massage simultaneously. There are many exercises that can help to develop palpatory awareness; a few of them are listed below but you will also benefit by making up some of your own. Make a habit of touching objects that are a part of your daily life. While you are doing so, describe the sensations to yourself; try giving words to what you feel so that you begin to differentiate – lots of things feel 'like' something else, but try to find the subtle differences between them. Palpate with the pads of your fingers and thumbs, which are highly innervated:

- Take two small bowls and put refined white flour into one and wholewheat flour into the other. Simultaneously put one hand into each and rub the flour between your fingers. Describe to yourself the different sensations.
- Collect together a number of different grades of sandpaper. Close your eyes and attempt to sort the paper by grade.
- Compare the differences in the texture of water, cooking oil and a thick body lotion by rubbing a little of each between finger and thumb.

- Place some small objects on a table (e.g. grains of rice, a piece of string, a matchstick, a key, a paperclip). Cover them with a thin cloth and palpate; repeat with thicker coverings such as a blanket and a piece of foam. Distinguish the variation of sensations between the covers and note any differences in the pressure you have applied.
- With one finger stroke your cheek, your arm, your palm, your abdomen, your knee and the sole of your foot. Feel any varying texture, skin temperature and moisture in these parts of the body.
- Practise palpation in the area of your wrist and forearm. The anterior aspect of the wrist is a good place to start; here you can see and feel the tendons and blood vessels. Let the fingers of one hand rest as lightly as a feather on your contralateral wrist. Move them very gently over the skin without stretching and register what you feel. Now apply slightly more pressure, so that the skin moves with your fingers; this should give you more information about the structures under the skin. Apply more pressure still so that the subcutaneous structures are compressed on the underlying bone. With this heavy pressure the sensitivity of your palpation decreases and the structures will not be so easy to differentiate.
- Palpate your own thigh. Note the depth of pressure required to gain information about the tone of the muscles in this region. Using your whole hand pick up and stretch the muscles and register any changes you feel in the resistance of the tissues.

It is useful to perform specific exercises to increase the mobility of your hands before you begin to learn massage. Figures 5.1A,B and 5.2A,B show suggested exercises to stretch your fingers and wrists.

PALPATION TECHNIQUE

To palpate effectively, the pads – rather than the tips – of the fingers should be used. The fingers should be straight but relaxed, with movement coming from the arm, not the intrinsic muscles of the fingers.

Layer Palpation

As your hands progress from layer to layer, you should visualize each one in turn and mentally register differences in the quality of feeling that each layer has.

Epidermis

Rest your hands lightly on the surface of the skin of your patient/model. The first thing you should be aware of is the temperature. If you choose to compare the temperature of different parts of the skin, use the same hand (in case the temperature varies between your right and left hands), and it is best to use the dorsum rather than the palm. Slide the hand slowly over the skin, firmly enough not to tickle. Dryness, scaliness, sweating and smoothness will be immediately detectable. A visual reinforcement of palpation findings can be useful, so look for circulatory alterations in the skin. Any scarring will be pal-

FIGURE 5.1   *(A,B) Exercise to increase flexibility in the joints of the thumbs and fingers.*

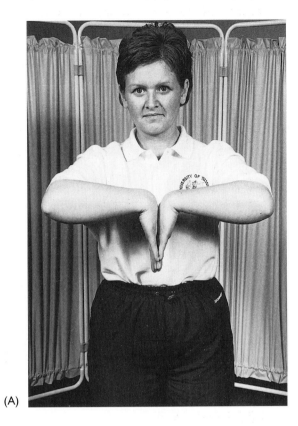

(A)

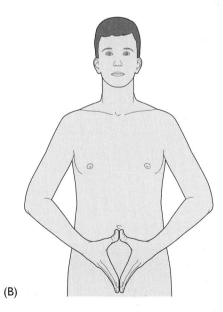

(B)

FIGURE 5.2   *(A,B) Exercise to increase wrist extension: with the elbows up, push the wrists down, keeping the heel of the hands together.*

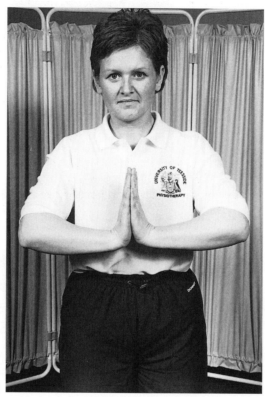

(A)

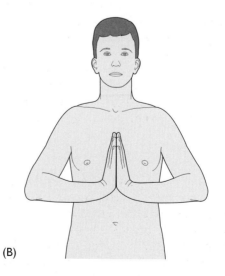

(B)

pable, as will any hot inflamed areas. You should note the patient's reaction to touch at this point: observe any alternations in facial expression (unless the patient is prone) and feel changes in underlying muscle tone. If the fingers remain at this depth but move *on* the skin, rather than *over* it, a wrinkle of skin will be formed around the fingertips, in front of the movement. This is because the epidermis is being pushed against the points of underlying adherence. A shear force is being created between the layers. As you push the epidermis, you almost immediately reach a point of resistance at which you will start to glide over the skin surface if your pushing continues. This is the *end-feel*, i.e. the feeling at the end of the movement (see below).

Dermis and Subcutaneous Layers

Next, ease a little further into the tissues by allowing the fingers to sink down a little. If done lightly, the fingers will come to rest in the subcutaneous layer. You should then ease off a little to feel the dermis.

Fascial Layer

To reach the fascia, you should find a place where muscle attaches to bone subcutaneously, or where a fascial intermuscular septum lies immediately under the skin. Elsewhere, from a position where the fingers have come to rest on the subcutis, push down slightly deeper to feel the final layer of tissue surrounding the muscles, but take care not to compress the tissues between your fingers and underlying bone.

Muscle

Knowledge of anatomy will inform you when you are sinking into muscle. This is firmer than subcutaneous tissue, and so offers more resistance to your fingers. It has specific tone. The fibre bundles may also be apparent, as the muscle will feel 'ridged'. In erector spinae, it may be possible to feel a thick rounded cord which can often extend several inches. This is a group of muscle fibres which have increased in tone over a period of time, common in such a postural muscle. If it has been present for any length of time, surrounding connective tissue will be tight or may be partly fibrotic, in which case it will feel hard and will be less readily responsive to massage. Slide your fingers right over the muscle and feel its edge and then its fascial attachment.

Other Structures

- *Tendon* feels like a thin firm cord which can often be moved or 'twanged'. This is easy to achieve on the tendons of the wrist which can be seen and palpated on the flexor aspect.
- *Ligament* is usually felt as a discrete flattened band of dense connective tissue. Careful palpation on the medial side of the knee will identify the edges of a band of slightly denser tissue, which is the medial collateral ligament. On the lateral aspect of the knee it is possible to palpate a cord-like rounded structure stretching from the head of the fibula to the femoral condyle. This lateral collateral ligament is much rounder than the ligament

on the medial side, but is denser than a tendon. Compare it with a tendon, which has a more mobile, elastic quality to it.

- *Joint capsules or synovium* can usually be palpated only if they are thickened. A capsule feels like a thickening over the line of the joint whereas a synovium has a more 'silky' feel.
- *Peripheral nerves* feel like small threads – much thinner than tendon, less elastic and difficult to feel because of their thinness. They are often fairly mobile and, if flicked, movement may be seen a few centimetres further along the course of the nerve.

END-FEEL

Recognition of the end-feel is essential for accurate localization of the technique and for pain-free massage. As defined above, it is the feeling at the end of the available movement and it can be identified at each tissue layer and in joints. Initially, movement in the tissues is effortless. As the tissues near their limit of movement, a little extra effort is required to move them. The resistance increases until movement stops. Pushing through this end-feel will create traction between this layer and the next, and will cause you to lose your layer localization. Continuing to push further will then cause discomfort to the patient. The quality of the end-feel varies with different tissues and will give information as to what has stopped the movement – whether it is the microstructure of the tissue itself, and therefore feels normal for that particular tissue, or whether it is altered because of an abnormality. In the epidermis, the fingers slide over the skin before any resistance is felt. In the dermis and subcutis, the end-feel is pliant. It is firm in fascia and elastic in muscle. Working *within* the end-feel will maintain but not increase mobility. Working *at* the end-feel will produce stretch in the tissues, which is necessary for mobilization. Stretching *beyond* the end-feel will be uncomfortable and may cause damage. If pain occurs before the end-feel, the tissues are hypersensitive and tender, and this should be respected, as normal movement or squeezing will be perceived as painful. In the absence of trauma or underlying pathology, the skin can be desensitized by gentle massage.

ABNORMALITIES

When palpating within a specific layer or structure, the therapist will encounter abnormalities which may be easy to find, but difficult to recognize. Very gentle palpation can detect a soft 'sponginess' which indicates excess tissue fluid in the superficial layers. Acute swelling in these layers is extremely soft and it is easily missed when it lies superficially. Very gentle palpation is required. A chronic swelling is more dense and resistant, but still soft in feel. A very superficial sogginess can sometimes be detected, which creates a *peau d'orange* effect, where the skin looks like orange peel when squeezed. Tiny indentations made by something as small as a matchstick will leave tiny pits. Gunn (1989) refers to this reflex effect as trophoedema. A long-standing pitting oedema will compress to leave a 'pit', the size of the palpating fingertip or thumb, which remains after the pressure is removed. A rapidly occurring

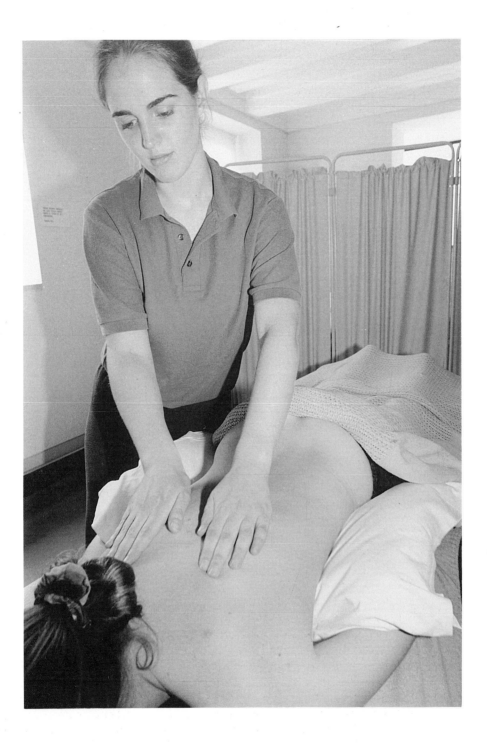

very 'boggy' swelling around a joint may indicate haemarthrosis, which requires further investigation.

When fluid in the tissues is discovered, the therapist should decide:

● whether it is lymphoedematous or hydrostatic (from its history and quality) (see Ch. 3)
● which tissue layer it is in
● whether it is acute, chronic or organized (fibrous).

Occasionally a small area in the tissues will be felt to 'pop' and disappear. This is thought to be a patch of enclosed fluid which dissipates under pressure. It can happen under the plantar fascia and should not be confused with crystal formation.

Crepitus can be felt or heard in the soft tissues if chronic fibrosis is present. This is a friction effect due to loss of lubrication and fibrosis in an area of tissue.

Cellulite is seen as an uneven surface and felt as tiny dimples and sectioned tissue. It may be moist, in which case it is enlarged (often perceived by the patient as increased fat) with swelling in the subcutaneous layer. If chronic, collagenous separation of groups of fat cells can be shortened and the tissue will feel hardened.

Any fibrous structure (e.g. aponeurosis) can be thickened as a result of continued tension on an adherent structure. A common example is the insertion of levator scapulae at the superior angle of the scapula. Knowledge of anatomy will indicate that what is felt is a thickened structure.

Myofascial trigger spots (Travell & Simons 1992) can be felt as a hardening in the muscle and diagnosed by the 'twitch' test. The spot is exquisitely tender and, when a finger is slid over the muscle fibre, it is seen to twitch.

Abnormality of the tissue interfaces can be felt as a loss of mobility. The normal glide between the interfaces is restricted and produces a sensation of being stuck together; rolling the tissues is impaired. In chronic situations the end-feel can be reached before movement has occurred.

Nodules are sometimes palpated in muscles. They can be herniations of fat through the fascia (Grieve 1990) or ischaemic fibrotic muscular lesions. They may be mobile or adherent, and are often painful on pressure. Their tenderness reduces when circulation and mobility are increased following massage.

With practice, you will become familiar with the feel and behaviour of normal tissues. This will enable you to get the most out of your experience of palpating and treating abnormal tissues, ensuring that your palpation and assessment skills become refined enough for effective practice.

KEY POINTS

- ◆ Palpation should be undertaken using the pads, not the tips, of the fingers.
- ◆ Exercises will help you to develop manual sensitivity.
- ◆ Different anatomical structures have their own unique feel.
- ◆ Working within the end-feel of a tissue maintains mobility; working at the end-feel will stretch the tissues; and stretching beyond the end-feel will cause discomfort and possible damage.
- ◆ Abnormalities in the tissues can be recognized by their own distinctive feel.

REFERENCES

Grieve G P 1990 Episacroiliac lipoma. Physiotherapy 76(6): 308–310

Gunn C C 1989 Treating myofascial pain: intramuscular stimulation for myofascial pain syndromes of neuropathic origin. University of Washington, Seattle

Travell J G, Simons D G 1992 Myofascial pain and dysfunction: the trigger point manual, vol. 2. Williams and Wilkins, Baltimore, MD

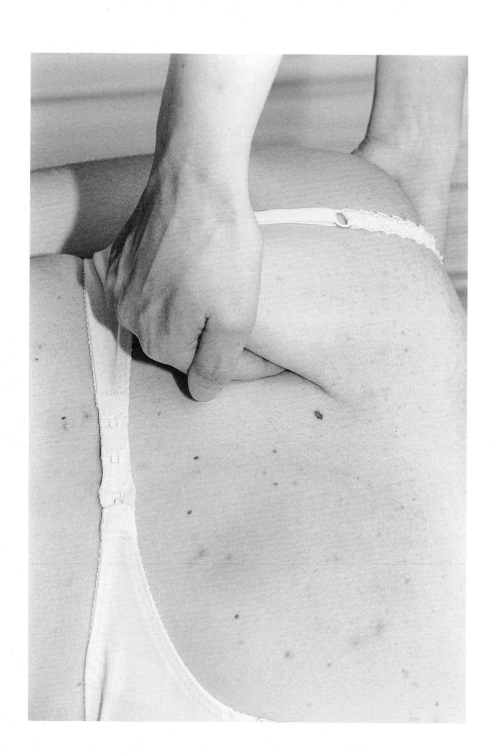

6 Assessment and Treatment Planning

Therapeutic massage, when practised at a professional rather than a technical level, is influenced by a number of intellectual activities. It should be *directed* by the initial assessment of the patient, *modified* to suit the needs of the individual and *adapted* in the light of the individual's responses to it. Thus, the actual carrying out of a treatment intervention such as massage is only a part – albeit a highly significant one – of the whole process. The intellectual reasoning that precedes, accompanies and follows the treatment is essential but complex, and the quality of the decisions made about treatment depends on the sophistication of this clinical reasoning.

CLINICAL REASONING

Clinical reasoning is the process by which clinical decisions are made. This *clinical decision-making*, a continuous event that begins before treatment, is applied and maintained through the treatment programme in an ongoing evaluation of its effects, leading to any necessary adaptation. It culminates in discharge or re-referral of the patient. A wider reflection is also appropriate, whereby the therapist evaluates a series of patient interventions and the service she provides as a whole, both on a personal and a wider professional level. A useful approach to treatment is a *problem-based approach* which ensures that the essential cognitive steps are followed. With this approach, the thinking begins with the recognition and identification of the problem; essential information is acquired to help with analysis of the problem; and then decisions can be made to meet all the stages of problem-solving. For clinical reasoning to occur at its highest level, the therapist must develop the related intellectual skills; this is just as important as the acquisition of the psychomotor skills which enable the therapist to act on any clinical decisions made. Intellectual skills are divided into *cognitive* and *metacognitive* (Henley 1994). *Cognitive* skills are knowledge, understanding, synthesis, analysis and evaluation, which is known as Bloom's taxonomy (Bloom 1956). This is an acknowledgement of the hierarchical nature of intellectual functioning. The first step is to gain knowledge as this provides the foundation that underpins useful clinical thought. This knowledge can be applied to different situations only if it is understood. It must then be placed in a wider context so that aspects of previously acquired knowledge are selected if judged to be relevant, or temporarily disregarded if considered irrelevant. The new knowledge is then made to fit comfortably with previously gained knowledge in a synthesis which enhances the understanding of any individual component. At a higher level, this synthesis can be analyzed, when a deeper interpretation, deconstruction and judgement takes place. Finally, the material can be evaluated when it is further examined critically in the light of other knowledge bases, experience, personal judgement, acknowledged opinion and so on. The total process occurs throughout undergraduate study and should continue when an individual acquires new knowledge, either experiential or theoretical. However, of interest here is the fact that, experientially, the same process occurs throughout the assessment and treatment of patients. The *metacognitive* skills involved in clinical reasoning include reflection, in which an awareness and monitoring of our thinking processes (asking how and why) takes place (Henley 1994).

Payton (1985) applies this to the clinical situation and identifies the *stages of clinical reasoning* as follows:

- *Cue acquisition*, whereby information is gathered from a variety of sources to provide 'clues' to the problem
- *Hypothesis generation* – an experienced clinician will often formulate a hypothesis as to what the problems are very early on in an assessment
- *Cue interpretation*, which is an essential step in which the 'clues' are interpreted in detail
- Hypothesis evaluation.

Put more simply, these are the steps involved in patient interviewing and examination, assessment of findings and evaluation of the opinions formed, and the establishment of a diagnosis or problem list, as appropriate.

The order in which the therapist travels through these stages may vary as ideas and thoughts are mentally checked and revisited. This occurs to satisfy the need to ensure that the decisions made are valid. Mattingley & Fleming (1994) term this hypothetical reasoning *procedural reasoning*. This is an additional category of reasoning which is interactive. The exact style varies, depending on the individual patient the therapist is working with, but it reflects the relationship between therapist and client and the impact this interaction has on the reasoning process. The same authors suggest that a holistic approach requires a further stage in reasoning, *conditional reasoning*, in which the problem is seen in its widest context.

The theory of 'fuzzy traces' assumes that experiences are organized in the memory and retrieved in both verbatim and gist representations. These two types are encoded and stored independantly. It is thought that gist representations support pattern recognition and verbatim memories assist in explaining things to others (Lloyd & Reyna 2001).

So, how do we go about this? Clearly, the central activity is assessment of the patient.

PATIENT ASSESSMENT

Thorough assessment of the patient includes a *subjective* assessment, in which the patient is interviewed, and an *objective* examination. The findings from these two components must then be evaluated. The purpose is to identify any problems caused by the condition and to devise an intervention strategy to resolve them. Detailed discussion of patient assessment for the many and varied conditions for which massage may be used is outside the scope of this book and is covered in other texts. It is suggested that before massaging a patient, a full assessment is carried out in the usual way, depending on the patient's presenting condition and the preferred individual approach of the therapist. For example, a patient presenting with back pain should have a full assessment. A British physiotherapist will usually base this on the Maitland, McKenzie or orthopaedic medicine (Cyriax) approach. On the other hand, a patient with learning disabilities will be assessed in a completely different way, attention being focused, for example, on functional ability, mental processes, developmental stage, the presence of contractures, behavioural problems, communication and social skills.

In addition, once it is thought that massage may be appropriate, the therapist may incorporate other factors into the usual assessment to assist with the clinical decision-making specific to massage.

Assuming, then, that each therapist has a preferred assessment approach, we will highlight factors which relate specifically to massage and which can be adapted to many types of clinical situation and incorporated into a wider assessment method. If the patient is being assessed specifically for massage midway through a treatment programme, or has consulted the therapist specifically for massage, then the assessment outlined below may be sufficient.

When assessing a patient for massage, it is important that the therapist is clear about what the main assessment principles are. We are trying to establish:

- what the patient's problems are
- whether massage can help these problems
- what the limitations of massage will be in this particular set of circumstances
- the presence of any dangers or contraindications
- any factors that will necessitate modifications to the preferred method of application
- which massage techniques will be most effective
- which media should be used
- how the patient is likely to respond to the massage.

Subjective Assessment

Subjective assessment involves interviewing the patient to establish what symptoms the patient has noticed, what her/his perceptions are, and to extract detailed information which will assist in decision-making. It is also useful to identify a subjective marker by which progress can be monitored (for example severity of pain). The interview should consist of a mixture of open and closed questions. Open questions are those that invite a patient's free expression. Prompting should be minimal, merely to invite expression but not to direct or constrain ('How do you feel about that?'; 'Tell me about your stress').

It is also important to employ the use of closed questions to ensure that specific and necessary information is obtained ('Do you ever experience pins and needles?' 'How *exactly* do you sit when typing?'). These can be 'search' questions which are very specific, or 'scan' questions which are somewhat wider and attempt to pick up further cues (Henley 1994). It is sometimes necessary to control a verbose patient tactfully, especially if time is restrained ('Could we leave that for the moment – I need to ask you some specific questions about your thumb stiffness'; 'I understand, but where *exactly* is the sharp pain? Could you point to it with one finger?').

The following is a checklist of information required from the patient:

1. *Symptoms*
    Pain
        location
        area to which it spreads
        type, quality (sharp, stabbing, ache)
        severity (rate on a scale of 0–10 where 0 = no pain, 10 = unbearable pain)
        irritability (i.e. how easily it is provoked and how long it lasts, once provoked)
    Paraesthesia
        tingling
        numbness
        dullness
        hypersensitivity
        normal stimulus experienced as pain
    Tenderness
    Behaviour
        provoking factors such as pressure and stretch
        easing factors such as a change of position
    Functional difficulties
    Biomechanical adaptation
        posture
        gait
        range of joint movement
    Muscle spasm
        presence
        tenderness
        position
        muscles involved
    Emotional factors
        anxiety
        depression
        fear
    Autonomic changes
        tissues
        sympathetic dominance
        parasympathetic dominance
2. *Previous medical history*
3. *Other medical problems* (alertness to possible contraindications)
4. *Palpation* (see Ch. 5).

PROBLEM IDENTIFICATION

Once the assessment is complete, the therapist should draw up a list of problems and, in partnership with the patient, try to prioritize them. There may be a difference between the therapist's objective prioritizing and the patient's subjective perceptions. For example, it may seem clear to the therapist that the tissues must be mobilized first, to produce the outcome of pain reduction if tissue adherence is causing pain. The patient, however, may feel that some soothing pain relief itself is the first priority. It can also be discussed with the patient that a combination of techniques may be appropriate: some initially painful ones to loosen the tissue and treat the cause, but also some that will reduce pain and spasm. Explanation and discussion of this type of difference in perception will enhance communication between therapist and client and facilitate patient participation in the treatment programme.

Effective therapists have long been skilled at clinical problem-solving, but this has been difficult to learn other than by experience. In more recent years, there have been attempts to formalize the problem-solving and decision-making processes through identification and analysis of the steps involved, despite the fact that individual styles of problem-solving vary. It is worth bearing in mind that effective problem-solving demands a flexible approach so that skills are transferable to a variety of situations. The more specialized the therapist becomes, the less this characteristic is demanded of them.

STAGES OF PROBLEM-SOLVING

1. Problem Recognition

Some problems are more obvious than others and will be readily expressed by the patient – severe pain, for example. Others are more subtle and require highly developed interviewing or examination skills. Autonomic imbalance may be detected by asking the patient searching questions about sleep patterns, energy levels, urine output and so on, whereas slight autonomically induced changes in the tissues may be detected only by skilled palpation as the patient may be unaware of them. Thus, a systematic process of information gathering is essential to ensure that a stage is not omitted (May & Newman 1980), or problems will remain unrecognized. Both subjective and objective collection of information (sometimes referred to as clinical signs and symptoms, or patient data) from the patient is essential for this stage, which demonstrates the necessity for an effective thorough procedure.

2. Problem Definition

The next stage is the interpretation of all the information received in stage 1. Data collected through listening, observing, palpating, testing and reading (the patient's medical notes or a referral letter) must then be analyzed. Knowledge of the meaning of the information collected, and understanding of the implications of certain combinations of it occurring together, are essential prerequisites for effective decision-making. The therapist is, at this stage, defining the boundaries of the individual and collective problems. It is important that this is discussed with the patient. If, for example, a patient has a condition that is beyond the scope of the therapist, then it must be made clear that symptoms arising from that problem cannot be helped by massage and cannot be treated. Alternatively, the therapist may define several separate problems in unravelling the symptoms; for example, pain in the leg may reveal an arthritic knee but may also be referred from the lower back. In relation to massage, the source of pain may be perceived to be arising from local muscle spasm but the spasm may be found to be caused or perpetuated by biomechanical abnormalities, as a result of extensive tight scar tissue (following internal fixation of fracture, for example). Obviously, problem diagnosis at this level is possible only if a sensitive assessment method is used. The patient may identify some problems, for example back pain, and the therapist may discover associated or causative problems, for example adherent scar tissue. Thus, the problem list is more than a list of symptoms and should contain functional achievements to which the patient can directly relate (for example, the length of time the patient is able to sit without discomfort). This process often begins as soon as contact is made with the patient, but it is important that the therapist does not jump to conclusions based on experience or on some new information just learned. Final decisions must be left until the end of the assessment process, otherwise inaccuracies can occur.

3. Problem Analysis

An analytical procedure involves organization of all the data collected and determination of relationships between the separate pieces. This is where decisions will be made about whether past medical history is relevant: is this problem a new one, or a recurrence of an old problem? Possible outcomes can be discussed and agreed between therapist and client at this stage.

4. Goal Formulation

The data collected in the assessment are used to identify and analyze problems. Goal-setting depends on theoretical knowledge and previous experience, which informs the therapist as to which interventions are likely to help the problems, what the likely outcomes are, what the prognoses for solving the problems are and what is a realistic time span within which the outcomes can be achieved. In addition, psychosocial factors (the patient's personality, practical difficulties in following advice, personal feelings about any particular treatment methods, the acceptability of the treatment and associated psychological factors such as depression, anxiety, stress, etc.) must all be taken into account; this is especially important when predicting the length of a course of treatment. It is essential that the therapist and patient agree on desired outcomes and goals, otherwise conflict could occur and the two parties involved will not be working towards the same ends. It is also essential that the patient is aware of exactly what the therapist can offer and what the limitations of the therapist or therapy are, so that he/she can decide whether or not to continue with treatment. The goals should be measurable (preferably objectively, although subjective measurement also has a place), or it is not possible to evaluate outcome.

5. Data Management

The data referred to here are basically information, that is, any information that is of relevance to the patient. By this stage, the therapist has collected a great deal of data from the patient but, having analyzed the problem, may decide that further information is required in order to *solve* the problem. First, then, it has to be decided which methods of data collection are required. This may involve looking something up in a book; for example, if some thickened painful tissue is found in an unexpected place, the therapist may need to look up the anatomy of the region. If the patient is on an unfamiliar drug, does this require researching? Is the problem obscure or complex, and would the therapist benefit from discussion with fellow professionals? Is there a query concerning certain contraindications to treatment which warrants discussion with the patient's doctor? Thus, a complete picture can emerge by which the problems can be solved satisfactorily.

6. Development of the Solution

Data Analysis

Once complete, the data must be organized and relationships established. This may necessitate classification of complex data, either mentally or on paper, and the formulation of short-term goals which must be met if the eventual long-term goal is to be reached.

Alternative Solution Determination

Once this stage is reached, the therapist then has to identify, from her 'toolbag' of techniques, which ones are appropriate to this situation.

Solution Selection

Often, there seem to be several possible appropriate techniques and it is the selection of those optimally suitable for the individual situation which is difficult. This decision is often based on the experience and beliefs of the therapist, and the accuracy of this decision can shorten the treatment programme. Where possible, it should be based on sound research findings.

7. Solution Implementation

This is the point at which treatment is carried out. Here, technical skill and competency are important. If the massage is to be performed by a technician, this is the only stage with which she is involved. Specific treatment is ordered and should be carried out skilfully. The referring practitioner carries out all the other stages, with or without consultation with the technician. In professional practice, however, this is only one stage of many. The preceding stages are intellectual and not apparent to the patient. It is asserted here that, when massage is used therapeutically, it should be used by a therapist who is as competent in problem-solving and clinical reasoning as in the psychomotor skills of massage.

8. Outcome Evaluation

The outcome of the treatment is assessed in relation to the stated desired outcomes: in other words, the therapist checks that the goals are being met. If so, it may be appropriate to progress treatment by introducing a new treatment intervention aimed at achieving another goal. Alternatively, if it is unlikely that further progress will be made, the treatment may be terminated and the patient discharged. If the goals are not being met, but it is thought that this should be possible, the treatment may be modified in some way.

Goals that may be identified for which massage may be useful include the following:

- reducing pain
- reducing swelling
- reducing muscle spasm
- increasing extensibility of tissues
- reducing tension in tissues
- improving skin condition
- increasing mobility at tissue interfaces
- stretching adhered tissue
- mobilizing scar tissue
- increasing local circulation
- increasing general circulation
- assisting post-exercise recovery
- aiding removal of metabolites from muscle
- promoting remodelling of tissue
- removing toxins and waste products from the tissues
- promoting lymphatic drainage
- facilitating general relaxation
- promoting physiological relaxation
- inducing a feeling of well-being
- enhancing communication through touch
- promoting behavioural change
- facilitating a feeling of caring and security
- providing sensory distraction to assist drug tolerance or withdrawal
- increasing sensory threshold
- reducing hypersensitivity
- reducing feelings of stress
- enhancing body image
- increasing body awareness
- enhancing sense of self
- providing caring through touch.

As already stated, the therapist will collect information regarding the patient's condition and examine the tissues through observation and palpation. It may also be necessary to take measurements, for example when tight or adherent tissue is restricting the joint range of movement. A problem list is identified and goals are set, both short-term and long-term. It must be clear in the therapist's mind what she is trying to achieve and whether the massage is aimed at prevention (for example in an athlete before competition, or to assist relaxation at the end of a hectic day at work), treatment (in mobilizing scar tissue, for example, or in improving communication skills through touch), or maintenance (in a situation where muscles have a tendency to go into spasm because of an underlying joint problem that cannot be resolved). Change must be measured both subjectively and objectively; for example, does the patient feel better and is this accompanied by the tissues being looser or less swollen?

It is important to be organized so that the total process is facilitated in an efficient and effective manner. This can be achieved through the process of the *problem-oriented medical record* (POMR). In particular, the method of recording the assessment and treatment plan can be helpful. SOAP notes (see below) were introduced as a part of POMR by Weed (1971) and are now in wide use.

There are various modifications and interpretations of the method in common use and the principle of SOAP is popular among physiotherapists and medical students. Once the assessment findings are summarized, recording of the thought processes is as follows:

Subjective findings (e.g. movement in knee limited by painful feeling of stretch over scar)
Objective findings (e.g. knee flexion 90 degrees)
Assessment: summary, impressions of situation, problem list, short-term and long-term goals
Plan: treatment plan to match the set goals.

Some practitioners prefer to begin the SOAP list with a problem list. An example of an assessment chart with SOAP recording is given in Figure 6.1 and readers are recommended to consult Kettenbach (1990) for further reading on the topic.

The intellectual and practical processes must be in the context of reflective practice. Reflection should occur throughout an individual treatment session, must provide continuity throughout a course of treatment, and must also take a wider view of the overall quality of service provided by the practitioner. In this way, the therapy offered will be of the highest quality and, more importantly, will remain so over the years. Reflection also guides continuous personal and professional development, necessary to maintain competence over time and to improve practice. Learning needs and the impact of learning on practice must be explored for learning to be effective. Clinical reasoning can be developed through the use of the script concept (networks of knowledge linked to clinical goals, Charlin et al 2000), teaching interventions (Round 1999) and fuzzy-trace theory (Lloyd & Reyna 2001).

Wolf (1985) has identified the principles underlying clinical decisions. These are helpful and are reproduced here:

1. Effective treatment must be based upon a plan.
2. Effective treatment forsakes empiricism as a primary guide.
3. The cornerstone of effective clinical decisions is the ongoing acquisition of knowledge.
4. Effective treatment is based upon integrative and often multiple treatment approaches.
5. Re-evaluation of treatment efficacy must be an ongoing process.
6. The body of knowledge that characterizes physiotherapy practice is growing exponentially and promotes specialization.

FIGURE 6.1 *An example of a problem-oriented assessment chart.*

PROBLEM-ORIENTED
ASSESSMENT CHART

Personal details:

Name:_____Address _____ Age____

Occupation:_____ Hobbies: _____

Medical Practitioner:_____

Relevant Social History:_____

_____

History of Present Complaint:
(onset, site, spread, etc.)

Behaviour of Symptoms:	
24-hour pattern:	
Aggravated by:	
Eased by:	
Medication	
Other treatments:	
Past Medical History:	
Contraindications:	Severity Irritability Nature
Observations: Posture	Gait:
Muscle Power:	
Muscle Length Tests:	
Range of Joint Movement:	

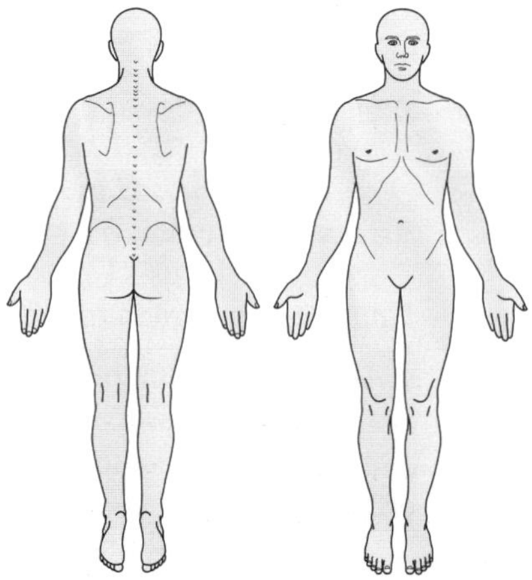

Summary: Problem list	P1	P2	P4	P4
Subjective				
Objective				
Assessment				
Plan				

7. Enhanced clinical expertise comes from knowing when you do not know; clinical wisdom is born from knowing with whom to consult and when to effect the best treatment.
8. The more chronic a patient's condition, the more time will be required to make decisions and treat effectively.

REFLECTIVE PRACTICE

The importance of professional reflection has been discussed above. Here are some points that may help to develop these reflective skills. The headings are in no way absolute or definitive as many other topics would fit into a number of these categories equally well.

Interpersonal

- Do I communicate well with my patients?
- Do my patients seem to understand what I am explaining to them?
- Are my patients usually happy to go along with my suggestions?
- Do I listen thoroughly to my patients and hear what they are saying?
- Do my patients and I have good eye contact and a relaxed, but professional, relationship?
- Am I aware of my body language?
- Do my patients feel I have time for them?

Cognitive

- Am I making the right decisions about which techniques to use?
- Do patients respond quickly to the massage: are there objective and subjective improvements within, on average, two treatment sessions?
- Do I progress my treatments gradually in response to improvement?
- Do I swap and change techniques because I am not very sure about which to use?
- Do I use the same techniques through the whole course of treatment?
- Am I creative but cautious about the media I use?

Psychomotor

- Do my patients relax when having massage or do they feel tense?
- Am I able to feel the changes in the tissues and the whole person as I massage?
- Do I always know which tissue or tissue interface I am working on?
- Are my techniques comfortable and enjoyable to receive?
- Is my massage effective?

Philosophical

- Do I have a holistic approach?
- Am I primarily satisfying the needs of my patient or of myself?
- Are the treatment methods and course of treatment negotiated with patients?
- What exactly is my personal philosophy for the use of massage and patient care?

Professional

- Are my patients satisfied with the treatment they receive?
- How do I monitor that?
- Do my treatments work?
- Have I done all I can to ensure the environment in which I massage is conducive and pleasant?
- Do I have superb health and safety mechanisms in place?
- Do I respect my patients' dignity and privacy (e.g. by leaving the room while they undress and dress)?
- Do I keep up to date with new developments?

Start your reflective practice now by making your own list.

A thoughtful therapist is more likely to be a good therapist. This process can be furthered by setting clinical standards and by auditing practice.

KEY POINTS

- ◆ Clinical reasoning is the process by which clinical decisions are made.
- ◆ The essential intellectual skills are knowledge, understanding, synthesis, analysis and evaluation (cognitive), and reflection (metacognitive).
- ◆ Clues are found, hypotheses generated, cues interpreted and hypotheses evaluated in clinical reasoning.
- ◆ A problem-based approach is central to clinical practice.
- ◆ Detailed and thorough subjective and objective assessment of the patient's problem is necessary.
- ◆ Treatment goals should be set and outcomes evaluated.

REFERENCES

Bloom B S 1956 Taxonomy of educational objectives. David McKay, New York

Charlin B, Tardif J, Boshuizen H P 2000 Scripts and medical diagnostic knowledge: theory and applications for clinical reasoning instruction and research. Academic Medicine 75(2): 182–190

Henley E C 1994 The clinical reasoning process – how can we maximize it? Journal of the Singapore Physiotherapy Association 15(1): 16–21

Kettenbach G 1990 Writing SOAP notes. F A Davis, Philadelphia, PA

Lloyd F J, Reyna V F 2001 A web exercise in evidence-based medicine using cognitive therapy. Journal of General Internal Medicine 16(2): 94–99

Mattingley C, Fleming M H 1994 Clinical reasoning: forms of enquiry in a therapeutic practice. F A Davis, Philadelphia, PA

May B J, Newman J 1980 Developing competence in problem solving: a behavioural model. Physical Therapy 60(9): 1140–1145

Payton O D 1985 Clinical reasoning process in physical therapy. Physical Therapy 65(6): 924–928

Round A P 1999 Teaching clinical reasoning – a preliminary controlled study. Medical Education 33(7): 480–483

Weed L L 1971 Medical records, medical education, and patient care. Year Book Medical, USA

Wolf S 1985 Clinical decision making in physical therapy. F A Davis, Philadelphia, PA

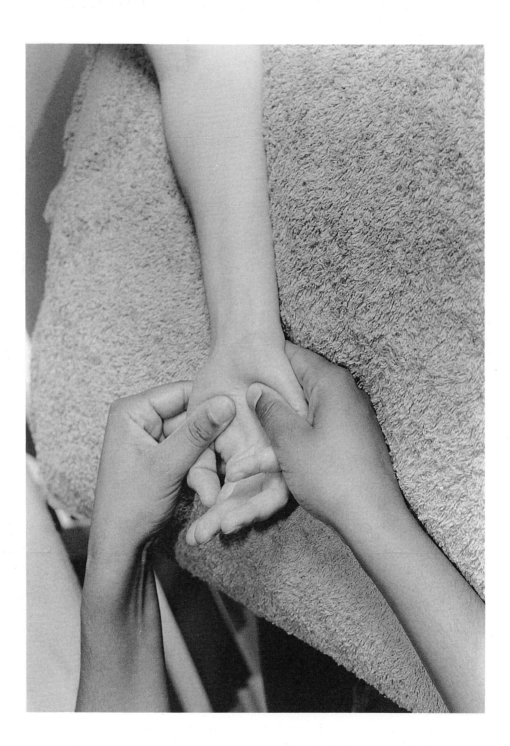

7 Massage Techniques

The first section of this chapter contains information about the lubricants and essential oils that may be used in massage. Stance, posture, movement and safety issues, in relation to both the therapist and the patient, are also addressed. The second section describes the techniques and manipulations of classical massage, and also includes those of neuromuscular technique and deep transverse frictions.

LUBRICANTS (MASSAGE MEDIA)

Massage may be performed either with or without a lubricant; both methods have ardent supporters who are prepared to dispute the merits of the opposing point of view. To enable the therapist to form her own opinion on this question, some of the most common points for and against are presented here.

Points for Massage with a Lubricant

- Reduces friction on the skin.
- Protects fragile skin from being stretched.
- Protects very hairy skin from being pulled.
- Some oils (e.g. wheatgerm, olive) are said to aid skin nutrition.
- Perspiration can be absorbed by a powder lubricant.
- The gliding effect of some massage manipulations is enhanced.
- Perfumed oil has a beneficial psychological effect on the patient.
- Essential oils can be selected for their therapeutic properties.

Points for Massage without a Lubricant

- Massage can be applied more deeply in the tissues.
- Oil is messy to use and easily spilled.
- A lubricant may cause an allergic reaction.
- Oils may stain clothing.
- Lubricants create an increased risk of infection.
- The tissues are more easily palpated.
- The massage can be more stimulating.
- Tissues are more easily manipulated if they are not slippery.
- Commercial massage oils are over-priced and highly scented.

A balanced approach to these opposing viewpoints is recommended. Clearly there are occasions when a lubricant is desirable and times when it is not. The following factors may be taken into account when deciding whether the use of a lubricant is appropriate to a specific treatment:

Condition of the Skin

On hairy, fragile or scaly skin a lubricant will aid patient comfort and prevent irritation.

Possibility of Allergic Reactions

Some people are allergic to nuts and will have an anaphylactic reaction (which causes shock, an acute fall in blood pressure and bronchospasm, and can be fatal) if they are exposed to oil derived from nuts. Peanuts are the most common allergen: about 1 in 500 of the population are affected (Demain 1996). Arachis oil is derived from peanuts and many commercial massage lotions use a nut oil, such as almond or hazel, in their preparation. The therapist should always question the patient concerning allergies before using any lubricant and be fully aware of the constituents of any lubricant she has not prepared herself.

Safety

Talc can be inhaled into the lungs where it can cause irritation. It is no longer in use in the UK National Health Service for this reason.

Necessity for Skin Traction

Massage manipulations that grasp and lift the superficial tissues are ineffective if too much lubricant is used, making the surface of the skin slippery, and a highly viscous oil can cause excess skin traction. A small amount of oil or powder can, however, make these techniques more comfortable for the patient and prevent friction. It is not appropriate to use a lubricant for massage manipulations where the therapist's hand does not glide on the skin, but specifically moves the skin on underlying tissue. For these manipulations it is important for there to be traction between the massaging hand and the patient's skin; a lubricant would not serve any purpose.

Categories of Lubricant

The literature contains many examples of lubricants that have been used in massage, some of which have waned in popularity in recent years.

Lubricants of Vegetable Origin

Oils: corn, safflower, sesame, soyabean, sunflower, wheatgerm, coconut, almond, hazel, grapeseed, arachis (peanut), olive, avocado. *Powder*: corn starch.

Lubricants of Mineral Origin

Baby oil, petroleum jelly, liquid paraffin, french chalk, talc, cold cream.

Lubricants of Animal Origin

Wool fat, lanolin, soap solution, neat's-foot oil (*neat* is an old Saxon word meaning animals of the ox kind), hog's lard.

Other Categories

Commercial preparations of oils, creams and lotions. Many of these use petro-chemicals as a base; some use vegetable oil; and some are water based and easily removed from clothing by washing. Many commercial products do not list the ingredients and it is therefore impossible to determine whether they are suitable for use on a patient with specific allergies.

Comments

It is advisable for the therapist to sample a variety of the available lubricants and to try using them on her own skin. This will enable the therapist to judge their suitability for massage and experience the type of sensation that a patient may feel when they are used. (N.B. The authors do not recommend the use of hog's lard.)

Oils of vegetable origin are generally the most pleasant to use and are suitable as a carrier with essential oils. Mineral oil does not penetrate the skin well and is therefore unsuitable for carrying volatile oils into the tissues. The lack of this property does, however, convey an advantage for general massage purposes, as it tends to stay on the surface of the skin and less is needed. There is some controversy concerning the use of mineral oil. Taken internally in large quantities it can interfere with the absorption of fat-soluble vitamins, but there is no evidence to suggest that it is detrimental when used as a massage lubricant (Skiba 1993). Some vegetable oils are more viscous than others (e.g. olive, wheatgerm) and should be added in small quantities to a lighter oil. Vegetable oils can become rancid; keeping supplies refrigerated in a well-sealed container slows this process, as does the addition of 5% wheatgerm oil, which has antioxidant properties. A therapist with sweaty palms may find that powder is a more suitable lubricant as it absorbs some of the moisture. A fine non-perfumed talc has traditionally been a useful addition to the therapist's equipment; some patients prefer it to oil and it does not degrade. Consent should be obtained from the client before using talc and great care should be taken to ensure it does not invade the atmosphere and that it cannot be inhaled by either the client or the therapist.

ESSENTIAL OILS

The medium used in massage can be therapeutic in its own right. Although oils can be used solely as lubricants for massage, they can also be the vehicle for the absorption of a particular substance, selected for its own therapeutic properties, into the body. Liniments, for example, have long been rubbed into the skin to affect the underlying tissues.

Aromatherapy is the name given to application of *essential oils*, which are the oils that provide the scent and/or flavour to flowers, fruit and herbs. They have been extracted from the plants and used for this purpose for thousands of years (Tisserand 1994), either as herbal medicines, inhalations or compresses. Pure oils can be extracted from the leaves, flowers or seeds of plants and used for specific therapeutic purposes. Many have a pleasant smell which produces a psychological effect, a feeling of well-being. Inhalation also ensures that they enter the bloodstream quickly through the highly vascular lung and respiratory tract fields; a popular method of inhalation entails heating the oils in an aromatherapy burner. Alternatively, they may be added to a warm bath for inhalation and skin absorption. They can therefore be self-administered, used simply to create a pleasant smell and atmosphere in a room, or can be skilfully prescribed and blended by an aromatherapist. Detailed discussion of each oil, sufficient to guide professional aromatherapy prescription, is beyond the scope of this book. However, the principles are described here to a sufficient depth to assist massage therapists to select a limited number of oils for safe use as a therapeutic or pleasantly scented medium.

Massage is a particularly popular way of applying essential oils, and results in a slow penetration. The oils are dissolved in a carrier oil and used as the medium for massage, allowing the effects of the oils to combine with the therapeutic effects of the massage. Relaxation massage should be used (see, for example, the one described in Ch. 10). As with any therapeutic substance that enters the body, dangers and side-effects may be present and anyone using these oils for any purpose should be aware of them. This applies particularly to a therapist using oils in health care settings where clients may have a variety of health problems. Unfortunately, research into the effects of the oils is patchy and knowledge is based predominantly on oral tradition. Where research has been undertaken, it has often focused on the main chemical constituents of the oils, so pure oils should be used in which the constituents are known. Good quality oils from professional suppliers are the purest, and inexpensive ones should be avoided. Air, heat and light can cause degradation of oils. This results in a changed chemical composition which may be less effective or more toxic; therefore oils should be kept in a cool, dark environment and not kept for longer than 6 months once opened unless in a fridge. This safety advice is important as degradation and oxidation may make the oils more likely to become carcinogenic, although the transfer of research conducted on rats to humans is not straightforward (Tisserand 1996).

Any therapy which has been used throughout history becomes refined through experience and often the knowledge surrounding its use is accurate. Present-day researchers are attempting to deepen this knowledge of essential oils in the light of current scientific methods by isolating specific constituents of the oils and testing their effects. Albert-Puleo (1979) reviewed the literature concerning the oestrogenic properties of fennel and anise, as identified by numerous animal experiments conducted in the 1930s and 1940s. He suggested that the oestrogenic active ingredients are anethole polymers. Work by Taylor (1964) has shown fennel to have low toxicity and no demonstrable carcinogenicity. Thyme (*Thymus capitatus*) has been found to have strong fungitoxic properties (Arras & Usai 2001).

Other researchers have attempted to define the effects of individual oils and isolate their mechanism of action. An example is the work by Aqel (1991) in which he applied oil of rosemary to rabbit and guinea-pig tracheal muscle samples. The oil inhibited muscular contractions induced by histamine and acetylcholine. Aqel suggested that the oil is a calcium modulator. Hills & Aaranson (1991) agreed with this suggestion, following similar work on the effects of peppermint oil on smooth muscle. Oil of orange diffused through a dental waiting room was found to have a relaxant effect (Lehrner et al 2000). Cooke & Ernst (2000) conducted a systematic review and concluded that aromatherapy massage has a mild, transient anxiolytic effect, useful for relaxation but not strong enough for the treatment of anxiety. Anderson et al (2000) found that tactile contact between mother and child in the form of massage improved childhood ectopic eczema but that adding essential oils was not more beneficial.

There is concern about the possibility of adverse effects of oils. Research in this area has often been conducted on animals using huge dosages of the oil, so transferability of findings to humans is difficult. Elliot (1993) reported a case of tea-tree oil poisoning, but suggested it may have been an allergic reaction. This does, however, highlight the fact that ingestion of these oils can carry some risk, the extent of which is unknown where there has been insufficient research. Studies into microbiological effects are easiest to conduct under controlled, scientifically valid conditions. Bassett et al (1990) found tea-tree oil to be as effective as 5% benzoyl peroxide in the treatment of acne, with fewer side-effects. Carson & Riley (1994) found that terpinen-4-ol was the main antimicrobial component of tea-tree oil. It was tested against 12 organisms, including *Staphylococcus aureus*, *Candida albicans* and *Lactobacillus acidophilus*, and only one of the 12 (*Pseudomonas aeruginosa*) was found to be resistant to the oil. A detailed literature review of essential oils will not be undertaken here, but the clinically based studies are often inconclusive, conducted on animals, and not readily transferable to humans. Caution is therefore needed and external application is safer than internal use. Aromatherapists should understand as much as possible about the oils they prescribe, and attempts are being made to examine and address safety issues (Tisserand & Balacs 1995).

Use of Essential Oils in Massage

Choice and prescription of oils can be interesting. The principles of perfumery and medicine are used: asking what types of scents the patient prefers and blending from a base note (fixative), middle note (relates to bodily functions, with a longer-lasting scent) and top note (volatile and stimulatory, often smelled immediately the top is removed from a bottle). Medical history and present complaints are examined in detail to identify any contraindications or potential sensitivities to a particular oil (for example: Are migraine attacks provoked by strong odours? Is the individual epileptic?) and to use the blend to specific effect. The exact amount of carrier oil required varies with the absorptive properties of individual skin, but blending 3–12 drops of essential oil in 30 ml carrier oil is a useful guide. To ensure a pleasant blend, essential oil should be added to the carrier drop by drop, using as little as is required. Blending should only be undertaken by those qualified in aromatherapy. It should be noted that drop size differs between manufacturers and therefore dosage is approximate. The therapist cannot be sure of the exact dose administered (Olleveant et al 1999).

The massage is usually a full body massage as this ensures that a good dosage is absorbed into the bloodstream. The oils are volatile and evaporate readily, so more is blended than is actually absorbed into the skin. None the less, a full body massage administers a good dose and should therefore not be given more than once per week. The therapist should be aware of the potential dose she is receiving herself: four massages are regarded as maximal in any one day. Both therapist and client should drink plenty of water after massage as the oils have a diuretic effect and can lead to dehydration and headaches: they can often be tasted after a massage, so encouraging clients to drink is not difficult.

Contraindications

There are few specific recorded contraindications to general aromatherapy, although individual oils have their own specific contraindications and cautions. Obviously, the contraindications for massage should be respected and allergic reactions guarded against. On no account should essential oils come into contact with the eyes. If they do, the eyes should be douched with water and medical help sought. Tea-tree oil should not be used in chidlbirth as it has been found to reduce uterine contractions in rats (Lis-Balchin et al 2000).

Users of aromatherapy should be aware of a recent study reported in the journal *Food and Chemical Toxicology* which examined the toxic effects of dill, peppermint and pine (Lazutka et al 2001). To summarize: all three oils were found to cause cytotoxic genetic mutations on human lymphocytes. These are worrying findings which raise concerns across all essential oil use. Until more is known about safe doses in humans, it would be wise not to use dill, pine or peppermint oils in massage.

Precautions

Precautions for each oil should be understood. In general (in relation to massage), certain oils should not be used in pregnancy as they have been found to cross the placental barrier in high doses. Oils that contain bergapten (bergamot) can produce ultraviolet sensitization and phototoxic reactions have been

Continued

TABLE 7.1   Oils in common use

Oil	Principal constituents	Main actions	Common uses	Precautions	Examples of research
Bergamot (*Citrus bergamia*) Base note	Linalyl acetate, limonene, bergapten	Analgesic, antiseptic, lifts mood, sedative, diuretic, aids digestion	Wound care, infections, anxiety, depression, stress, digestion	Photosensitivity, photocarcinogen (max. 0.4%)	Young et al. (1990)
Chamomile (*Chamaemelum nobile* (Roman)) Middle note	Esters of angelica, tiglic acid	Analgesic, anti-inflammatory, sedative, antispasmodic, digestive	Musculoskeletal pain, menstrual and menopausal problems, skin problems, headache, insomnia	Slight risk of dermatitis	Patzelt-Wenczl & Ponce-Poschl (2000)
Cedarwood (*Cedrus atlantica* (Atlas)) Base note	Atlantone, caryophyliene, cedrol	Antiseptic, diuretic, expectorant, sedative	Skin conditions, arthritis, chest problems, stress	Avoid during pregnancy	None found
Geranium (*Pelargonium graveolens*) Middle note	Citronelleol, geraniol, linalol	Haemostatic, antiseptic, analgesic, diuretic, tonic	Dry sore skin, oedema, poor circulation, throat infections, PMT	Slight risk of sensitivity	Clerc et al. (1934)
True lavender (*Lavandula angustifolia*) Top note	Linalyl acetate, linalol	Antiseptic, analgesic, hypotensive, diuretic, anti-depressive	Skin conditions, joint problems, chest problems, aids digestion, menstrual problems, headaches, stress	Some types of lavender can cause convulsions True lavender generally safe	Atanassova-Shopova et al. (1973), Saeki (2000)
Lemon (*Citrus limonum*) Top note	Limonene, bergamotene	Antiseptic, diuretic, stimulant, antirheumatic, haemostatic	Muscle problems, respiratory problems, skin problems, infections	Phototoxic (use 2% max) Some skin reactions	Roe & Field (1965)
Rosemary (*Rosemarinus officinalis*) Middle note	Pinenes, camphene, cineol	Analgesic, stimulant, antiseptic, diuretic, low dose hypotensor, high dose hypertensor	Musculoskeletal pains, fatigue, menstrual problems, digestive and liver problems, respiratory problems	Avoid if pregnant or epileptic due to camphor content	Craig & Frase (1953)

TABLE 7.1 *Oils in common use—cont'd*

Oil	Principal constituents	Main actions	Common uses	Precautions	Examples of research
Tea-tree (*Melaleuca alternifolia*) Top note	Terpinene-4-ol, cineol, pinene	Bactericidal, anti-inflammatory, expectorant, immunostimulant, antifungal	Skin infections, thrush, chest problems, colds and flu	Slight risk of skin reaction	Carson & Riley (1994), Hills & Aaranson (1991), Aqel (1991), Bassett et al. (1990), Albert-Puleo (1979), Lis-Balchin et al. (2000)
Ylang-ylang (*Cananga odorata genuina*) Base note	Methyl benzoate, methyl salicylate, terpenes	Antiseptic, antidepressant, hypotensive	Raised pulse rate and blood pressure, insomnia, depression, stress	Can cause headaches or nausea	None found

Sources: Lawless 1992, Tisserand & Balacs 1995, Varman & Walker 1995.

reported (Kaddu et al 2001), so care should be taken, particularly in summer. Oils can cause contact dermatitis. Increased use of lavender flowers around the home and in pillows has been found to cause contact dermatitis (Sugiura et al 2000). Lavender, jasmine, rosewood, laurel, eucalyptus and pomerance have been reported to cause skin reactions (Schaller & Korting 1995). Severe contact dermatitis reactions to tea-tree oil have also been reported (Khanna et al 2000). Great care should be taken to ensure that susceptibility to adverse reactions is assessed prior to massage. It should also be noted that chemical constituents often behave differently when combined together, so the therapist should be aware that research on individual oils will not provide a total picture. Damaged skin is best avoided except when the practitioner is highly experienced; oils that may provoke sensitivity should not be used on babies and young children.

Table 7.1 lists the oils in common use, together with their constituents, main actions and uses. It also summarizes the precautions for each oil.

APPLYING THE LUBRICANT

- *The lubricant should be at skin temperature.* Oil in a sealed container can be warmed by standing it in hot water. Talc can be warmed by being left close to a heat source.
- *Avoid spillages.* Oil can be transferred into a small squeeze bottle; this is probably the safest method. Alternatively it can be put into a shallow dish and placed on a surface close to the treatment couch but where it is not likely to be upset.
- *The therapist's hands should be washed before beginning the massage.*
- *The patient's clothing should be protected.*
- *Application.* The lubricant, be it oil or talc, is first rubbed onto the therapist's hands and then transferred to the skin of the patient. This method safeguards against applying too much lubricant or spilling it on the patient's clothing; it also protects the patient from the unpleasant sensation of feeling a sudden dollop of oil.
- *The lubricant is spread on the skin by stroking or effleurage.*
- *Reapplication.* During the massage treatment it may be necessary to reapply the lubricant and sometimes it is desirable not to lose physical contact with the patient. The technique is achieved by keeping the dorsum of one hand in contact with the patient so that the palm is upwards and can receive the lubricant from the other hand. The hands are rubbed together, maintaining patient contact, and the lubricant is then reapplied to the skin in the usual way. To achieve this method gracefully the lubricant should be within easy reach of the treatment couch.
- *Hygiene.* To ensure there is no risk of cross-infection, at the end of treatment the therapist should dispose of any oil that may have become contaminated and thoroughly wash her hands.

STANCE, POSTURE AND MOVEMENT

Therapists who perform massage regularly are aware that the activity places demands upon their physical capacities. Unless stance, posture and movement are addressed initially by the student therapist she will find that giving massage treatments is fatiguing. The therapy also has the potential to induce overuse syndrome. To achieve maximum effectiveness the therapist should comply with ergonomic principles. This means giving attention to the safety of her stance and posture and to the economy of her movements. Although this may seem complicated when first learning how to massage, the student therapist should not feel disheartened. As with any other psychomotor skill, the refinements of the technique are achieved with practice; expect less than perfect coordination when you first begin.

Base of Support

The position of the feet is important for three reasons. First, correct foot positioning enables the therapist to reach all parts of the patient's body without strain. The joints of the hands, arms and spine can be held in a stress-free position if body-weight is transferred from one foot to the other, thus reducing the need to reach.

Second, the direction in which the feet face is important to enable weight transference without trunk rotation. The knee to which the weight is transferred flexes, resulting in a lunge posture.

Third, foot position is important for balance. The body relies on the feet for its base of support – the area that encloses the feet and includes the space between them. The further apart the feet are, the wider the base of support. The weight of the body is transferred to the ground through the line of gravity; the body is most stable when the line of gravity falls in the centre of the base. If the line of gravity falls outside the base, the body will not be able to balance; this displacement is unlikely to occur when the base of support is large. Stability and balance enable the body to remain relaxed and free the muscles to perform the massage without strain on the therapist.

Stance

The therapist faces the direction of the massage manipulations. This varies according to the area of the body that is to be treated. The following examples can be adapted to encompass other massage techniques.

Long Manipulations

For effleurage to the back, for example (Fig. 7.1A), the therapist stands close to the left of the treatment couch where she can place her hands at the start of the stroke with no trunk rotation. The left foot is a comfortable stride forward of the right one; the left foot points towards the head of the treatment couch and the right foot is angled. At the start of the stroke there is more weight on the right foot than on the left; the therapist is using some body-weight to create the pressure of the stroke. As the stroke progresses up the back, weight is transferred from the right foot to the left; the left knee flexes so that a lunge position is adopted.

| **FIGURE 7.1** | *Foot positions for (A) long manipulations (e.g. effleurage of the back); (B) transverse manipulations (e.g. wringing to the back) (exposed area); (C) small-range manipulations on specific structures (e.g. transverse frictions).* |

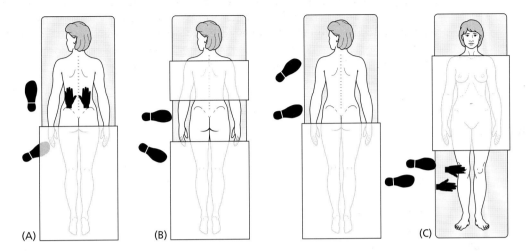

(A)   (B)   (C)

Transverse Manipulations

For wringing the back, for example (Fig. 7.1B), the therapist stands close to the treatment couch facing across the patient's back. The left foot is on a level with the thoracolumbar junction, which is where the manipulation begins. The right foot is angled so that the right lumbar segment can be treated with no trunk rotation. As the strokes move towards the buttocks, the therapist transfers weight to her right leg and flexes the knee. To massage the right thoracic region, the therapist adjusts her foot position so that the right foot is now on a level with the thoracolumbar junction. The procedure is repeated.

Small-range Manipulations on a Specific Structure

For frictions, for example (Fig. 7.1C), the therapist faces the structure to be treated; the left foot is forwards of the right. The left hand is supporting the patient's thigh while the right hand performs the manipulation. There is more weight being taken through the right foot than the left and, as this is a deep manipulation, there is substantial weight transference to the patient through the therapist's arms to exert pressure on the tissues.

Posture and Movement

The therapist should apply the same general principles of safe posture when giving massage as she would with any task that has an element of risk to the musculoskeletal system. The major areas of risk are identified below and suggestions are made about prevention:

- Excessive reaching causes unsafe trunk movements and is linked with muscle fatigue and soft tissue injury.

Prevention: The therapist should stand close to the treatment couch. The correct stance will ensure that she is able to reach all parts of the area to be treated. When a small therapist is treating a very tall patient, it may be helpful to divide the treatment area into sections so that the therapist can change position between segments.

- Prolonged elevation of the arms necessitates static loading of the shoulder girdle muscles and is fatiguing, causing soft tissue damage and compromise to peripheral nerves.

  Prevention: Ensure the height of the work surface is correct. This should be just below waist level so that it is rarely necessary to flex the shoulders beyond a 45-degree angle from the therapist's body.

- Excessive compressive forces can cause joint injury. The wrist and joints of the fingers and thumbs are those at greatest risk when massaging.

  Prevention: Avoid prolonged repetition of movements and hyperextension of these joints. When performing manipulations that require compressive forces, keep the joints in a near-neutral position.

- Prolonged muscular activity of the arms and hands causes muscle fatigue.

  Prevention: Avoid using muscles to create pressure. This is best achieved by transferring body-weight to the patient through the massaging hands. The therapist's shoulder, arm and hand should be free of tension. All movements should be kept to the minimum necessary to achieve the desired effect.

- Poor balance leads to faulty movement.

  Prevention: Adopt the correct stance. A wide base of support lowers the centre of gravity and so aids equilibrium. Dynamic balance is achieved by a transfer of weight, at the correct time, from one foot to the other.

ENVIRONMENT AND SAFETY

The safety and comfort of the patient are paramount and it is the therapist's responsibility to ensure that high standards are maintained.

The Environment

This should be tidy with equipment moved away from the area so that there is nothing the patient or therapist could bump into or trip over. For sedative massage, noise should be kept to a minimum if possible and, if not, as in a busy hospital department, it may be helpful to play music if the patient likes it. If music is played it should be relaxing and appropriate to the patient. It is always worth enquiring whether the chosen piece of music is acceptable to the patient, as associations triggered by particular music may produce unwanted effects that conflict with the aim of the massage.

The temperature of the environment should be comfortable for the patient. Steps should be taken to ensure that there is no interruption during the treatment session. Protecting the patient's privacy and dignity is essential.

All the equipment needed for the massage, such as lubricants, covers and pillows, should be placed near to the treatment couch. The couch should be prepared with fresh linen and be ready to receive the patient.

The Therapist

If a uniform is not worn then the mode of dress is optional, provided it is appropriate to the task. Appropriate, in this context, means that the therapist should be professional in appearance and that her clothing should not constrain her movements. The therapist should remove any jewellery that could come into contact with the patient, for example long necklaces, watches, bracelets and rings. Long hair should be tied back. Fingernails should be trimmed so that they do not protrude beyond the fingertips. Before each treatment the therapist should wash her hands and ensure they are warm.

Infection Control

The therapist who works in a hospital or clinic will find that there are existing infection control policies and she should familiarize herself with these. The following are the minimum standards that should be applied to protect against the transmission of infections or viruses borne by blood or body fluids:

- Practise high standards of basic hygiene, with regular hand-washing; the minimum frequency of hand-washing is between each client.
- Cover all skin wounds or lesions with a waterproof dressing.
- Protect the mucous membranes of the eyes, mouth and nose from blood or body fluids.
- Wearing rubber gloves, clear up blood, urine, vomit and faeces immediately; disinfect surfaces.
- Dispose of contaminated waste by burning.

PATIENT POSITIONING AND DRAPING

Adhere to the following principles:

- The patient must be comfortable and warm.
- The body part to be massaged should be free from clothing and jewellery.
- The body part to be massaged and the joints distal and proximal to it should be supported.
- Extra supplies of linen, pillows, blankets and towels should be nearby in case they are needed during the treatment.

The ideal patient position is lying on a treatment couch of adjustable height. For treatment to the arm and hand it is equally convenient to have the patient seated with the upper limb supported on a small table, with the therapist seated opposite. Massage to the neck and upper back can be performed with the patient sitting on a seated massage chair or seated at a table or on the couch. Pillows are piled up to a height that allows the patient to be supported anteriorly, with the upper limbs resting on the table. If the patient is not comfortable in any of these positions, the therapist should devise a suitable position which supports the body part to be treated and is also comfortable for the therapist.

Patient Supine-Lying on a Treatment Couch

- The patient may require one or two pillows under the head.
- A pillow or rolled towel may be placed behind the patient's knees.
- The patient is covered with a sheet; a blanket may also be required.
- The body part to be massaged is exposed by drawing back the cover from that area.

Patient Prone-Lying on a Treatment Couch

- The couch should have a removable section for the face; if it does not, two pillows can be placed in an inverted 'V' shape so that there is a space for the patient to breathe.
- A folded sheet may be placed under the patient's chest. This can be wrapped around the back, or, when that area is being treated, it can be draped over the upper arms.
- A female patient who has large breasts may require a pillow under her chest.
- A pillow may be placed under the abdomen to reduce lumbar lordosis.
- A rolled towel or small pillow is placed under the ankles so that they are not in an extreme range of plantarflexion and the knees are slightly flexed.
- The patient is covered with a sheet; a blanket may also be required.
- The body part to be massaged is exposed by drawing back the cover from that area.

Patient Side-Lying on a Treatment Couch

- The patient may require one or two pillows under the head.
- The upper arm and upper leg are supported anteriorly by pillows.
- A heavily pregnant woman may require pillows to support her abdomen.
- The patient is covered with a sheet; a blanket may also be required.
- The body part to be massaged is exposed by drawing back the cover from that area.

TECHNIQUES AND MANIPULATIONS

This section of the chapter describes the techniques and manipulations of classical massage, together with neuromuscular technique and deep transverse frictions. Specialized techniques such as myofascial release, manual lymphatic drainage and acupressure are covered in Chapter 9.

TECHNIQUE: STROKING

Categories: Long Stroking; Thousand Hands

Purpose

To apply the massage medium.
To habituate to touch.
To facilitate regression of sensory analgesia.
To sedate (slow stroking).
To stimulate (brisk stroking).
To decrease muscle tone (slow stroking).

Features

A unidirectional manipulation.
Usually applied from proximal to distal.

Manipulation: Long Stroking

Procedure

The manipulation begins at the most proximal part of the area to be treated.
The therapist places the whole of her hands in contact with the skin (Figs 7.2A,B).
A gentle but firm pressure is maintained.
The hands are drawn towards the therapist, leading the movement with the heel of the hand (Figs 7.2C,D).
An even depth of pressure is maintained while the hands mould to the body contours.
The hands are lifted off smoothly at the distal region of the treatment area without trailing the fingers.
The following stroke overlaps the first, continuing until the whole of the body region is covered.
The manipulation may be adapted for small areas by the therapist using only one hand, the fingers or thumbs.

Manipulation: Thousand Hands

Procedure

The therapist places one hand in contact with the skin at the proximal part of the area to be treated.
The therapist strokes distally for about 15 cm.

FIGURE 7.2   *Long stroking: (A,B) start of stroke; (C,D) direction of movement.*

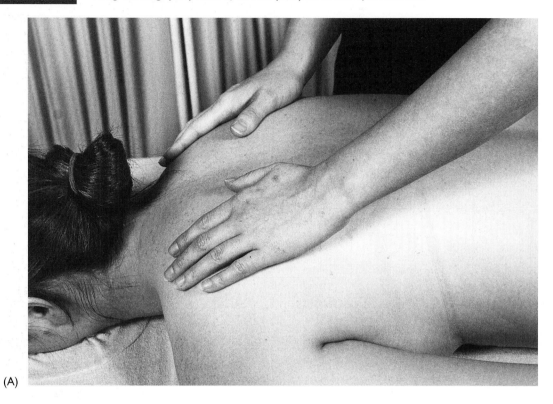

(A)

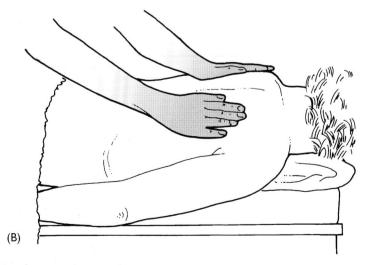

(B)

(Figure cont'd)

(Figure 7.2 cont'd)

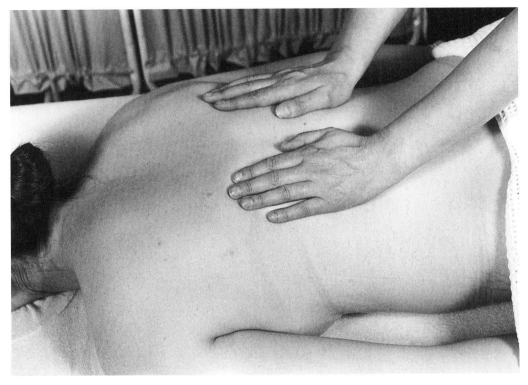

(C)

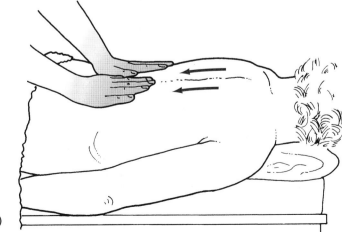

(D)

FIGURE 7.3   *(A,B) Thousand hands. The arrow indicates the direction of movement of the short overlapping strokes.*

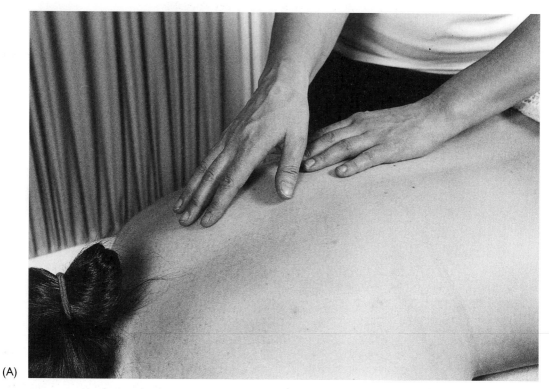

(A)

(B)

The alternate hand begins an overlapping stroke, along the same line of treatment, before the first hand is lifted off (Figs 7.3A,B).

There is always one hand in contact with the skin.

The fingers should not trail on the skin when lifting off.

The strokes are continued to the distal part of the treatment area.

The manipulation is repeated on an adjacent area until the whole of the region has been covered.

TECHNIQUE: EFFLEURAGE

Purpose

To aid venous and lymphatic return.

To aid interchange of tissue fluid.

To aid removal of chemical irritants.

To restore mobility at tissue interfaces.

To stretch muscle fibres passively.

To increase muscle tone (deep effleurage).

To decrease muscle tone (light effleurage).

Features

The manipulation is commonly utilized at the start and end of a massage treatment and often between the various petrissage manipulations.

On fragile or hairy skin, oil or talc is applied liberally to avoid stretching the tissues or dragging the hair.

The manipulation is always performed towards the lymph glands.

Depending on the size and shape of the body region to be treated, the therapist may use one or both hands, fingers or thumbs.

Manipulation: Effleurage

Procedure

The stroke begins at the distal part of the area to be treated.

The therapist contacts the skin and applies an even pressure to sink into the superficial tissues.

A sweeping movement is made to the proximal part of the treatment area, moulding to the body contours and maintaining the same depth of pressure throughout the stroke (Figs 7.4A,B).

The stroke is rhythmic and slow to facilitate the movement of fluid.

The stroke is completed, over the site of lymph glands, with a slight pause and overpressure which is almost imperceptible to the patient.

The hands are lifted and repositioned at the start of the next stroke which overlaps the previous one.

The strokes are continued until the whole of the body segment has been covered (Fig. 7.4C).

FIGURE 7.4   *(A,B) Effleurage of the back in the direction of the lymphatic flow; (C) suggested direction and sequence of effleurage strokes across the back; (D,E) effleurage of the forearm.*

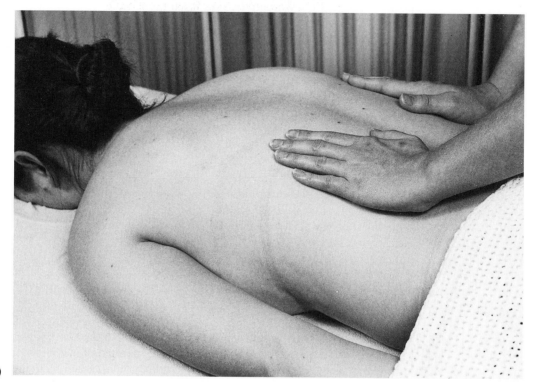

(A)

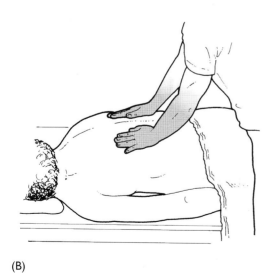

(B)

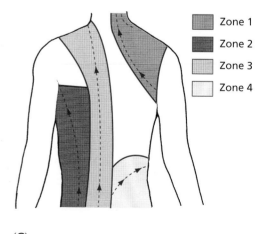

(C)

Zone 1

Zone 2

Zone 3

Zone 4

(Figure continued)

(Figure 7.4 cont'd)

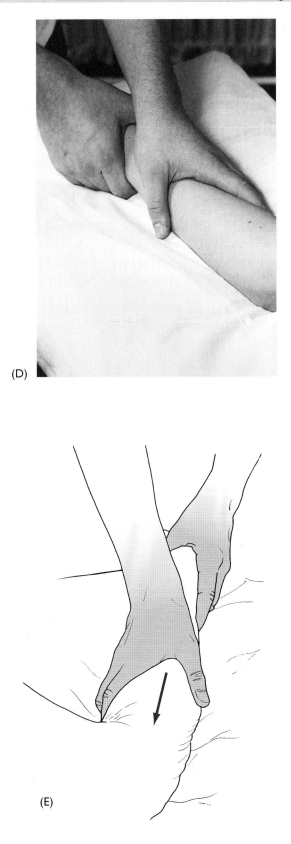

(D)

(E)

If there are no lymph glands in the body segment, effleurage is then continued to the site of the nearest lymph glands.

On cylindrical body segments, the hands or fingers are wrapped around the treatment area to perform the manipulation (Figs 7.4D,E).

TECHNIQUE: PETRISSAGE

Categories: Kneading; Wringing; Rolling; Picking Up; Shaking

Purpose

To aid venous and lymphatic return.
To aid removal of chemical irritants.
To increase mobility and length to fibrous tissue.
To restore mobility between tissue interfaces.
To aid interchange of tissue fluid.
To improve the appearance and mobility of subcutaneous tissue.
To increase extensibility and strength of connective tissue.
To provoke somatovisceral reflex effects.

Features

Petrissage manipulations first compress the soft tissues, they are then lifted, squeezed or rolled, and taken to the tissue end-feel.
The manipulation is performed on superficial tissue, muscles or ligaments.
Petrissage manipulations should be avoided on sensitized tissue, where they may be painful.
Care should be taken not to overwork any treatment area.

Manipulation: Kneading

Procedure

The manipulation is performed with one or both hands (Figs 7.5A,B), or the pads of fingers or thumbs, depending on the size and shape of the area to be treated.
The stroke begins at the proximal part of the area to be treated and moves distally.
The therapist contacts the skin and compresses the tissues.
The skin is moved on the underlying tissues; there is no glide.
The hands or digits are moved in a circular motion, which causes skin wrinkling ahead of the movement and a slight stretch behind it.
When both hands are used to perform the stroke they are moved alternately: the right hand moves clockwise and the left hand in an anticlockwise direction.

Hands can be placed on opposite aspects of the limb to apply extra compression ('box' kneading).

There is a pressure phase when the tissues are compressed on to the deeper structures.

The position of hands for the pressure phase requires a slight adjustment for flat and cylindrical body segments (Figs 7.5C,D).

After the first circular stroke a light glide is effected on the skin to reposition the massaging hand at the start of the next stroke.

The strokes are continued on adjacent areas, overlapping the previous stroke, until the whole of the treatment area has been covered (Fig. 7.5E).

When extra compression is required the manipulation is performed with one hand on top of the other to give reinforcement.

The therapist should take care to maintain finger and thumb joints in a near-neutral position when using the digits to perform the manipulation.

Manipulation: Wringing

Procedure

Wringing may be performed on skin and superficial tissue using the pads of the fingers and thumbs (Figs 7.6A,B).

Wringing may be performed on muscle using the whole of the hands (Figs 7.6C,D).

The therapist places her hands on the skin with the fingers adducted and the thumbs abducted.

The tissues are compressed.

The fingers and thumbs are squeezed together so that a roll of tissue or muscle gathers between them.

The therapist pushes one hand away and draws the other hand towards her; the roll of tissue is twisted (Figs 7.6E,F).

The twist is then applied in the opposite direction by changing the position of the hands.

The manipulation progresses along muscle in the direction of the fibres, beginning at one end and finishing at the other.

On superficial tissue the manipulation progresses forwards across the body region and then adjacently until the whole of the area has been covered.

Manipulation: Rolling

Procedure

Rolling of small muscles and superficial tissue is performed with the pads of the fingers and thumbs.

Rolling of large muscles is performed with the whole of the hands.

The therapist places her hands on the skin with the fingers adducted and the thumbs abducted.

The index fingers and thumbs of opposite hands are in contact to create a diamond shape between them (Figs 7.10A,B).

FIGURE 7.5   *(A,B) Whole-handed kneading of the back: (C,D) kneading a cylindrical body segment (upper arm); (E) direction and overlap of kneading manipulations of the back – pressure phase shown by the thickened line.*

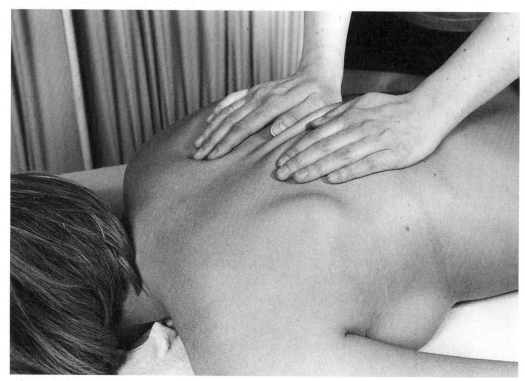

(A)

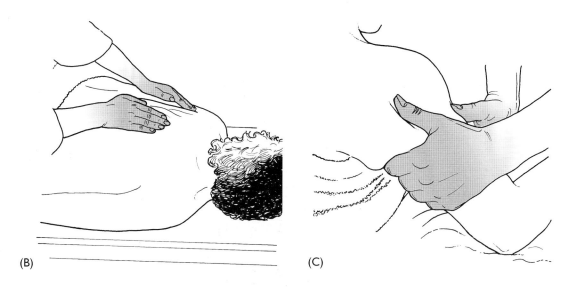

(B)   (C)

(Figure cont'd)

(*Figure 7.5 cont'd*)

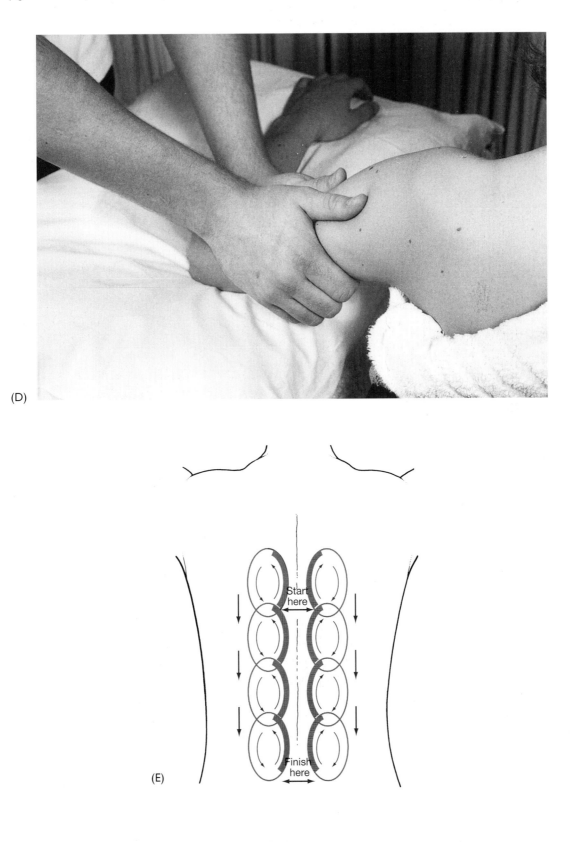

(D)

(E)

FIGURE 7.6 *(A,B) Wringing the Achilles tendon; (C,D) muscle wringing the back of the thigh; (E,F) wringing the back.*

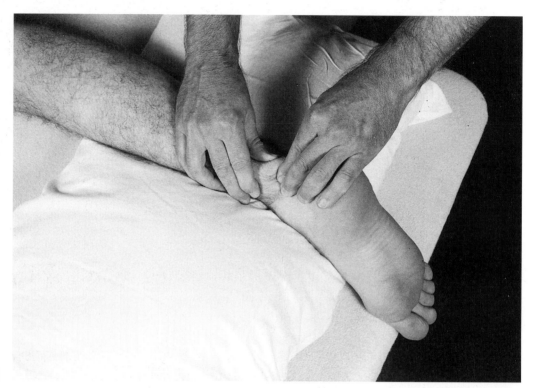

(A)

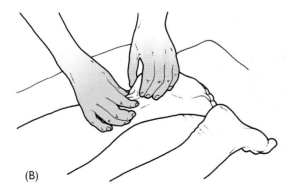

(B)

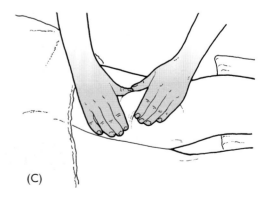

(C)

(Figure cont'd)

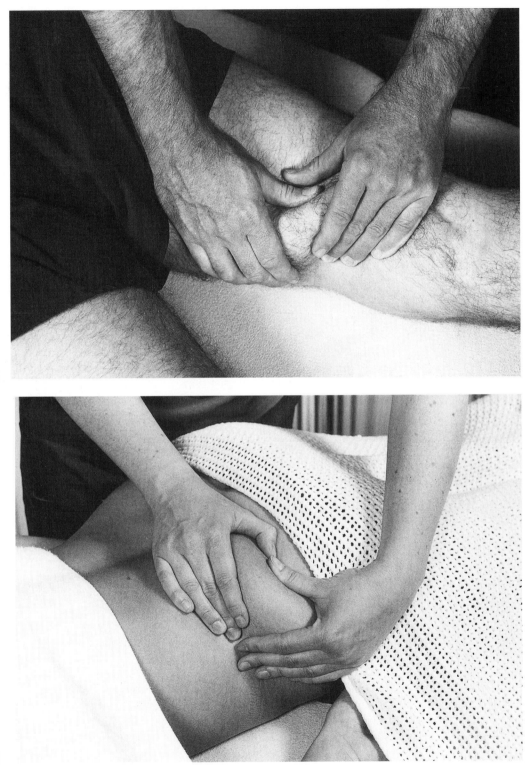

(D)

(E)

(*Figure 7.6 cont'd*)

(Figure 7.6 cont'd)

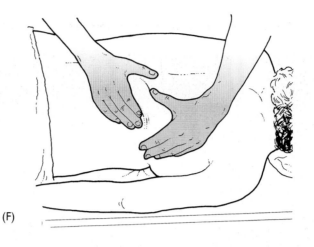

(F)

The tissues are compressed.

Keeping contact with the skin, the fingers are pulled towards the thumbs, creating a roll of tissue (Figs 7.10C,D).

The thumbs are pushed forwards while the fingers travel backwards so that the tissue rolls away from the therapist (Figs 7.10E,F).

Care must be taken to avoid pinching the tissues.

The roll of tissue gradually diminishes in size towards the end of the stroke where the fingers and thumbs of each hand make contact.

The following stroke is begun on an adjacent area of tissue and continues until the whole of the area has been covered.

On muscle, the manipulation is applied across the fibres beginning at one end and finishing at the other.

Manipulation: Picking Up

Procedure

Picking up may be performed with one hand or with two hands working alternately.

The therapist places her hand on the skin with the fingers adducted and the thumb abducted.

The tissues are compressed.

The therapist makes a scooping motion with the massaging hand (Figs 7.7A,B), at the same time bringing the fingers and thumb together to lift the tissues and gently squeeze them (Figs 7.7C,D).

The resultant roll of tissue is then pulled in the opposite direction and taken to the tissue end-feel.

FIGURE 7.7   *(A,B) Picking up – the direction of the scooping stroke; (C,D) lifting the tissues.*

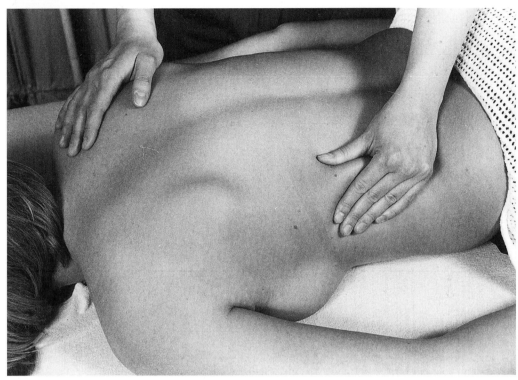

(A)

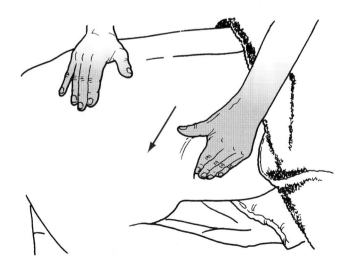

(B)

(Figure cont'd)

(*Figure 7.7 cont'd*)

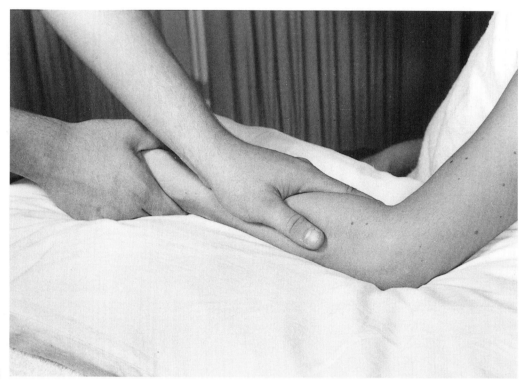

(C)

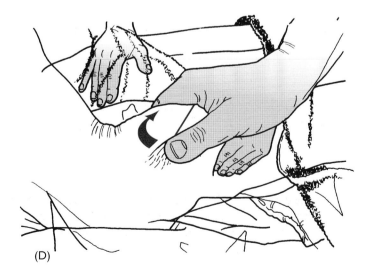

(D)

The tissues are released and the next stroke begun in the adjacent area, progressing until the whole of the treatment area has been covered.

Manipulation: Shaking

Procedure

Shaking is performed on muscle.

Small muscles may be shaken between the pad of the index finger and thumb.

On large muscles the manipulation is performed with the whole length of the fingers and thumb.

The patient is positioned so that the muscle is in mid-range.

The therapist grasps the belly of the muscle between fingers and thumb and lifts it away from the underlying bone (Figs 7.8A,B).

The muscle is shaken quickly from side to side.

TECHNIQUE: FRICTION

(*Cyriax* friction technique is described later in this chapter.)

Purpose

To stimulate local circulation.

To aid removal of chemical irritants.

To restore mobility between tissue interfaces.

To restore mobility to specific anatomical structures.

Features

There are two distinct manipulations in this category:

Manipulation 1

Performed with the whole hand, moving the skin back and forth on the underlying tissues (Figs 7.9A,B).

Manipulation 2

Performed with the tip of the thumb or fingers making small rotary movements, the pressure being appropriate to the desired tissue interface.

Lubricant is not used as there is no glide on the skin.

FIGURE 7.8   *(A,B) Muscle shaking the calf.*

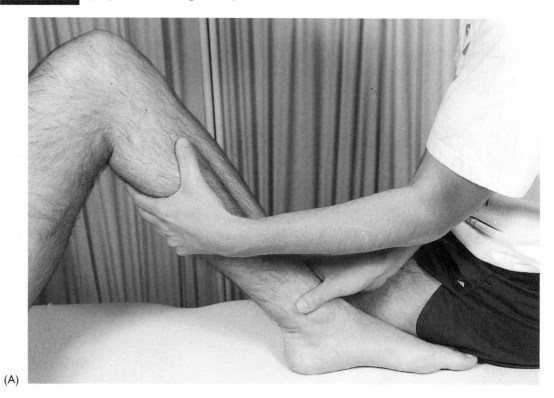

(A)

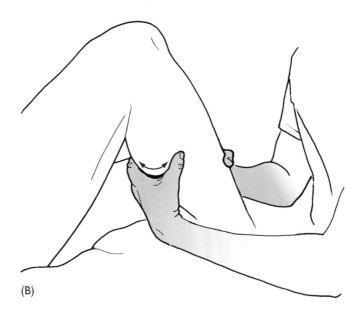

(B)

FIGURE 7.9   *(A,B) Frictions to the lower leg: manipulation 1.*

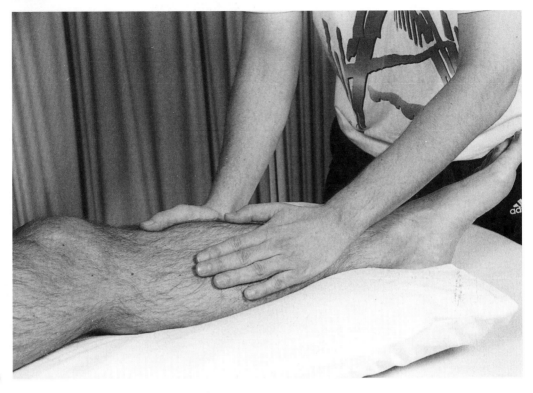

(A)

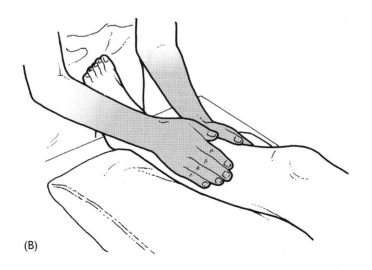

(B)

FIGURE 7.10 *(A,B) Rolling – the start of the manipulation; (C,D) creating a roll of tissue; (E,F) thumbs pushing the roll of tissue away.*

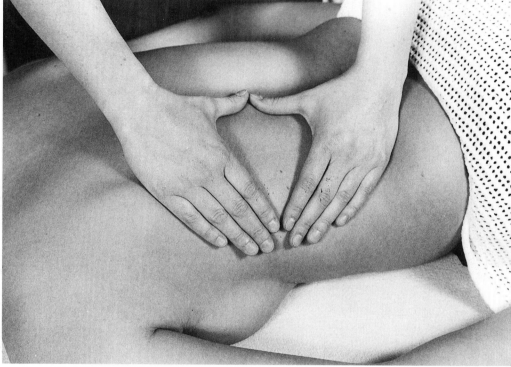

(A)

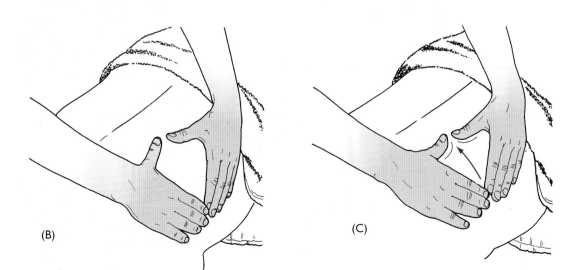

(B)

(C)

(Figure cont'd)

(*Figure 7.10 cont'd*)

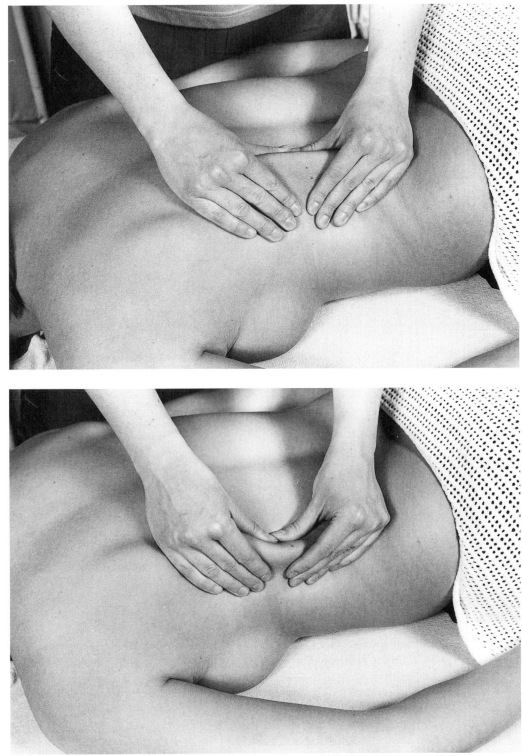

(D)

(E)

(*Figure cont'd*)

(*Figure 7.10 cont'd*)

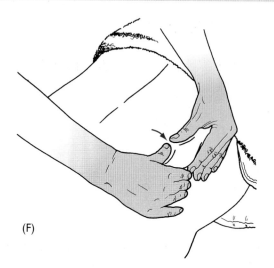

(F)

Manipulation: Friction

Procedure

Manipulation 1

The manipulation may be performed with one hand or two hands working alternately.

The therapist places her hands on the skin with thumb and fingers adducted (Figs 7.9A,B).

The therapist moves her hands back and forth repeatedly and briskly.

The following stroke begins adjacently and is continued until the whole of the treatment area has been covered.

Manipulation 2

The therapist places the tip of her thumb or finger(s) on the skin over the structure to be treated.

The tissues are compressed to the depth of the structure to be treated.

Small rotary movements are performed on the structure while maintaining a constant pressure.

There is no glide on the skin.

The superficial tissues are moved on the underlying structures.

TECHNIQUE: TAPOTEMENT

Categories: Clapping; Hacking; Pounding; Tapping; Vibration

Purpose

To stimulate local circulation.
To provoke muscle and tendon reflexes.
To provoke a general stimulatory effect.
To aid peristalsis (vibration).
To stimulate muscle tone.

Features

Light tapotement has an effect on the superficial tissues.
Heavy tapotement penetrates to deeper layers and should not be used over
organs unless this treatment is specifically indicated.
The area to be treated may be covered with a sheet or thin clothing to ensure
patient comfort.

Manipulation: Clapping

Procedure

The therapist's fingers and thumbs are adducted, with the thenar and
hypothenar eminences in opposition so that a cup shape is formed by the
relaxed hand (Figs 7.11A,B).
The therapist's elbows are flexed and the arms abducted.
The arms are alternately flexed and extended so that the borders of the hands
and fingers strike the skin.
The strokes are rapid, light and brisk.
Air is trapped between the hands and the skin, and produces a hollow sound
as contact is made.
The whole of the treatment area is covered.

Manipulation: Hacking

Procedure

The therapist's arms are abducted and her elbows flexed to near 90 degrees
(Figs 7.12A,B).
Her wrists are fully extended and the fingers relaxed (Figs 7.12C,D).
Her hips are flexed so that the shoulders are over the area to be treated.
The medial borders of the hands and fingers strike the skin alternately, lightly
and rapidly.
The movement is at the radio-ulnar joint, which pronates and supinates.
Very light hacking is performed by the fingers only striking the skin.

FIGURE 7.11   *(A,B) Clapping the deltoid.*

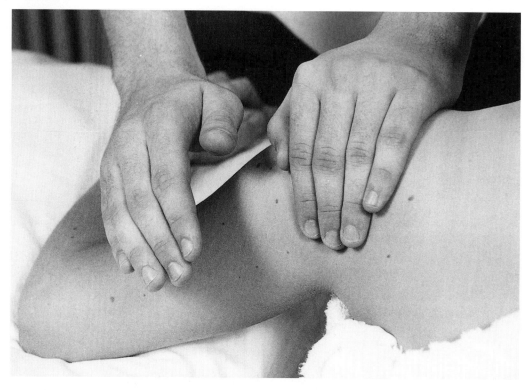

(A)

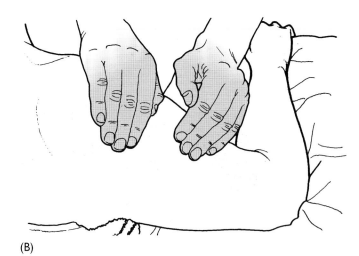

(B)

FIGURE 7.12   *Hacking (A,B) the back and (C,D) the forearm.*

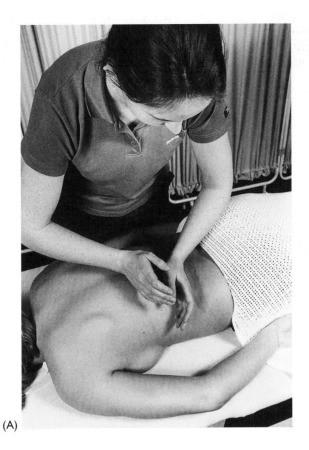

(A)

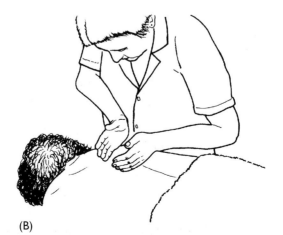

(B)

(Figure cont'd)

(Figure 7.12 cont'd)

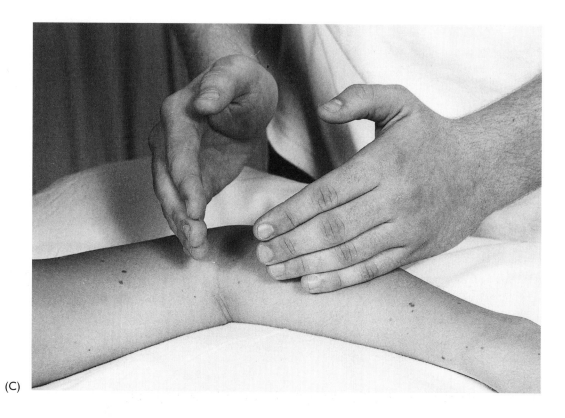

(C)

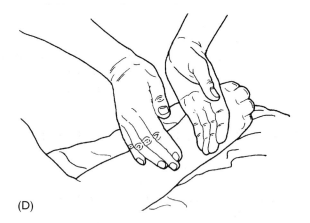

(D)

Manipulation: Pounding

Procedure

The therapist's arms are abducted and her elbows flexed to near 90 degrees.
Her wrists are extended and the fingers flexed loosely into a fist (Figs 7.13A,B).
Her hips are flexed so that the shoulders are over the area to be treated.
The medial borders of the fifth fingers strike the skin alternately and rapidly.
The movement is at the radio-ulnar joint, which pronates and supinates.

Manipulation: Vibration

Procedure

The manipulation is performed with one hand.
The therapist's shoulder is abducted and the elbow is slightly flexed.
The hand is placed on the skin with fingers adducted (Figs 7.14A,B).
The tissues are alternately compressed and released while performing small oscillations by movement of the whole arm, which produces a trembling effect.
The vibration travels through the patient's tissues.
When working in small areas, the fingertips may be used to perform the manipulation.

TECHNIQUE: NEUROMUSCULAR TECHNIQUE

Purpose

To identify and treat abnormalities of soft tissue.
To stretch and smooth thickened and fibrosed tissues mechanically.
To exert a reflex effect on underlying reflex points.
To reduce pain and restore function.

Features

This is an examination and treatment technique that is characterized by a stroking palpation of the soft tissues.
On finding any thickenings, indurations or nodules, the palpatory technique or pressure is used repetitively to treat the lesion.
A cream lubricant can be used if required.

Manipulation: Neuromuscular Technique

Procedure

The web space between the therapist's thumb and index finger should be stretched.
The therapist's finger and thumb tips should be placed on the patient's skin.

FIGURE 7.13 *(A,B) Pounding the covered gluteal area.*

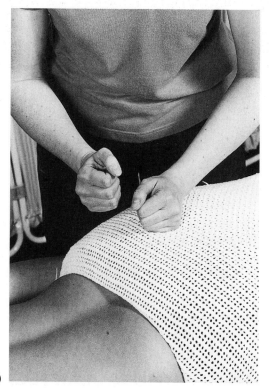

(A)

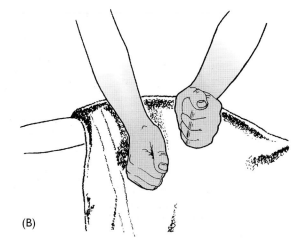

(B)

FIGURE 7.14   *(A,B) Vibration to the calf.*

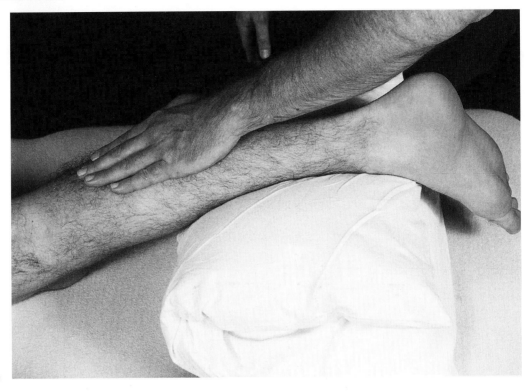

(A)

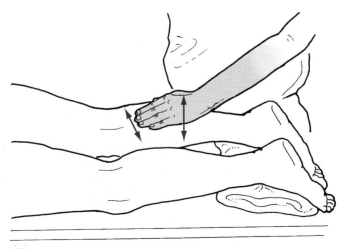

(B)

FIGURE 7.15   *(A,B) Neuromuscular technique.*

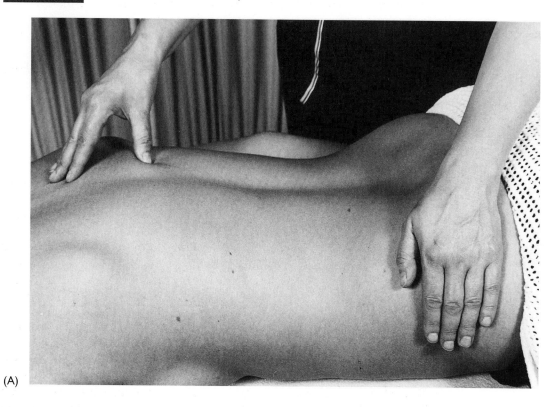

(A)

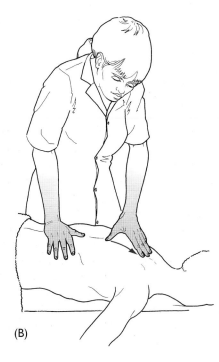

(B)

The thumb should be slid slowly 5–8 cm towards the fingers (Figs 7.15A,B).

The fingers are then lifted off the skin and moved away from the thumb.

The stroke is then repeated, overlapping with the previous one.

Lesions found are treated by a repetitive application of the stroke or other appropriate techniques.

The stroke can be applied with the fingers if the thumb is too large for any area.

TECHNIQUE: DEEP TRANSVERSE FRICTIONS (CYRIAX FRICTION MASSAGE)

This is a specialized technique developed by Dr James Cyriax for the treatment of soft tissue lesions. It is a very specific, localized technique that is applied to the point of injury of a structure. It is aimed at producing a widthways stretching across the fibres, separating them to lengthen the cross-bridges between collagen fibres, restoring interfibre mobility. This has the effect of restoring longitudinal stretch and widthways expansion to the structure, allowing the broadening of a contracted muscle. The stress applied by this technique ensures that remodelling of connective tissue is stimulated appropriately by precipitating plasticity of molecular bonding in the linear region of the stress–strain curve. Frictions are said to produce a reactive hyperaemia (Chamberlain 1982), which can be useful in healing and chronic scarring.

Frictions should be applied at the correct phase of healing. If they are used too early (within 48 hours of injury), the delicate fibrous network may be disturbed. However, beyond that stage, movement is important as it helps to limit adhesions and scar formation by encouraging proteoglycan synthesis and stimulating new collagen fibres to be aligned in the direction of stress.

The technique is well described in orthopaedic medicine textbooks (Cyriax & Cyriax 1993, Ombregt et al 1995). In addition, there is a limited amount of research literature on the subject. De Bruijn (1984) assessed the onset and duration of the analgesic effects by treating 13 patients with a variety of soft tissue injuries by deep transverse frictions (DTFs). He reported that the range in duration of friction massage was 0.4–5.1 (average 2.1) minutes before analgesia was achieved. In 10 sessions with five patients, the post-massage analgesia lasted between 0.3 minutes and 48 hours (mean 26 hours). It is postulated that the analgesic effect is useful as it facilitates earlier movement following soft tissue injury. Troisier (1991) used DTFs to the common extensor tendon below the epicondyle in 131 patients suffering from tennis elbow. 'Good and excellent' results were achieved in 63% of patients. Unfortunately the English abstract of this French paper does not give further detail of the study or method of measuring improvement. A further study (Pellechia et al 1994) compared two regimens in the treatment of patellar tendinitis. The first comprised iontophoresis (movement of a drug through the skin by the application of an electrical current) of dexamethasone and lidocaine (lignocaine). The second protocol consisted of transverse frictions, moist heat and phonophoresis (movement of a drug through the skin by the application of ultrasound) of 10% hydrocortisone and a cold pack. Some 17 men and nine women were studied, age range 14–43 years. Symptoms had been present between 3 days and 10 years. They received six sessions and were changed to the other protocol if the symptoms persisted at session 7. Iontophoresis showed significant improvement in measures of a visual analogue pain scale, a functional index questionnaire, a rating of palpation tenderness and the number of step-ups needed to elicit pain. Only the last measure improved significantly following the combination treatment protocol. The conclusion reached was that iontophoresis is the most effective treatment. Obviously, this study did not examine the separate components of the combined treatment. Further work to analyze this programme would be useful. A more curious study was undertaken in which changes in biting force were measured following deep transverse frictions to the masticatory muscles of 10 cerebrovascular accident victims. The improvement in bite was primarily attributed to facilitation of muscle tone (Iwatsuki et al 2001), although there were no differences between affected and non-affected sides.

Other research has attempted to demonstrate the exact effects of DTFs. Walker (1984) studied the effects of frictions on the healing of a minor sprain in the medial collateral ligament of the rabbit. Twelve rabbits received a sprain on the right side; the left sides were used as healthy controls. A further six rabbits were additional untreated controls. Tissue samples showed no differences between treated and untreated ligaments. Unfortunately, there were no clinical signs of inflammation following the sprains. The earliest any of the tissues was examined following injury was 11 days, in which case healing would be well advanced in a small animal. As there were no differences between sprained and unsprained ligaments, the injuries may have been too negligible to have been influenced by this technique. Unfortunately, then, this study does not enhance our knowledge of the effects of DTFs.

A Cochrane systematic review concluded that there is no evidence of clinically important benefits of DTFs for treating iliotibial band syndrome, but acknowledged that more studies are needed before any conclusions relating to practice can be drawn (Brosseau et al 2002). (See Ch. 13 for discussion of the use of DTFs in bursitis.)

Manipulation: Deep Transverse Frictions

Purpose

Produces local hyperaemia, aiding the resolution of inflammation.
Reduces pain as a result of a counterirritant, pain-gate effect and the resorption of metabolites.
Promotes movement and remodelling of healing tissue.
Stretches fibrous tissue.
Prepares the structure for manipulation.

Features

Must be applied accurately to the exact site of damage.
Must be applied at 90 degrees to the direction of the fibres, across the structure.
Must take the tissues through their full sweep, i.e. to their end-feel.
The skin must move with the therapist's fingertips.

FIGURE 7.16   *Cyriax friction technique to (A,B) tendon of infraspinatus, with patient's shoulder in lateral rotation; (C,D) coronary ligaments, right knee – the knee is laterally rotated to place the ligaments on a stretch; (E,F) left common extensor and flexor tendon.*

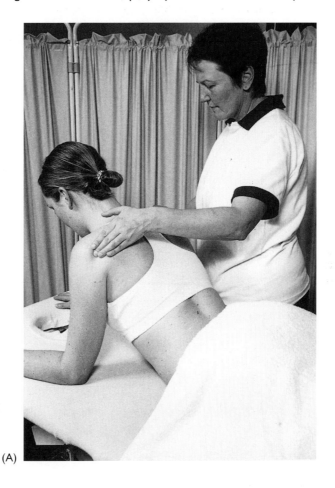

(A)

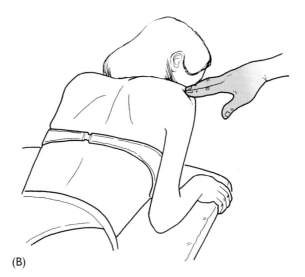

(B)

(Figure cont'd)

(*Figure 7.16 cont'd*)

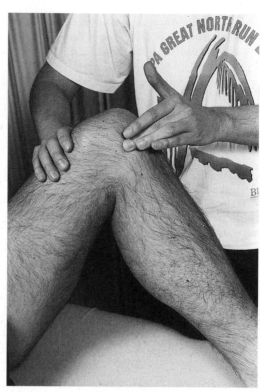

(C)

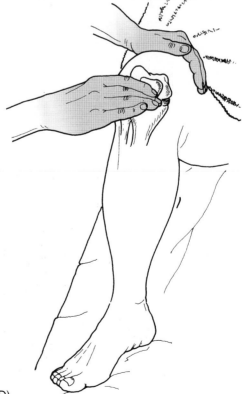

(D)

(*Figure cont'd*)

(Figure 7.16 cont'd)

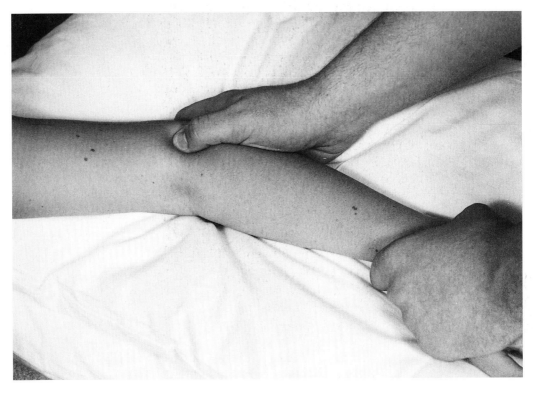

(E)

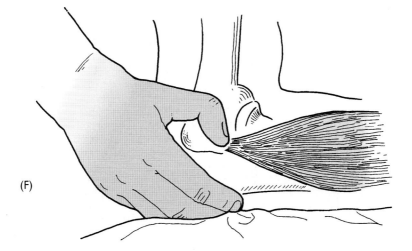

(F)

The patient must be warned that the technique will be painful until numbing is achieved (after approximately 2 minutes).

Should be applied within the patient's pain tolerance.

Position

Patient

Comfortable, fully supported, body position.

Limb fully supported.

Structure exposed, e.g. shoulder laterally rotated for infraspinatus tendon (Figs 7.16A,B); internally rotated for supraspinatus.

Ligaments – on stretch (Figs 7.16C,D).

Tendons in sheath – on stretch.

Tendons without sheath – either taut or short (Figs 7.16E,F).

Muscle – shortened.

Therapist

Close to structure.

Comfortable position.

Joints of the arm in a neutral position.

Procedure

Contact made between pad of index or middle finger.

Reinforce with adjacent finger.

Apply counterpressure with the other hand.

Sweep back and forth across the lesion using the large muscles of the arm.

Ensure the therapist's fingertips and patient's skin move together.

A full sweep should be achieved – to the end-feel of the tissue.

Continue for up to 15 minutes (expect a numbing effect after about 2 minutes).

REFERENCES

Albert-Puleo M 1979 Fennel and anise as estrogenic agents. Journal of Ethnopharmacology 2: 337–344

Anderson C, Lis-Balchin M, Kirk-Smith M 2000 Evaluation of massage with essential oils on childhood ectopic eczema. Phytotherapy Research 14(6): 452–456

Aqel M B 1991 Relaxant effect of the volatile oil of Romarinus officinalis on tracheal smooth muscle. Journal of Ethnopharmacology 33: 57–62

Arras G, Usai M 2001 Fungitoxic activity of 12 essential oils against four postharvest citrus pathogens: chemical analysis of thymus capitatus oil and its effect in subatmospheric pressure conditions. Journal of Food Protection 64(7): 1025–1029

Atanassova-Shopova S et al 1973 On certain central neurotropic effects of lavender essential oil. II. Communication: studies on the effects of linalool and of terpineol. Izvestiia Inst Fiziol Sof 15: 149–156

Bassett I B, Pannowitz D L, Barnetson R 1990 A comparative study of tea tree oil versus benzoylperoxide in the treatment of acne. Medical Journal of Australia 153: 455–458

Brosseau L, Caslmiro L, Milne S et al 2002 Deep transverse friction massage for treating tendinitis: a systematic review. Cochrane Library, issue 1, Oxford

Carson C F, Riley T 1994 The antimicrobial activity of tea tree oil [letter]. Medical Journal of Australia 160: 236

Chamberlain G J 1982 Cyriax's friction massage: a review. Journal of Orthopaedic and Sports Physical Therapy 4(1): 16–22

Clerc A et al 1934 Experiments on dogs with certain substances which lower the surface tension of the blood. Current Reviews of Society of Biology 116: 864–867

Cooke B, Ernst E 2000 Aromatherapy: a systematic review. British Journal of General Practice 50(455): 444–445

Craig J O, Frase M S 1953 Accidental poisoning in childhood. Archives of Disease in Childhood 28: 259–267

Cyriax J H, Cyriax P J 1993 Cyriax's Illustrated manual of orthopaedic medicine, 2nd edn. Butterworth-Heinemann, Oxford

De Bruijn R 1984 Deep transverse friction: its analgesic effect. International Journal of Sports Medicine 5: 35–36

Demain S 1996 Departmental danger of death [letter]. Physiotherapy 82(1): 71

Elliot C 1993 Tea tree oil poisoning [letter]. Medical Journal of Australia 159: 830–831

Hills J M, Aaranson P I 1991 The mechanism of action of peppermint oil on gastro-intestinal smooth muscle. Gastroenterology 101: 55–65

Iwatsuki H, Ikuta Y, Shinoda K 2001 Deep friction massage on the masticatory muscles in stroke patients increases biting force. Journal of Physical Therapy Science 13(1): 17–20

Kaddu S, Kerl H, Wolf P 2001 Accidental bullous phototoxic reactions to bergamot aromatherapy oil. Journal of the American Academy of Dermatology 45(3): 458–461

Khanna M, Qasam K, Sasseville D 2000 Allergic contact dermatitis to tea-tree oil with erythema multiform-like id reaction. American Journal of Contact Dermatitis 11(4): 238–242

Lawless J 1992 The encyclopaedia of essential oils. Element, Shaftesbury, Dorset

Lazutka J R, Mierauskiene J, Slapsyte G, Dedonyte V 2001 Genotoxicity of dill (Anethum graveolens L.), peppermint (Menthaxpiperita L.) and pine (Pinus sylvestris L.) essential oils in human lymphocytes and Drosophila melanogaster. Food and Chemical Toxicology 39(5): 485–492

Lehrner J, Eckersberger C, Walla P et al 2000 Ambient odor of orange in a dental office

reduces anxiety and improves mood in female patients. Physiology and Behaviour 71(1–2): 83–86

Lis-Balchin M, Hart S L, Deans S G 2000 Pharmacological and antimicrobial studies on different tea-tree oils (Melaleuca alternifolia, Leptospermum scoparium or Manuka and Kunzea ericoides or Kanuka), originating in Australia and New Zealand. Phytotherapy Research 14(8): 623–629

Olleveant N A, Humphris G, Roe B 1999 How big is a drop? A volumetric assay of essential oils. Journal of Clinical Nursing 8(3): 299–304

Ombregt L, Bisschop P, ter Veer H J, Van de Velde T 1995 A system of orthopaedic medicine. W B Saunders, London

Patzelt-Wenczler R, Ponce-Poschl E 2000 Proof of efficacy of Kamillosan® cream in atopic eczema. European Journal of Medical Research 5(4): 171–175

Pellechia G L, Hamel H, Behnke P 1994 Treatment of infrapatellar tendinitis: a combination of modalities and transverse friction massage versus iontophoresis. Journal of Sport Rehabilitation 3: 135–145

Roe F J C, Field W E H 1965 Chronic toxicity of essential oils and certain other products of natural origin. Food and Cosmetic Toxicology 3: 311–324

Saeki Y 2000 The effect of foot-bath with or without the essential oil of lavender on the autonomic nervous system: a randomized trial. Complementary Therapies in Medicine 8(1): 2–7

Schaller M, Korting H C 1995 Allergic airborne contact dermatitis from essential oils used in aromatherapy. Clinical and Experimental Dermatology 20(2): 143–145

Skiba B 1993 The mineral oil myth. Massage 44: 40–41

Sugiura M, Hayakawa R, Kato Y et al 2000 Results of patch testing with lavender oil in Japan. Contact Dermatitis 43(3): 157–160

Taylor J M 1964 Fennel. Toxicology and Applied Pharmacology 6: 378–387

Tisserand R 1994 The art of aromatherapy. C W Daniel, Essex

Tisserand R 1996 Essential oil safety. I. International Journal of Aromatherapy 7(3): 28–32

Tisserand R, Balacs T 1995 Essential oil safety: a guide for health professionals. Churchill Livingstone, Edinburgh

Troisier O 1991 Les tendinites epicondyliennes. La Revue du Praticien 41(18): 1651–1655

Varman S, Walker A 1995 Introduction to aromatherapy for physiotherapists [course notes]. University of East Anglia, Norwich

Walker J M 1984 Deep transverse frictions in ligament healing. Journal of Orthopaedic and Sports Physical Therapy 62: 89–94

Young A R, Walker S L, Kinley J S et al 1990 Phototumorigenesis studies of 5-methoxypsoralen in bergamot oil: evaluation and modification of risk of human use in an albino mouse skin model. Journal of Photochemistry and Photobiology 7: 231–250

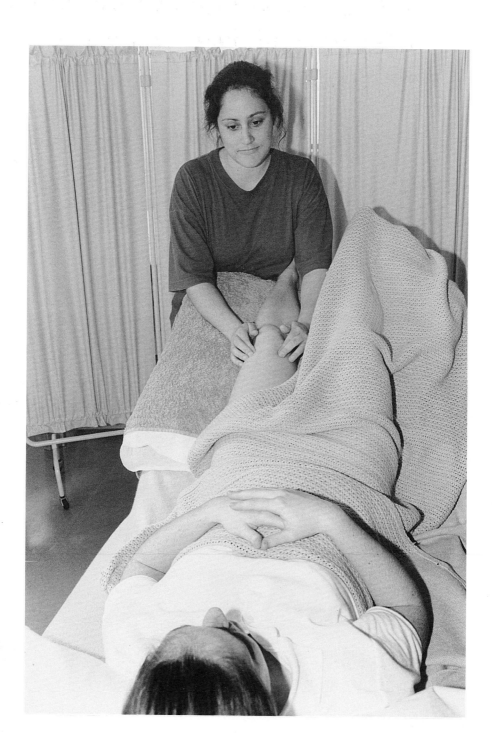

8 Regional Application of Classical Massage Techniques

The basic massage strokes must be adapted to the contours of the body and guided by the underlying anatomy (Fig. 8.1). In this chapter, we suggest a format for each region.

UPPER LIMB: THE ARM

Positioning of the Patient

Sitting, arm supported on a table.
Lying, arm supported on a pillow, resting on the treatment couch.
Lying, arm elevated on pillows.

Special Anatomical Points

Lymph glands: in the cubital fossa at the front of the elbow and in the axilla.
Major muscle groups: trapezius, deltoid, triceps, biceps, brachioradialis, flexors and extensors of the forearm.

Manipulations

Stroking.

FIGURE 8.1   *Major muscles of the body.*

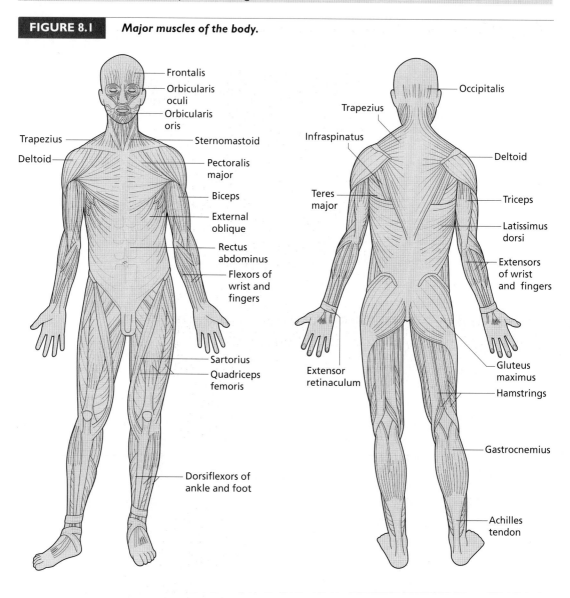

Effleurage: apply three overlapping strokes to the flexor aspect of the forearm with your right hand, repeat on the extensor aspect with your left hand (Figs 8.2A,B).

Kneading: trapezius, two-handed reciprocal kneading to deltoid (Figs 8.3A,B), biceps, triceps, forearm and hand.

Finger kneading: fibres of deltoid, between the forearm muscles, tendons of the wrist.

Picking up: deltoid, biceps, triceps (Figs 8.4A,B), brachioradialis.

Wringing: triceps (Figs 8.5A,B), biceps, brachioradialis.

Muscle shaking: biceps, triceps, brachioradialis (Figs 8.6A,B).

Clapping: flexor and extensor aspects of the arm and forearm (see Figs 7.11A,B).

Hacking: flexor and extensor aspects of the arm (Figs 8.7A–C) and forearm.

FIGURE 8.2   *(A,B) Finish of effleurage stroke along the extensor aspect of the arm. Note that the stroke ends in the axilla.*

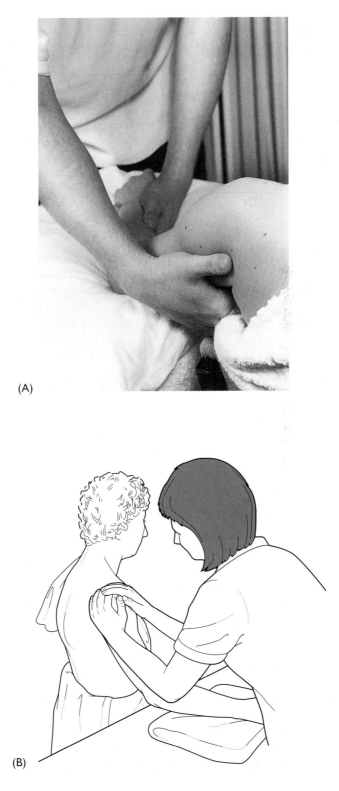

(A)

(B)

FIGURE 8.3   (A,B) Hand positions for reciprocal kneading of the deltoid.

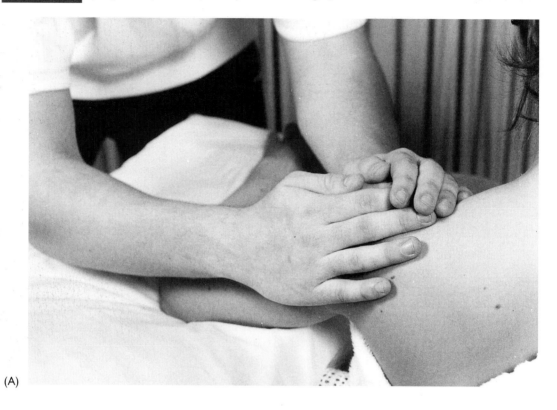

(A)

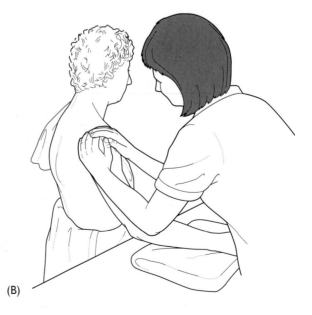

(B)

FIGURE 8.4   *(A,B) Picking up the triceps, the therapist's hand fully grasping the muscle.*

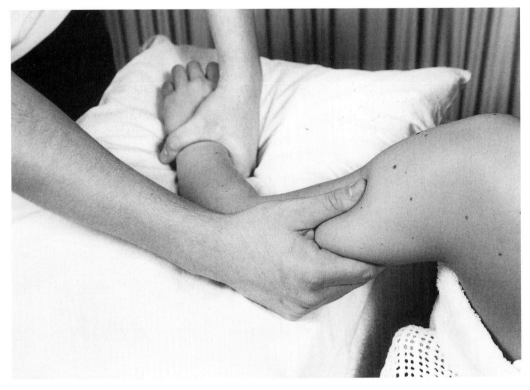

(A)

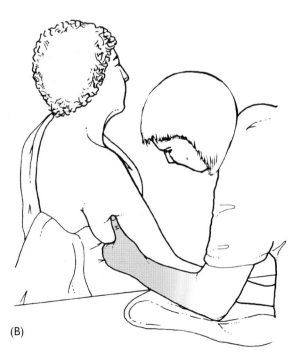

(B)

FIGURE 8.5 *(A,B) Wringing the triceps, the therapist's hands on the extensor aspect of the arm.*

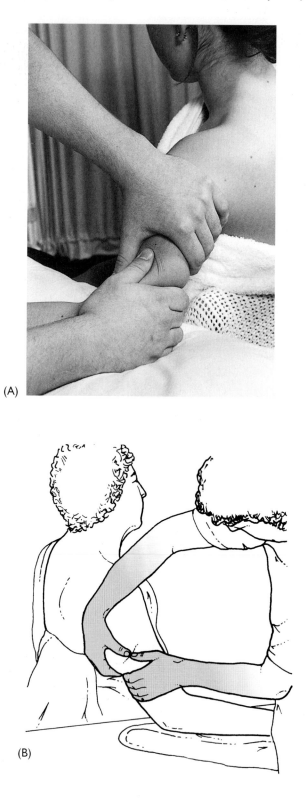

(A)

(B)

FIGURE 8.6   *(A,B) Muscle shaking the brachioradialis. Note the position of the therapist's supporting hand.*

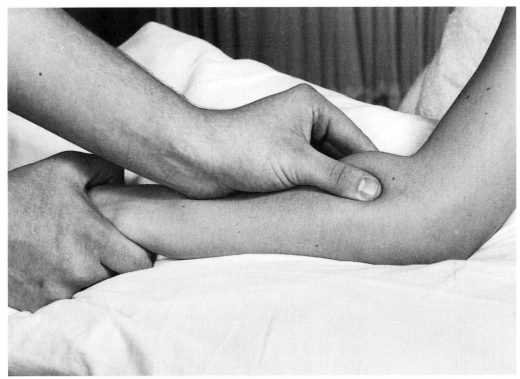

(A)

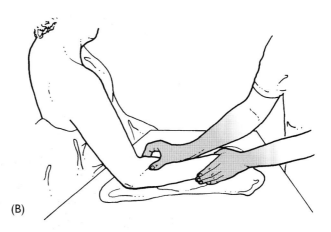

(B)

FIGURE 8.7   *(A–C) Hacking the biceps with the patient's forearm supinated. The therapist then asks the patient to pronate her arm and continues along the extensor aspect, avoiding bony prominences.*

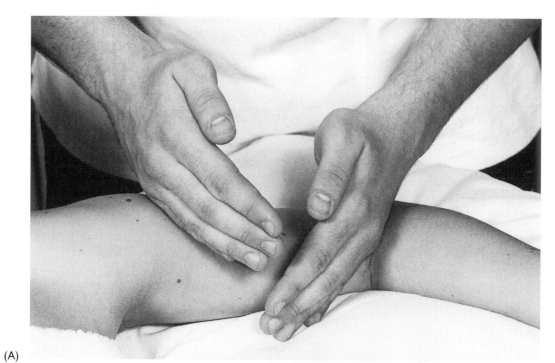

(A)

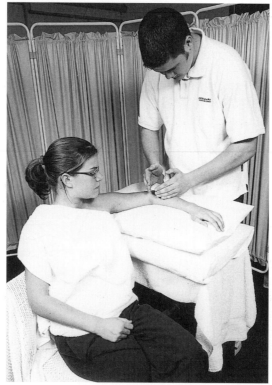

(B)

(Figure cont'd)

(*Figure 8.7 cont'd*)

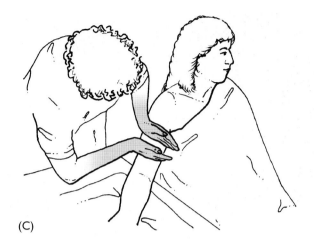

(C)

UPPER LIMB: THE HAND

Positioning of the Patient

Sitting, arm supported on a table.

Special Anatomical Points

Swelling is commonly trapped in the fibrous compartments of the hand.

The areas between adjacent metacarpal bones may need special attention.

Splintage or chronic swelling may lead to soft tissue contracture which will require petrissage manipulations.

The hand contains numerous muscles and tendons that can be implicated in burns and scarring. As resulting disability can be serious massage should be vigorous.

It is often desirable to include the wrist in a hand massage (see Figs 8.11A,B); manipulations may include thumb kneading to the carpal bones, petrissage to the flexor retinaculum.

Manipulations

Effleurage: to the nearest proximal lymph glands with the whole hand (Figs 8.8A,B), individual fingers (Figs 8.9A,B), between the metacarpals, thenar and hypothenar eminences.

Kneading: finger kneading to individual fingers, thumb kneading to the thenar eminence and hypothenar eminence (Figs 8.10A,B), between the metacarpals. (See also Figs 8.11A,B.)

FIGURE 8.8   *(A,B) Effleurage of the whole hand.*

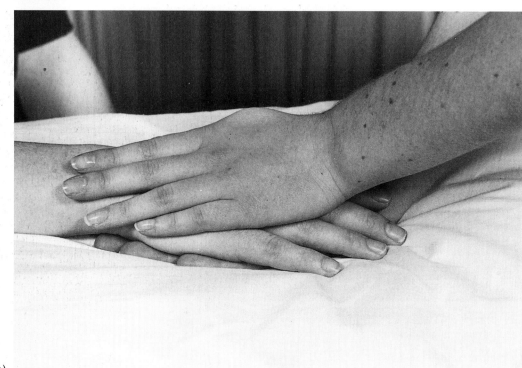

(A)

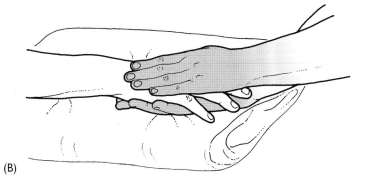

(B)

FIGURE 8.9   *(A,B) Effleurage of the fingers.*

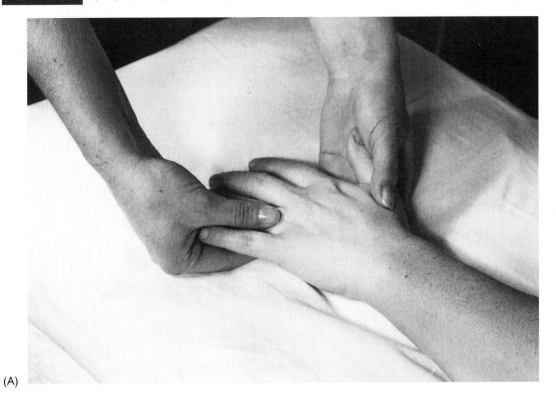

(A)

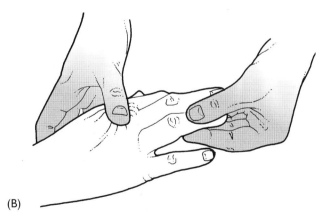

(B)

FIGURE 8.10   *(A,B) Thumb kneading the hypothenar eminence; the left hand of the therapist is supporting the patient's hand.*

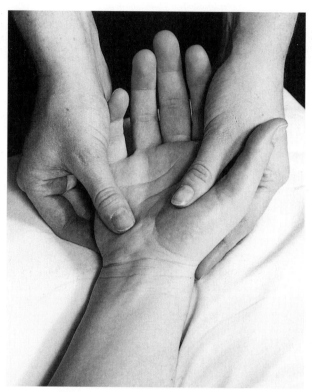

(A)

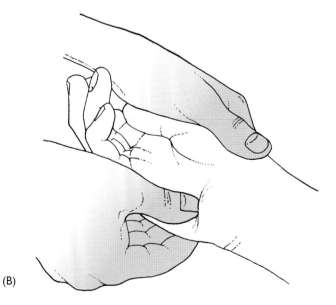

(B)

FIGURE 8.11   *(A,B) Position for finger kneading between the tendons of the wrist and along the tendon sheaths.*

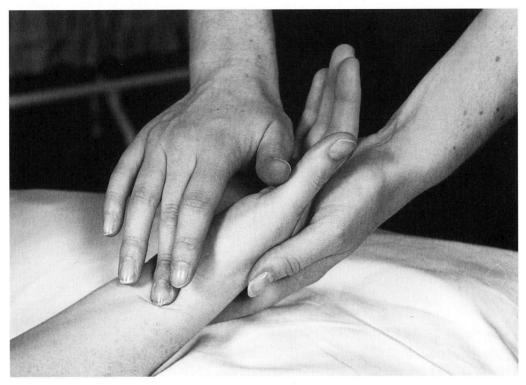

(A)

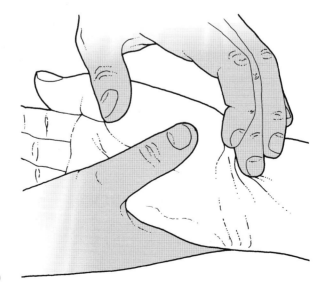

(B)

Wringing: skin on the dorsum of the hand (Figs 8.12), the muscles of the thenar eminence (Fig. 8.13) and hypothenar eminence.

Picking up: the dorsum of the hand, the thenar and hypothenar eminences.

FIGURE 8.12   *Wringing the skin on the dorsum of the hand.*

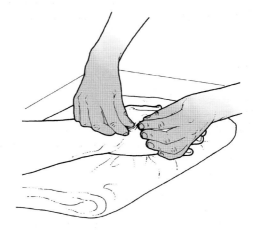

FIGURE 8.13   *Wringing the muscles of the thenar eminence.*

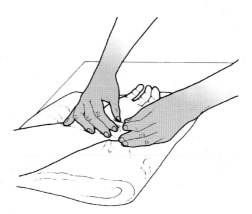

LOWER LIMB: THE LEG AND FOOT

Positioning of the Patient

Lying supine, with leg elevated.
Lying supine, with leg supported on pillows.
Sitting on the treatment couch, with leg supported on pillows.

Special Anatomical Points

Lymph glands: in the popliteal fossa behind the knee and in the groin.

Knee, patella and iliotibial band require special attention.

Anatomical spaces behind the malleoli and either side of the Achilles tendon can contain swelling.

The posterior aspect of the limb can be massaged with the patient lying prone.

Major muscle groups: quadriceps, hamstrings, adductors, anterior tibials, triceps surae, interossei and the layers of the foot.

Manipulations

The whole of the leg:

Stroking.

Effleurage: the whole leg; start at the toes and include the calf and anterior tibial area, around the patella (Figs 8.14A,B) and continue along the thigh to the groin (Figs 8.15A,B).

The thigh:

Kneading: medial and lateral aspects together, anterior and posterior aspects together.

Picking up: anterior aspect, adductors, posterior aspect (with leg laterally rotated).

Wringing: anterior aspect (Figs 8.16A,B), adductors, posterior aspect (with leg laterally rotated).

The knee:

Finger/thumb kneading around the patella, along the joint line, over the collateral ligaments.

The leg:

Kneading: single-handed and thumb kneading to the anterior tibials, reciprocal two-handed kneading to the calf (see also Figs 8.17A,B).

Picking up: the calf (Figs 8.18A,B).

The foot:

Kneading: whole-handed, finger/thumb kneading to the medial and lateral borders of the foot, the interosseous spaces (Figs 8.19A,B), around the malleoli, to the sides of the Achilles tendon.

In addition, if required, the following can be applied: *clapping, hacking, muscle shaking* to the thigh and calf (see Figs 7.8A,B), *vibrations* to the thigh and calf.

FIGURE 8.14 *(A,B) Effleurage around the patella. The manipulation continues into the popliteal fossa.*

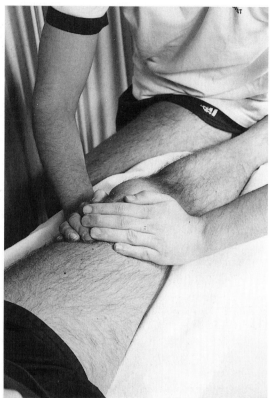

(A)

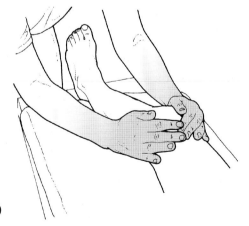

(B)

FIGURE 8.15   *(A,B) Finish of the effleurage stroke along the leg, over-pressure being applied to the lymph glands in the groin.*

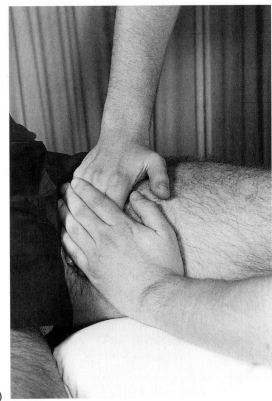

(A)

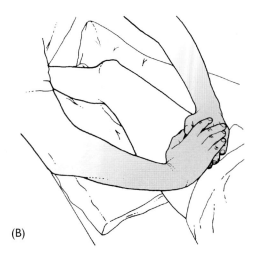

(B)

FIGURE 8.16   *(A,B) Muscle wringing the thigh.*

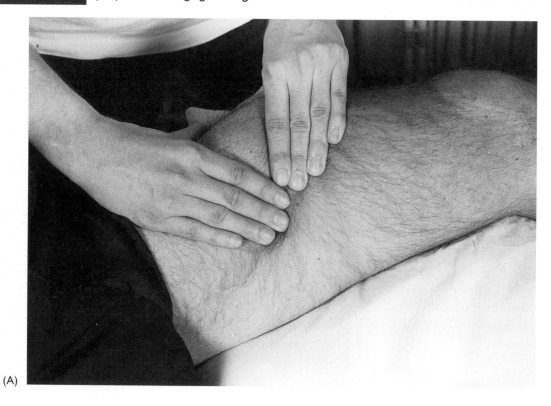

(A)

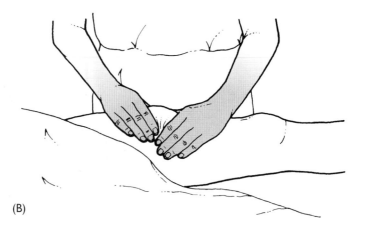

(B)

FIGURE 8.17   *(A,B) Skin rolling the medial aspect of the knee.*

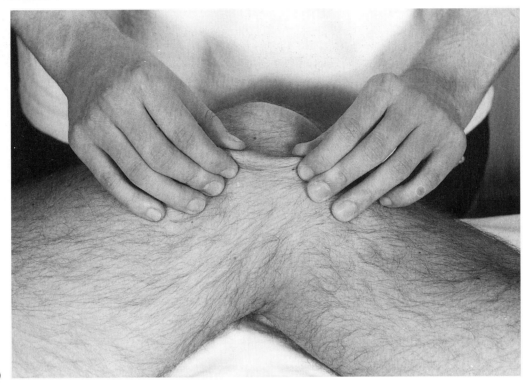

(A)

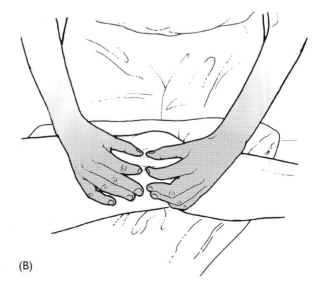

(B)

FIGURE 8.18   *(A,B) Reciprocal picking up of the calf muscles. Note the positioning of the patient's leg.*

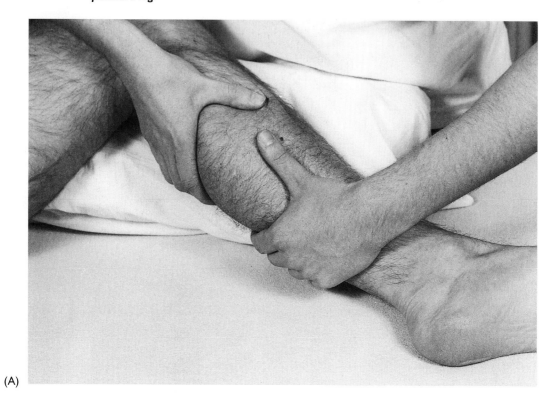

(A)

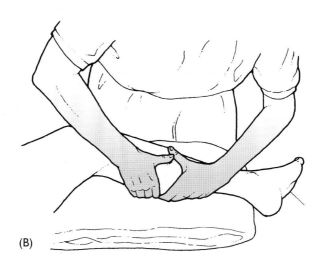

(B)

FIGURE 8.19   *(A,B) Thumb kneading the interosseous spaces of the foot; the therapist's hand supports the foot.*

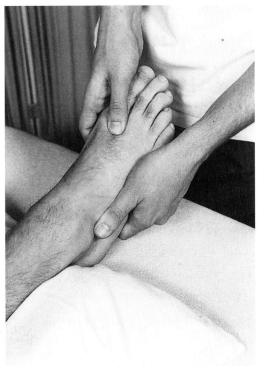

(A)

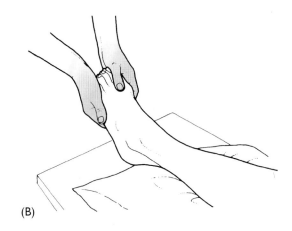

(B)

THE BACK

Positioning of the Patient

Patient supine, pillows underneath abdomen and ankles

Special Anatomical Points

Lymph glands: the lower back drains into the groin, the thorax drains into the axilla, and the neck and shoulder girdle drain into the anterior triangle of the neck.

The bony points which are tender are the spinous processes, the scapulae and the ribs.

There is considerable natural variance of skin mobility in different parts of the back.

The patient's arms should remain by her/his side; if they are above or under the head, the skin over the trunk becomes taut and therefore difficult to massage.

Major muscle groups: trapezius, rhomboids, supraspinatus, infraspinatus, erector spinae, latissimus dorsi, quadratus lumborum, the glutei.

Manipulations

Stroking: start at the shoulder girdle and work downwards.

Effleurage: start at the sacrum and work in sections towards the lymph glands (see Figs 7.4A,B).

Kneading: whole handed (see Figs 7.5A–E).

Finger/thumb kneading: along bony attachments – iliac crest (Figs 8.20A,B), vertebral border and spine of scapula. Attention should be focused on problem areas – insertion of levator scapulae at the superior angle of scapula (Figs 8.21A,B).

Reinforced kneading: glutei (Figs 8.22A,B), quadratus lumborum.

Skin rolling: thorax and lower back (see Figs 7.10A–F).

Picking up: latissimus dorsi (see Figs 7.7A,B).

Wringing: trapezius (Figs 8.23A,B), lower back, glutei (Figs 8.24A,B).

Tapotement: as required.

THE NECK

Positioning of the Patient

Prone, head and body supported, as described in Chapter 7.

Seated at table and supported anteriorly, as described in Chapter 7.

In a seated massage chair.

Supine on the treatment couch, head supported by pillows on the therapist's lap (for acute neck pain).

Side-lying, upper arm supported by pillows (acute neck and arm pain).

FIGURE 8.20   *(A,B) Finger kneading along the iliac crest.*

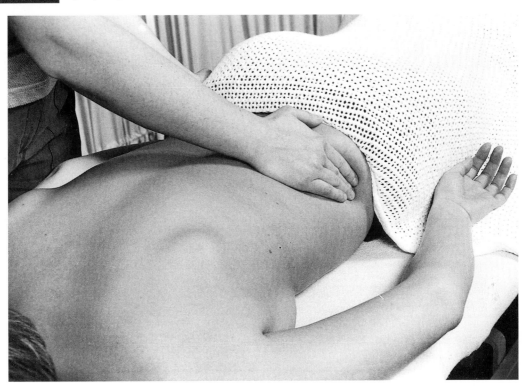

(A)

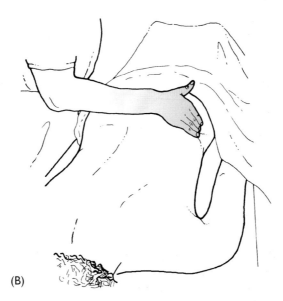

(B)

FIGURE 8.21   *(A,B) Thumb kneading the insertion of levator scapulae at the superior angle of scapula.*

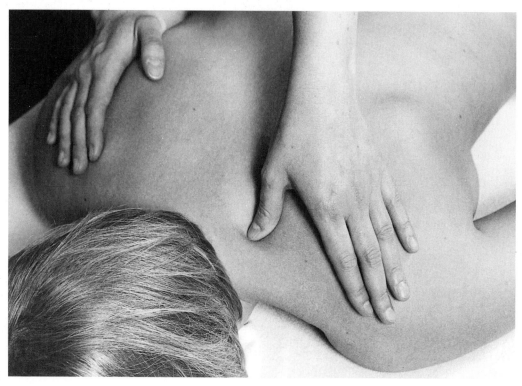

(A)

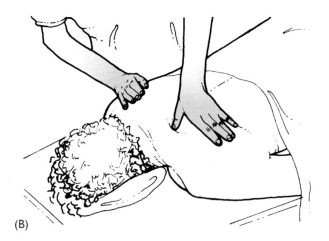

(B)

FIGURE 8.22   *(A,B) Reinforced kneading of the glutei.*

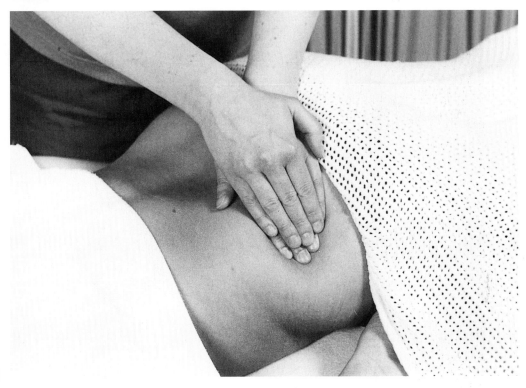

(A)

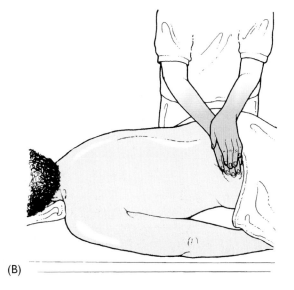

(B)

FIGURE 8.23 (A,B) Wringing the trapezius.

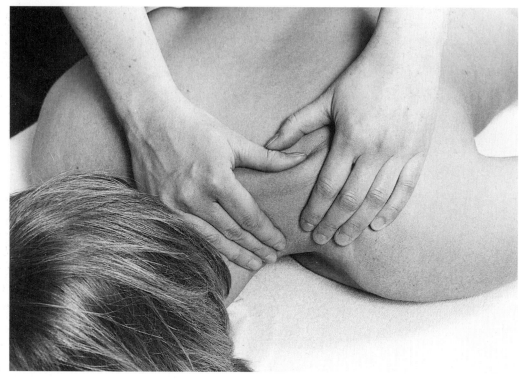

(A)

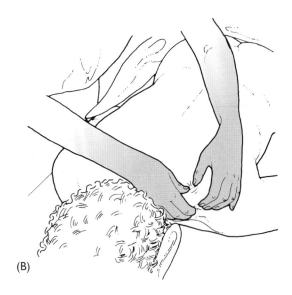

(B)

FIGURE 8.24   *(A,B) Wringing the glutei.*

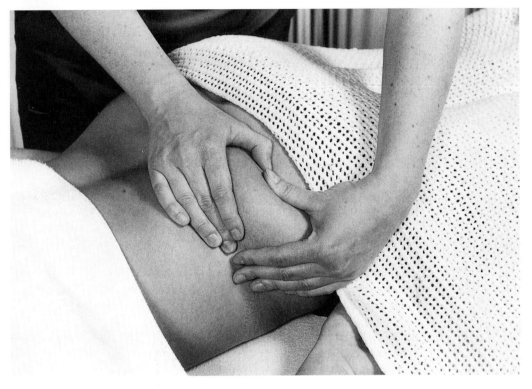

(A)

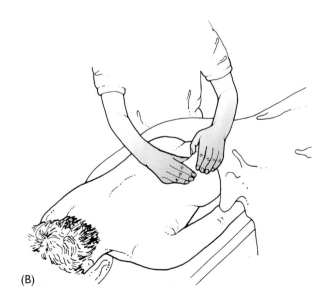

(B)

Special Anatomical Points

Lymph glands: in the anterior triangle of the neck.

The cervical spine should be maintained in a neutral position during the massage.

Deep massage should be avoided at the anterior aspect of the neck.

Avoid the vicinity of the thyroid gland (see Ch. 4).

Major muscle groups: paravertebral muscles, scalenes, sternocleidomastoid, trapezius.

Manipulations

Stroking.

Effleurage: from the occiput to the lymph glands, across trapezius to the lymph glands, along the scalenes to the lymph glands (Figs 8.25A,B and 8.26A,B).

Kneading: whole handed to the paravertebral muscles (Figs 8.27A,B) and trapezius.

Finger kneading: paravertebral muscles (Figs 8.28A,B), insertion of trapezius along the nuchal line of the occiput, scalenes (Figs 8.29A,B), sternocleidomastoid and problem areas – insertion of levator scapulae, nodules, trigger points.

Picking up: upper fibres of trapezius.

Wringing: upper fibres of trapezius, paravertebral muscles and sternocleidomastoid (Figs 8.30A,B).

Skin rolling: upper fibres of trapezius.

THE ABDOMEN

Positioning of the Patient

Supine, pillows under the knees to facilitate relaxation of the abdominal muscles.

Patient sitting on the treatment couch, its head section inclined at a 45-degree angle to support the patient's back.

Special Anatomical Points

Direction of strokes directed by the underlying visceral anatomy (note the ascending colon lies from the right iliac fossa to the ribs, the transverse colon runs transversely under the costal margin, arching below the ribs, and the descending colon runs down to the left iliac fossa; Fig. 8.31).

Depth of massage is dictated by the depth of the superficial tissue.

The colon should be palpable during the massage.

The organs may be displaced if trunk deformity is present.

FIGURE 8.25   *(A,B) Effleurage of the neck. Note the therapist's overlapped hands.*

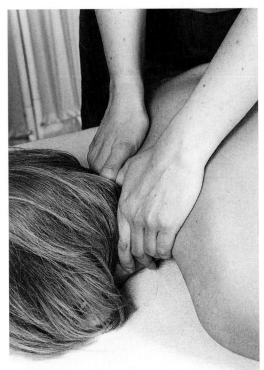

(A)

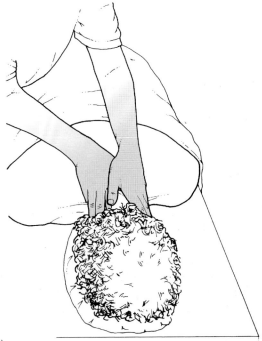

(B)

FIGURE 8.26 *(A,B) Finish of the effleurage stroke along the neck in the anterior triangle of the neck, above the clavicle.*

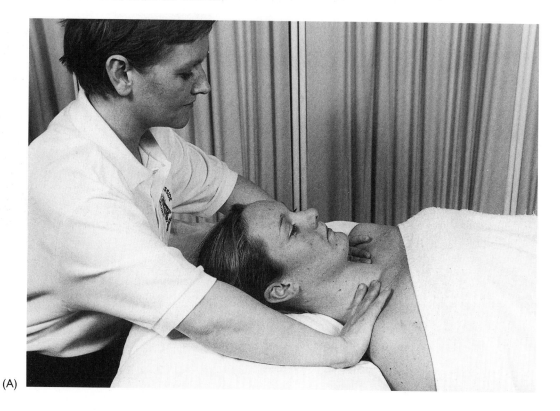

(A)

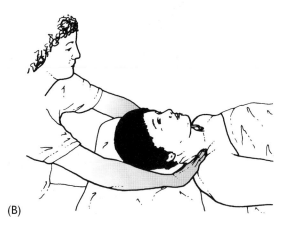

(B)

FIGURE 8.27   *(A,B) Whole-handed kneading of the paravertebral muscles of the neck. For acute neck pain the patient's head is supported on a pillow on the therapist's lap.*

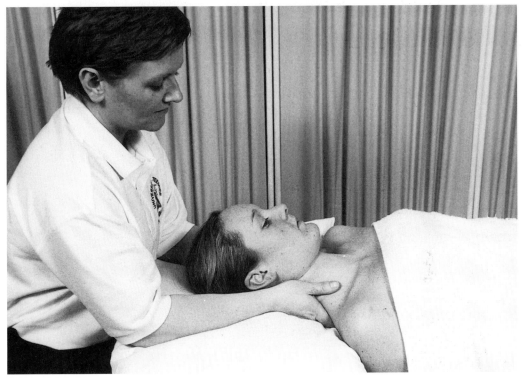

(A)

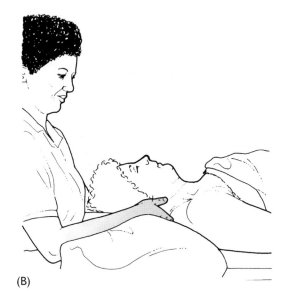

(B)

FIGURE 8.28　*(A,B) Finger kneading the paravertebral muscles.*

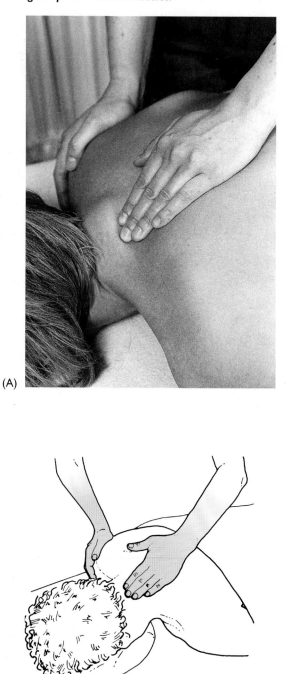

(A)

(B)

FIGURE 8.29   *(A,B) Finger kneading the scalene muscles using the pads of the fingers.*

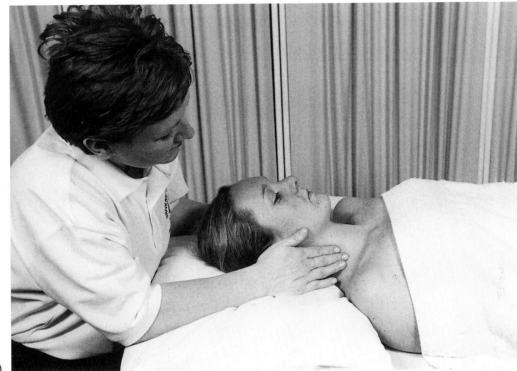

(A)

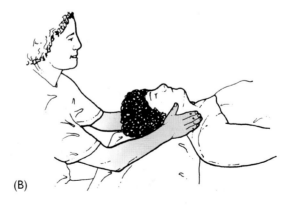

(B)

FIGURE 8.30   *(A,B) Wringing the sternocleidomastoid.*

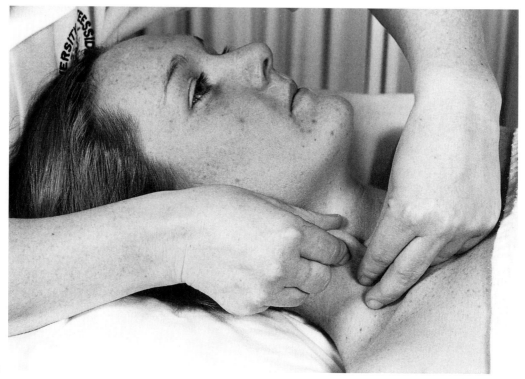

(A)

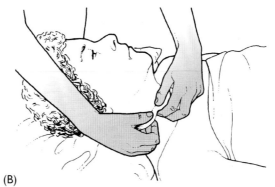

(B)

| FIGURE 8.31 | *Surface position of the intestines.* |

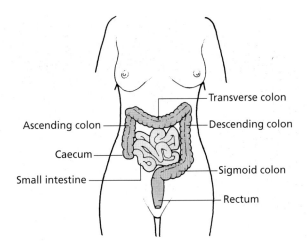

Manipulations

Stroking: across the abdomen (Figs 8.32A,B) until relaxation of the muscles occurs.

Small Intestine

Kneading: finger kneading and flat-handed kneading across the abdomen (Figs 8.33A,B).

Colon

Deep stroking along the line of the ascending, transverse and descending colon (Figs 8.34A,B).

Kneading: finger kneading (Figs 8.35A,B) and flat-handed kneading along the ascending transverse and descending colon or moving the colon sideways with fingertips, or on the abdominal wall at the start of massage, to dispel wind.

Vibrations: along the colon (Figs 8.36A,B).

FIGURE 8.32 *(A,B) Stroking across the abdomen.*

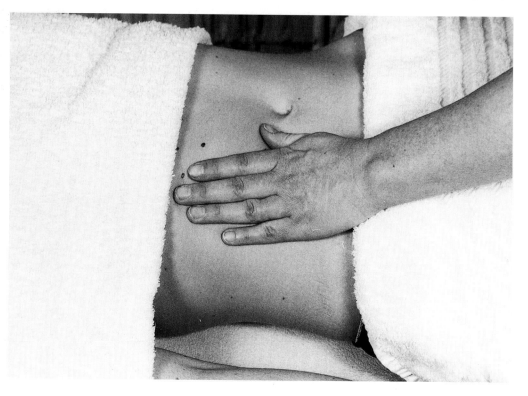

(A)

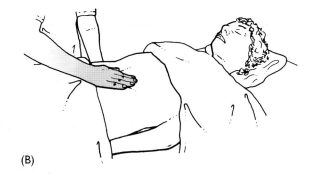

(B)

FIGURE 8.33   *(A,B) Kneading the small intestine with the heel of the hand.*

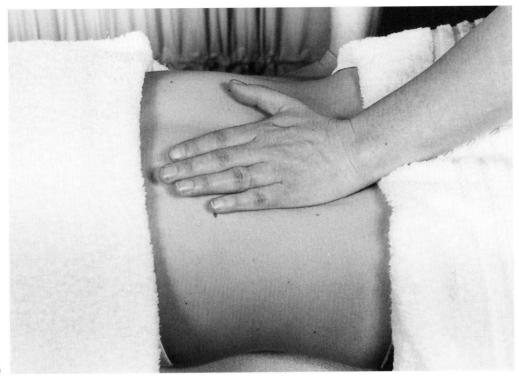

(A)

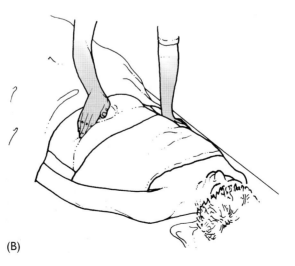

(B)

FIGURE 8.34   *(A,B) Deep stroking along the course of the colon.*

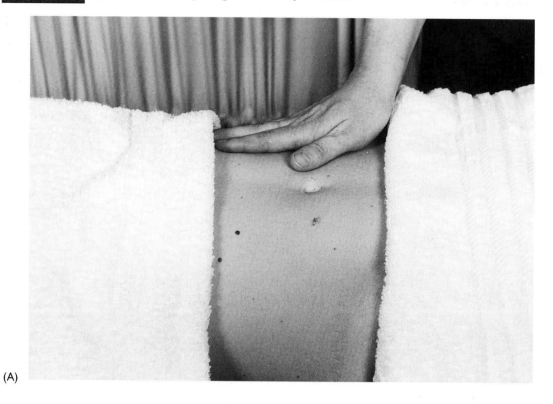

(A)

(B)

FIGURE 8.35   *(A,B) Reinforced finger kneading the colon.*

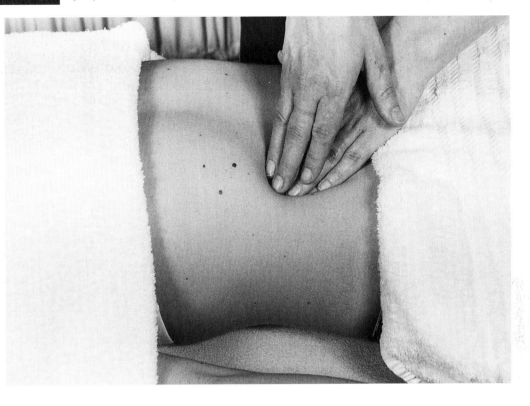

(A)

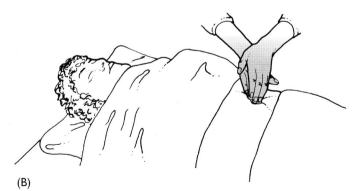

(B)

FIGURE 8.36   *(A,B) Vibrations along the course of the colon.*

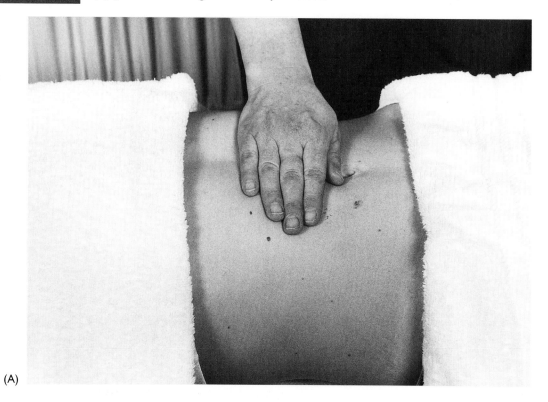

(A)

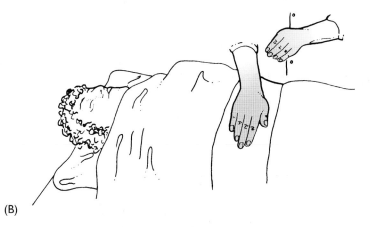

(B)

THE FACE

Positioning of the Patient

Supine on the treatment couch, head supported on a pillow.
Supine on the treatment couch, head supported on a pillow on the therapist's lap.

FIGURE 8.37   *Lymphatic drainage of the head and neck.*

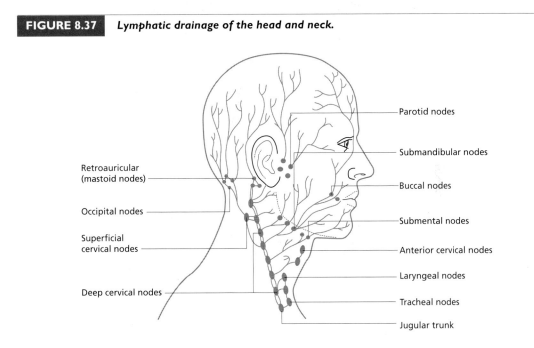

Parotid nodes

Submandibular nodes

Retroauricular (mastoid nodes)

Buccal nodes

Occipital nodes

Submental nodes

Superficial cervical nodes

Anterior cervical nodes

Laryngeal nodes

Deep cervical nodes

Tracheal nodes

Jugular trunk

FIGURE 8.38   *The muscles of facial expression.*

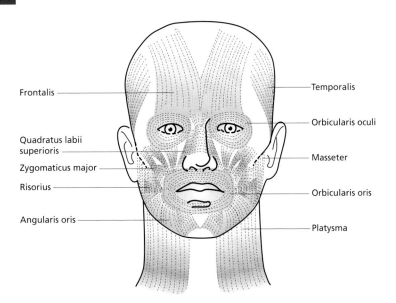

Frontalis

Temporalis

Orbicularis oculi

Quadratus labii superioris

Zygomaticus major

Masseter

Risorius

Orbicularis oris

Angularis oris

Platysma

FIGURE 8.39 *(A,B) Start of the effleurage stroke across the forehead.*

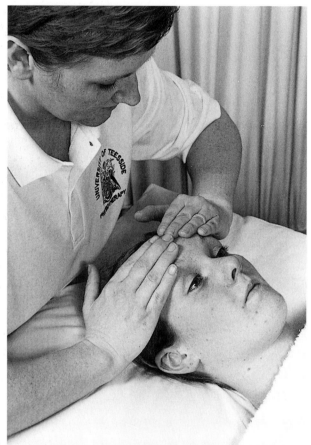

(A)

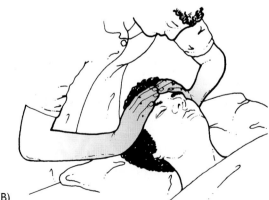

(B)

FIGURE 8.40   *(A,B) Finish of the effleurage stroke over the parotid lymph nodes.*

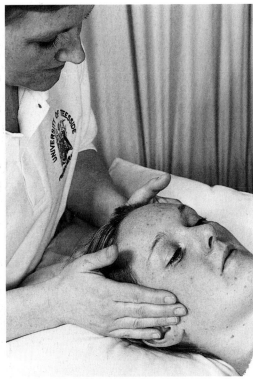

(A)

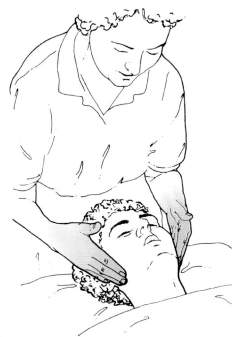

(B)

FIGURE 8.41   *(A,B) Plucking the tissues of the face.*

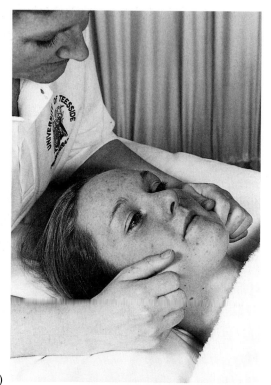

(A)

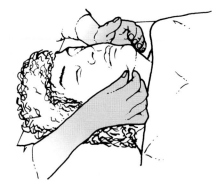

(B)

FIGURE 8.42   (A,B) Wringing the cheeks.

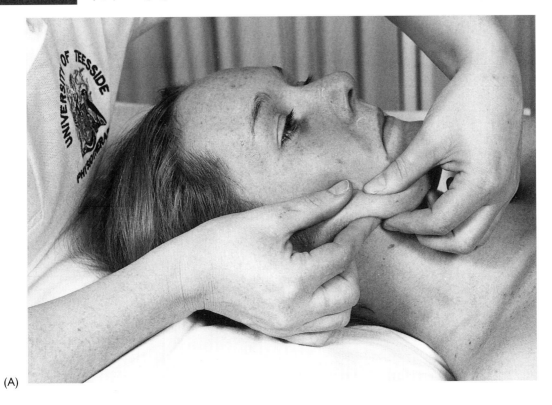

(A)

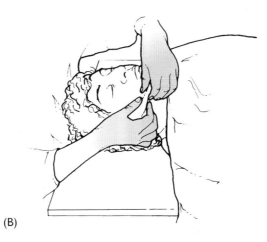

(B)

Sitting on a low-backed chair, head supported on a pillow against the therapist's chest.

Special Anatomical Points

Lymph glands: submandibular nodes drain the forehead and the anterior part of the face; parotid nodes (just below the ear) drain the lateral part of the face and eyelids; submental nodes (just below the chin) drain the chin. All these nodes drain into the deep cervical glands (Fig. 8.37).

The muscles of the face are supplied by the facial (7th cranial) nerve.

In facial (Bell's) palsy, massage should maintain the mobility of the facial muscles.

Major muscles: procerus, orbicularis oculi and oris, levator labii superioris, levator and depressor anguli oris, zygomaticus major, buccinator, occipitofrontalis, corrugator, depressor labii inferioris, mentalis, platysma, masseter, temporalis and the pterygoids (Fig. 8.38).

Manipulations

Effleurage: across the cheeks to the parotid glands, across the forehead (Figs 8.39A,B) down the sides of the cheeks to the submandibular nodes (Figs 8.40A,B).

Finger kneading: across the forehead, cheeks, upper lip and chin, following the facial muscles. Avoid over-stretching the muscles or the skin.

Plucking: pluck the tissues gently in the same areas as finger kneading (Figs 8.41A,B).

Wringing: gentle wringing in a continuous line over the forehead, cheeks (Figs 8.42A,B) and chin.

Tapping: over the muscles for stimulation, or the sinuses to aid drainage.

Vibrations: using the middle finger only, vibrate over the foramina where the ophthalmic (supraorbital foramen), maxillary (infraorbital foramen) and mandibular (mental foramen) nerves emerge and over the sinuses.

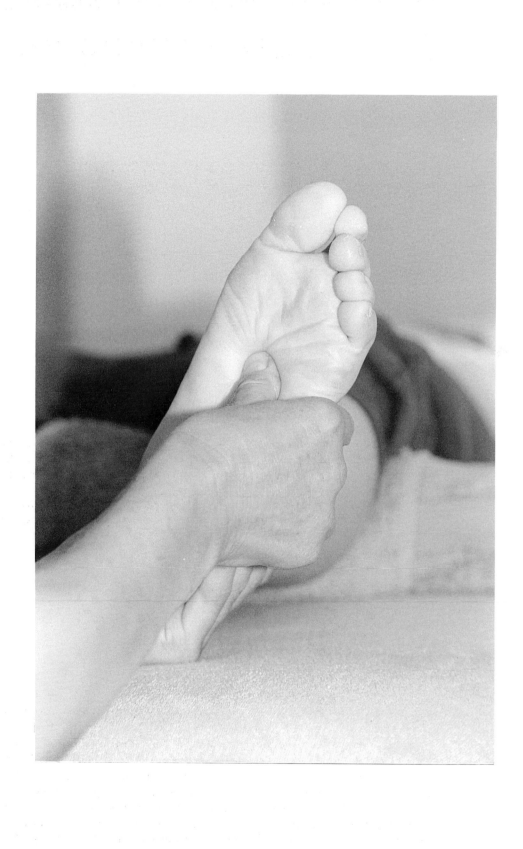

9 Specialized Techniques

This chapter introduces a variety of specialized techniques which are either employed for particular clinical situations or rather complex to use. While the techniques in themselves may not be difficult to learn, their safe application requires sophisticated clinical reasoning and the detailed conceptual framework for this is outside the scope of this book. It is important to emphasize that they are simply introduced here (some very briefly) and must be learned from an experienced practitioner.

TECHNIQUE: CONNECTIVE TISSUE MANIPULATION/BINDEGEWEBSMASSAGE

Features

Connective tissue manipulation (CTM) is a soft tissue manipulative therapy which is, conceptually, a reflex therapy. It influences cutaneovisceral autonomic reflexes (see Ch. 3) to induce balance between the sympathetic and parasympathetic nervous systems. It utilizes connective tissue (CT) zones derived from the skin zones of Head and the muscle zones of McKenzie. These are found principally on the back where they can be seen and palpated. The zones are both visible and palpable. Acute zones are seen as 'puffy' raised areas which feel soft to the touch, with underlying tension felt when superficial layers are moved on deeper layers. Chronic zones are recognized as drawn-in areas in which the tissues are palpated as tight and adherent (Haase 1962). They are often hypersensitive. The zones (see Fig. 3.7) are assessed to detect the level of autonomic balance and specific functional problems. For example, a positive liver zone may indicate recent drug therapy, heavy social drinking, or disease. The number of visible and palpable zones indicates the generality of autonomic imbalance. The zones can indicate the degree to which imbalance has occurred or can inform progression of treatment, location of strokes to be applied, or indicate cautions. A specific stretch manipulation is applied to the fascial layer and is thought to stimulate segmental and suprasegmental cutaneovisceral reflexes. All structures sharing the same spinal segmental innervation are stimulated via the autonomic nervous system (ANS), resulting in effects that include vasodilatation and alterations in smooth muscle tone. The suprasegmental effects are mediated in the medulla and wider physiological effects are achieved, such as improved balance between the two components of the ANS, endocrine and hormonal balancing and raised beta-endorphin levels. It produces a feeling of well-being and increased flexibility.

CTM must be applied skilfully at the correct tissue interface and must begin at the sacrum to avoid adverse autonomic reactions. The progression of the strokes depends on the aims of treatment and on clinical reasoning. The technique and its clinical application must be learned from an experienced practitioner.

Patients who may benefit from this treatment are those with:

- local mechanical musculoskeletal problems, for example scarring or shin splints
- hormonal problems, for example women experiencing menopausal or menstrual symptoms
- visceral problems, for example bowel disorders
- autonomic problems, for example complex regional pain syndrome, intractable nerve root pain.

Application of the different techniques depends on individual patient needs. Generally, the therapist is aiming to use the fascial technique. If this is used inappropriately, adverse reactions such as fainting can occur. The 'basic section' must be treated first to induce a parasympathetic response, to prepare the body for stimulation of sympathetic dermatomes. Superficial layers must be prepared first. The preparatory strokes are usually used initially and these are often clinically effective in their own right. Treatment is progressed by working superficial to deep and caudad to cephalad. Care must be taken not to overtreat, due to the possibility of producing adverse reactions. Treatment should always be comfortable, and never painful.

Categories – Preparatory Strokes: Fascial Technique; Skin Technique; Subcutaneous Technique; Flat Technique

MANIPULATION: FASCIAL (*FAZIEN*) TECHNIQUE

Purpose

To reduce fascial tension.
To reduce trophoedematous changes in zonal areas.
To improve visceral function.

To promote fluid level balance.

To achieve balance between the sympathetic and parasympathetic nervous systems.

To reduce sympathetically maintained pain.

To increase circulation.

To produce a feeling of well-being.

To increase local and general flexibility.

To enhance hormonal and endocrine function.

To increase circulation.

Procedure

This is CTM 'proper', which produces the strong autonomic reflex reactions.

The pad of the therapist's third finger makes contact with the skin (Fig. 9.1A).

The finger is reinforced by the ring finger.

The distal interphalangeal joint is flexed, to gather up the slack superficially in the tissues.

The therapist should then push into the end-feel using the hand and arm to exert a traction effect at the fascial layer.

Each stroke must be performed in the palmar or radial direction of the operating hand.

The stroke must be accurately aimed at the correct tissue interface.

The tissues must be adequately prepared by preparatory techniques to produce the desired effect.

Each stroke must produce a cutting sensation and a triple response, or adverse reactions will occur.

All strokes must be within the patient's tolerance of discomfort.

The strokes *must* begin at the sacrum.

Progression of the strokes depends on the individual patient's response and on the aims of treatment: they can be dictated by the zones, segmental relationships and understanding of the underlying pathological processes.

MANIPULATION: SKIN (*HAUT*) TECHNIQUE

Purpose

This is to be used during the fascial technique when most of the strokes produce the normal 'cutting' reaction, to ensure uniformity of reaction.

Skin technique is applied to a localized area where it becomes difficult to obtain a clear 'cutting' response.

Procedure

The therapist places all four finger*tips* on the skin where treatment is required (Figs 9.1C,D).

The fingertips are lightly and rapidly brushed over the surface of the skin.

The fascial technique is then retried, and should now produce the cutting sensation.

FIGURE 9.1 *Connective tissue manipulation: (A,B) fascial* (fazien) *technique; (C,D) skin* (haut) *technique; (E,F) shallow* (flashige) *technique; (G,H) subcutaneous* (unterhaut) *technique.*

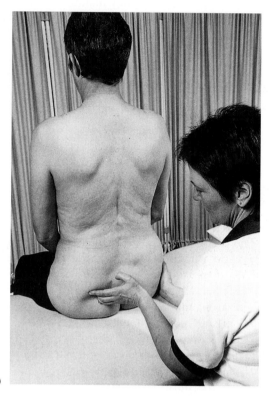

(A)

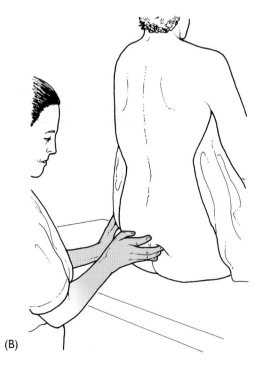

(B)

(Figure cont'd)

(Figure 9.1 cont'd)

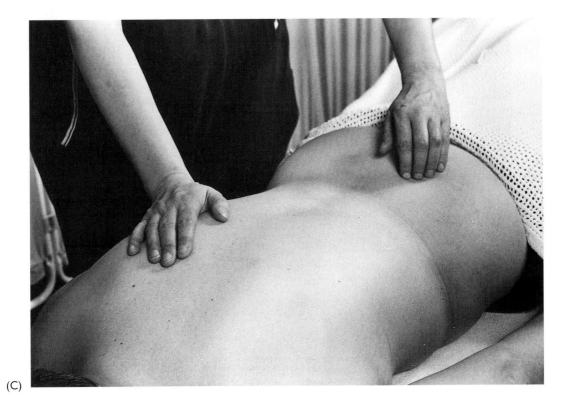

(C)

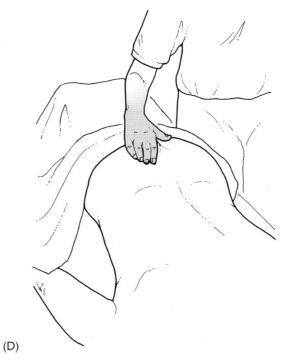

(D)

(Figure cont'd)

(Figure 9.1 cont'd)

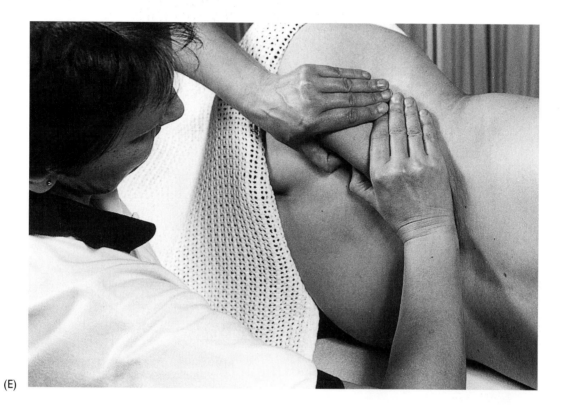

(E)

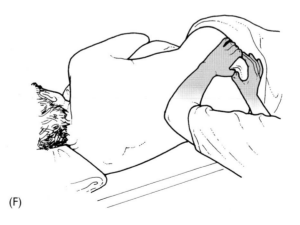

(F)

(Figure cont'd)

(*Figure 9.1 cont'd*)

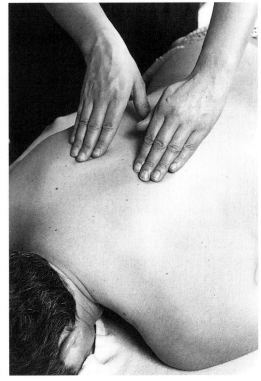

(G)

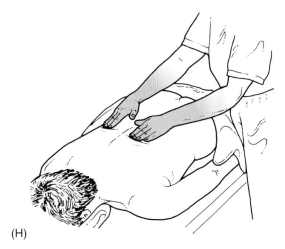

(H)

MANIPULATION: FLAT (*FLASHIGE*) TECHNIQUE

Purpose

To be used where there is subcutaneous swelling and the fascial technique is unable to produce the 'cutting' sensation.

Procedure

The patient should be side-lying.

The therapist sits behind the patient.

The therapist's thumbs are flexed, the nails placed together and the tips hooked under the subcutaneous tissues at their insertion into the sacral border (Figs 9.1E,F).

The therapist's fingers are spread over the skin, which they pull gently towards the thumbs.

The thumbs are pushed away, towards the fingers, applying a stretch to the fascia, *to* the end-feel of the movement.

Do not stretch *into* the end-feel by exerting an over-pressure, to produce a 'cutting' reaction.

Proceed the strokes in the following order: along the sacral border, along erector spinae (both edges), along the vertebral border of the scapula, and along the greater trochanter.

MANIPULATION: SUBCUTANEOUS (*UNTERHAUT*) TECHNIQUE

Purpose

This is to be used when the tissues are extremely tender and unable to tolerate other techniques.

Procedure

The patient lies prone.

The therapist stands to one side of the patient's trunk.

The therapist places the pads of the fingers of both hands lightly on the skin (Figs 9.1G,H).

The finger pads sink into the subcutaneous layer.

Small pushing movements are made in a cephalad direction.

The skin is moved with the fingers and the stimulus must remain in this layer.

The strokes can be progressed over the area requiring treatment or over an area implicated in a desired reflex effect.

TECHNIQUE: MYOFASCIAL RELEASE

Features

A stretching technique that recognizes and utilizes the craniosacral rhythm.

The craniosacral rhythm, believed to be a pulsing of the cerebrospinal fluid, is particularly involved with release of the cranial base, the dural tube and the pelvic and respiratory diaphragms.

Tightening of the myofascia is identified by palpation.

Passive stretching along the direction of the muscle fibres is followed by a hold, until release is felt and the process is repeated until there is no further release.

Somato-emotional release can occur, so it is important that the therapist is qualified to work with and support this release, or functions within a multidisciplinary team.

Procedure

A longitudinal stretch is applied along the direction of the muscle fibres by:

1. Applying the therapist's fingertips on the skin and moving the fingers and underlying skin apart.
2. Placing crossed hands on the skin, exerting pressure through the ulnar border of the hands and separating the hands to stretch the underlying skin (Figs 9.2A,B).
3. Firmly grasping the limb and pulling along its long axis, the muscle to be stretched dictating the position of the joints (e.g. internal rotation with adduction).
4. Increasing the localization of a longitudinal stretch by placing one hand on the proximal border of the muscle under stretch (Figs 9.2C,D).

TECHNIQUE: MANUAL LYMPHATIC DRAINAGE

This is the treatment of choice for lymphoedema. (See Ch. 11 for discussion.)

Features

Characterized by extremely light, superficial strokes.

The strokes are directed towards lymph glands along lymphatic channels.

Proximal areas must be cleared before distal areas.

Treatment may need to work across lymphatic watersheds from one area to another.

The trunk often needs clearing before the affected limb.

Progress should be made towards healthy lymph glands.

'The softer the tissue, the lighter the pressure' (Wittlinger & Wittlinger 1982).

All techniques should be done as stationary ones or continuous spirals; there is no glide over the skin.

FIGURE 9.2 *(A,B) Myofascial cross-handed release technique; (C,D) longitudinal myofascial release.*

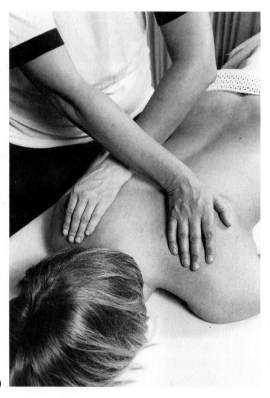

(A)

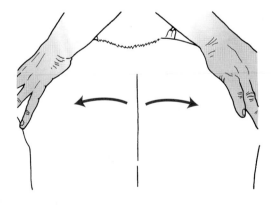

(B)

(Figure cont'd)

(*Figure 9.2 cont'd*)

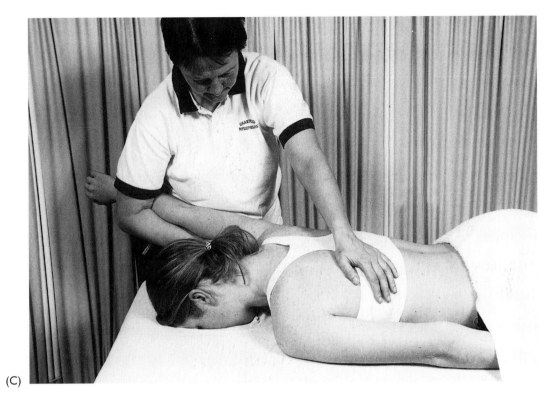

(C)

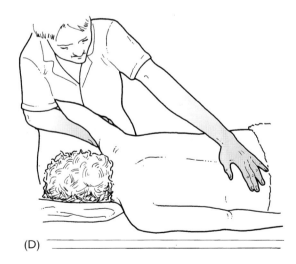

(D)

Purpose

To stimulate lymphatic drainage.
To increase lymphatic flow.
To stimulate the lymph glands.
To reduce lymphoedema.

MANIPULATION: PUMP TECHNIQUE

Procedure

The therapist's hand should be placed flat on the skin, palm down.
The wrist is lifted to pull the hand slightly backwards.
The wrist is then lowered to move the hands forwards, applying a slight forwards pressure (Figs 9.3A,B).
Hand movements should be controlled so that they follow a slight oval circular pathway.
The skin must move with the hand, which does not glide over the skin.

MANIPULATION: STATIONARY CIRCLES

Procedure

The therapist's fingers should be placed flat on the patient's skin.
The hands should be placed side by side or one on top of the other for reinforcement.
The hands should exert a light pressure in a circling motion (Figs 9.3C,D).
The skin should move with the hands, which do not glide at all on the skin.
The pressure should go on into the circle and come off out of the circle.
The circles should be applied in the direction of lymph drainage.
Stationary circles should be applied over the lymph nodes and face.

MANIPULATION: SCOOP TECHNIQUE

Procedure

The dorsum of the therapist's hand should lie on the patient's skin.
The arm should be rotated so that the carpometacarpal joint of the index finger bears the weight of the hand.
The wrist is then rotated from side to side by slight pronation and supination of the forearm.
The therapist's body position should be appropriate to minimize end-of-range wrist movements.
The skin should move with the therapist's hand.

MANIPULATION: ROTARY TECHNIQUE

Procedure

The therapist's hand should lie palm down on the patient's skin.

The fingers and thumb are separated to increase the web space between the thumb and index finger.

The wrist is raised.

As the wrist is lowered, pressure is applied downwards through the heel of the hand.

Pressure is then transferred from the base of the thumb across the heel of the hand to the little finger.

The skin is moved with each rotatory movement.

Each new stroke should begin slightly further along to overlap with the previous one.

TECHNIQUE: SEGMENT MASSAGE

Features

Effective as a reflex technique.

Works by stimulating the ANS via the skin by a mechanism similar to that of CTM.

It is particularly effective at the maximal tenderness points of CT zones.

It has a more gentle, gradual effect than CTM, working predominantly in the subcutaneous layer but also the fascial layer and the periosteum.

It produces a strong parasympathetic effect and is less likely to produce an adverse reaction.

A wide variety of techniques are included, some of which relate to spinal segments and others to the dermatomes in the limbs.

Assessment of the patient involves stroking segmentally with the thumb tips; a 'paradoxical reaction' is produced which leaves white lines rather than the triple response of CTM.

If the skin does not move or react appropriately, vibrations are performed.

Purpose

To produce a parasympathetic reaction, promoting a feeling of relaxation and well-being.

To influence other functions or structures within the same spinal segment and to stimulate cutaneovisceral reflexes.

To reduce pain.

To increase circulation.

FIGURE 9.3   *Manual lymphatic drainage: (A,B) pump technique in the axilla; (C,D) stationary circles.*

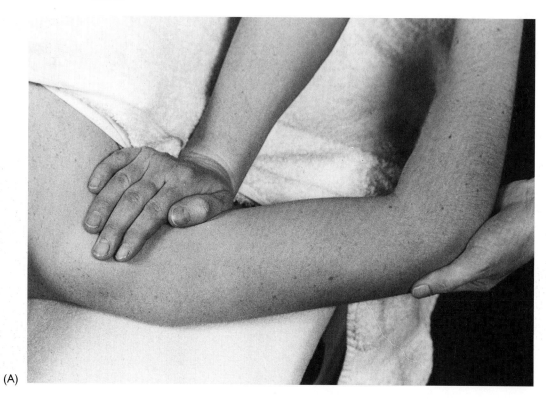

(A)

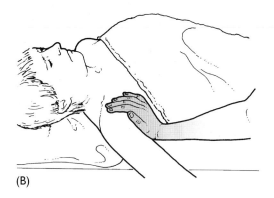

(B)

(Figure cont'd)

(Figure 9.3 cont'd)

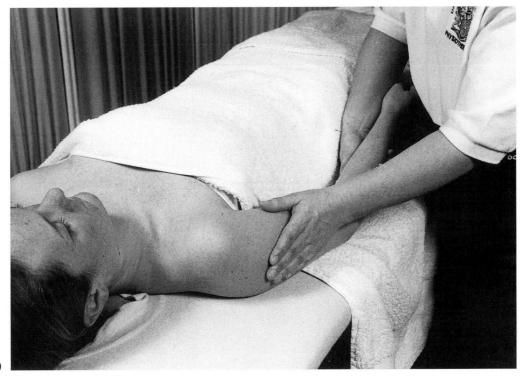

(C)

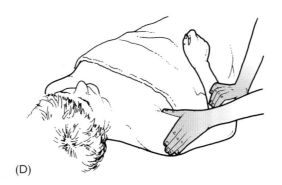

(D)

FIGURE 9.4   *Segmentmassage: (A,B) thumb circling; (C,D) of the forehead; (E,F) of the undersurface of scapula.*

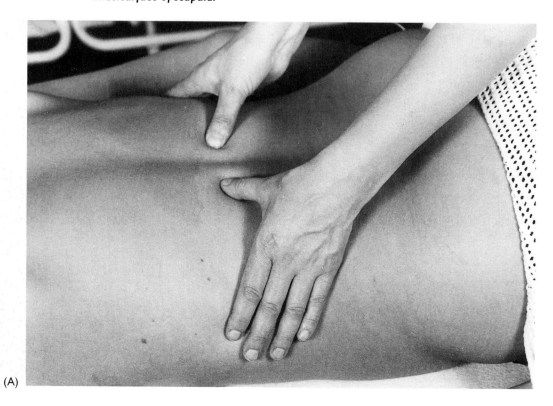

(A)

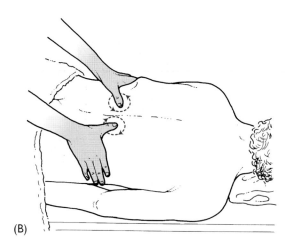

(B)

(Figure cont'd)

(Figure 9.4 cont'd)

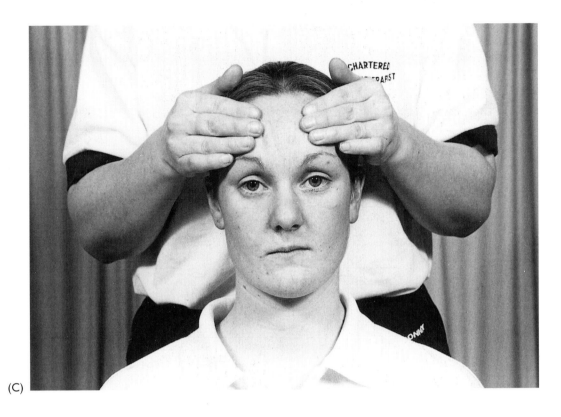

(C)

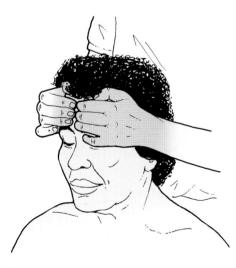

(D)

(Figure cont'd)

(*Figure 9.4 cont'd*)

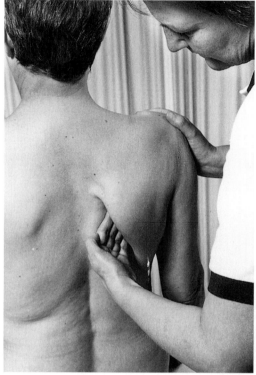

(E)

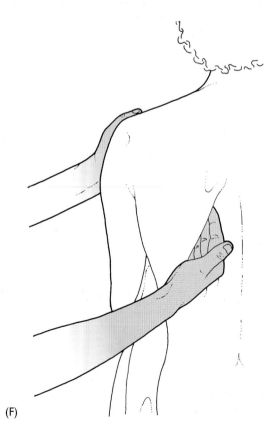

(F)

SEGMENTMASSAGE MANIPULATIONS

The names for these manipulations do not translate easily from the German and this will not be attempted here.

Procedure 1

The patient sits on a stool, pelvis tilted forwards to sit on the ischial tuberosities.

The therapist sits behind and places her hands around the patient's iliac crests.

The therapist's thumb tips are placed on the skin on the border of erector spinae and pushed into the muscle layer.

The thumbs are circled away from the spine (Figs 9.4A,B).

The hands gradually progress in a cranial direction, circling in each spinal segment.

Procedure 2

The patient sits on a chair and leans back on to the therapist, who is standing behind.

The patient's head is supported on the therapist.

The therapist places the tips of her fingers on the patient's forehead, with the fingernails of each hand back-to-back (Figs 9.4C,D).

Small light circles are followed with the fingertips.

The skin should move with the fingers; there should be no glide over the skin.

Procedure 3

The patient is sitting upright.

The therapist stands behind and grasps the point of the patient's shoulder.

The other hand slides underneath the scapula, with fingers on teres minor and the thumb under the scapula.

The length of the rhomboid attachment is thumb kneaded (on the periosteum) on the vertebral border of the scapula.

The technique is then modified so that the hand is turned round and small circular movements are applied to the undersurface of the scapula (Figs 9.4E,F).

TECHNIQUE: PERIOSTEAL MASSAGE

Features

Works very specifically on the periosteum.

Small stationary circles are circumscribed.

Utilizes a reflex effect.

Purpose

Reduces pain.

Stimulates the ANS through the maximal points of reflex zones.

Procedure

The therapist flexes all the joints of her index finger.

Contact is made between the ulnar border of the proximal interphalangeal joint of the index finger and the point to be treated.

Pressure is increased through this point until the periosteum is reached.

Tiny circular movements are performed with the hand, maintaining the pressure to ensure that the knuckle does not glide over the skin (2 minutes).

BIOENERGY THERAPIES

A growing number of therapists incorporate what has come to be known as 'bioenergy healing' into their preferred system of massage or touch therapy. This is probably due to an emerging collection of evidence about the biology of human energy. While, historically, more attention has been paid by the medical community to the chemical factors of human biological communication, it is now thought that electrical and electronic factors may be of equal importance (Oschman 2000a). Clearly, a therapeutic intervention in the nature of bioenergy healing is wholly different in character to the therapies traditionally used in orthodox medicine. It creates a new paradigm in relation to the boundaries of holism.

Very concisely, an accepted explanation of bioenergy healing is that a therapist's intentions can create specific patterns of electrical and magnetic activity in her own nervous system which may interact or influence the electrical and magnetic activity of the patient. The evidence for human energy fields is no longer in dispute. Seto and co-workers (1992) detected large biomagnetic fields emanating from human hands, confirming the earlier work of Zimmerman (1990). The fields are in the frequency range 0.3–30 Hz, the same frequency as brainwaves. It is well accepted that a 7 Hz frequency of pulsating magnetic fields can stimulate the growth of bone after fracture, an event which is initiated therapeutically by a medical device. It is thought that similar stimulation can occur with nerves (2 Hz), skin and fibroblasts (15 Hz) and ligaments (10 Hz) (Oschman 2000b).

Although the proposed mechanism for bioenergy healing is speculative, there are many types of healing intervention being practised where the focus is the therapist's intention to affect, for example in reiki, faith healing, spiritual healing, psi healing, bioenergy therapy and therapeutic touch. These therapies are becoming accepted in mainstream medicine, particularly in oncology and palliative care. Their use is justified because of the vast number of reported studies which have shown bioenergy therapies (or 'healing') to be effective, thus supplying an evidence base. Benor (1993, 1994) conducted a comprehensive literature review of 131 trials where the standards of research reached modern protocols. Of these trials, 59% reported a statistically significant outcome, considerably more than would have been expected to occur by chance.

ACUPRESSURE

Eastern therapies, in particular acupuncture, acupressure and shiatsu, use reflex effects to assist in diagnosis and treatment.

MERIDIANS

In Traditional Chinese Medicine there are 12 major channels (meridians) of the body in which *Chi* (energy or life force) circulates (Figs 9.5A,B). The meridians are paired and named after the organs with which they are connected: the Lung and Large Intestine; the Stomach and Spleen; the Heart and Small Intestine; the Urinary Bladder and Kidneys; the Pericardium and Triple Heater; the Gallbladder and Liver.

Of each pair, one channel is *yin* and the other is *yang*, reflecting the concept of balance between a negative and a positive state of energy. When yin and yang are in dynamic balance this is reflected by a healthy body and mind; if the yin and yang are out of balance this denotes a state of ill-health in the individual.

The channels link together the organs and interact with each other, and there are also regions where they run close to the surface of the body. These superficial regions often coincide with intermuscular or intertendinous depressions, which are easily palpated by a trained therapist. Acupoints are situated along the course of the channels; the points are believed to be three dimensional, that is, not only are they on the surface of the skin but also they extend to a varying depth into the underlying tissues. They also have a different electrical resistance to that of the surrounding tissue. The significance of the acupoints is that they offer a means of access to the channels, the energy of which can then be altered by the application of various treatment modalities, for example needling, finger pressure, electrical current, laser or moxibustion.

Although there is a lack of definitive evidence (in Western terms) for the existence or non-existence of the channels, there is a growing body of research which supports claims that stimulation of acupoints can cause neurohumoral and chemical changes. For example, it has been shown that stimulating acupoints produces significant analgesic effects when compared with non-acupoints (Chapman et al 1977); stimulating an acupoint near the wrist can reduce nausea and vomiting in postoperative patients (Dundee et al 1986).

Acupuncture is being used increasingly by Western orthodox medical practitioners to relieve pain. It is thought both to influence the pain-gate mechanism and to provoke the release of analgesic endogenous opiates.

It has been found that ohmic resistance is generally lower over acupoints in relation to surrounding areas of skin. The phenomenon is used by practitioners of Ryodoraku acupuncture therapy, based on the belief that the points of high conductance correspond with increased excitability of sympathetic nerves.

FIGURE 9.5

Major meridians of (A) the anterior and medial and (B) the posterior and lateral aspects of the body. In (A): short dashed line – lung; dash dotted line – pericardium; long dashed line – heart; solid line – spleen; dotted line – liver; dash treble dotted line – kidney. In (B) short dashed line – large intestine; dash dotted line – triple heater; long dashed line – small intestine; dash treble dotted line – stomach; dotted line – bladder; solid line – gallbladder.

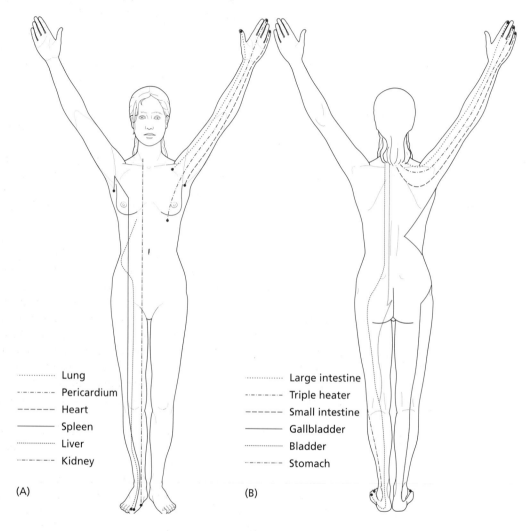

Lung
Pericardium
Heart
Spleen
Liver
Kidney

(A)

Large intestine
Triple heater
Small intestine
Gallbladder
Bladder
Stomach

(B)

There is, however, some disagreement as to the significance of the difference in electrical conductance, as this can also be influenced by autonomic arousal. (Chinese researchers have found a correlation between acupoints and nerves.)

Although complete mechanisms have not yet been found for the changes produced by stimulation of acupoints, there is a vast body of empirical evidence which supports its clinical effectiveness.

Practice

The therapist should at least be aware that there are many types of reflex points suggested by various schools of medicine; she should be wary of their presence and the possible effects of manipulating them. Alternatively, having assessed the individual patient and made decisions concerning treatment goals, she may choose a specific type of reflex massage with the intention of having a wider physiological and therapeutic effect, rather than a purely local mechanical effect. For example, she may also choose to incorporate their therapeutic power as an integral part of a massage treatment, as in massaging the reflex points of the feet (reflexology) for a combined local mechanical and broader reflex effect (Fig. 9.10).

Acupressure is another example of a therapy that was brought to the West from the East. Early Chinese texts indicate that the practice of applying finger pressure to points on the body predates the practice of acupuncture.

The technique is variously described as Chinese micromassage, pressing the Tsubo (shiatsu) or acupressure. Although the philosophies and practices differ, they all have in common a system of channels (meridians) and the manipulation of points along the channels to effect a change in the balance of energy. The different schools advocate various methods of manipulation and some propose that the channels should be tonified or sedated, depending on the diagnosis, which may be of either excess or deficient yin or excess or deficient yang. The yin–yang theory is based on the belief that all qualities contain the potential of their opposite. Yin is associated with such attributes as passivity, cold and rest, whereas yang is associated with activity, heat and stimulation (Kaptchuk 1983). When yin and yang are in balance, a person is presumed to be in an optimum state of health; conversely, a state of ill-health exists when they are out of balance. Most systems agree that, in a condition where yin is depleted, the treatment should be aimed at tonifying; this is done by working along the channel in the direction of the energy flow, using slow and gentle pressure. If the condition is thought to be yang, sedation is the aim of treatment; this is achieved by working against the flow of energy more quickly and with greater pressure.

The therapist usually uses the pad of a finger or thumb to apply the pressure. Some writers maintain that this is because there is a relative electrical neutrality at the end of the digit, being the location where yin and yang are in equilibrium (Lavier 1977). Whether or not this is so, the digits are clearly the tools of choice. However, on regions of the body that are covered by thick muscular or fascial layers, and which do not have a low pain threshold for pressure, an elbow or knuckle may be used to apply the pressure, which should always be within the tolerance of the patient. As with acupuncture, the aim of treatment can be to reduce pain, to alleviate symptoms of disease and to promote a balance to maintain or restore health. Acupoints should not be overtreated and it is generally recommended that local points be pressed for up to 1 minute, while more distal points may be held for up to 3 minutes.

Cautions and Contraindications

Caution is required when working with acupoints because of the potential reflex effects. If acupressure is used as a method of pain relief in musculoskeletal disorders, the therapist should be aware of the possibility of stimulating complex visceral and autonomic effects. For this reason, acupressure should not be used for patients with heart disease and other serious visceral disorders. Neither should it be used for the treatment of any disease state unless the therapist is appropriately qualified.

MANIPULATION: ACUPRESSURE

Procedure

There is no requirement for the patient to remove clothing for acupressure. However, if the therapist relies on palpation to find the points, clothing should be removed.

The patient is lying or seated in a comfortable position.

The body area to be treated is supported.

Method 1

The therapist contacts the skin over the acupoint with the tip of her finger or thumb. The digit is held stationary while the pressure is gradually increased. The pressure is kept within the tolerance of the patient.

Method 2

The therapist uses the pad of the finger or thumb and, keeping contact with the skin, makes very small rotary movements (Figs 9.7A,B).

Method 3

The therapist taps the acupoint with one or two fingers.

Method 4

Over thick muscular or fascial layers, the therapist may use a knuckle (Figs 9.6C,D) or the elbow (Figs 9.6E,F) to apply pressure.

LOCATION OF ACUPOINTS

Due to individual anatomical variation some of the location of acupoints are best described with reference to the *cun*. This is a unit of measurement based on the patient's anatomy. Thus, 1 cun is the distance between the creases of the distal and the proximal interphalangeal joint of the patient's middle finger (the length of the middle phalanx of that finger). The breadth of the index and middle finger, at the level of the distal interphalangeal joint when the fingers are adducted, is 1.5 cun. The breadth of the patient's four fingers, at the level of the proximal interphalangeal joint when the fingers are adducted, is 3 cun.

The following are points that are commonly used in acupressure massage.

FIGURE 9.6 *Acupoint stimulation: (A,B) with the thumbs making small rotary movements; (C,D) using the knuckle; (E,F) using the elbow.*

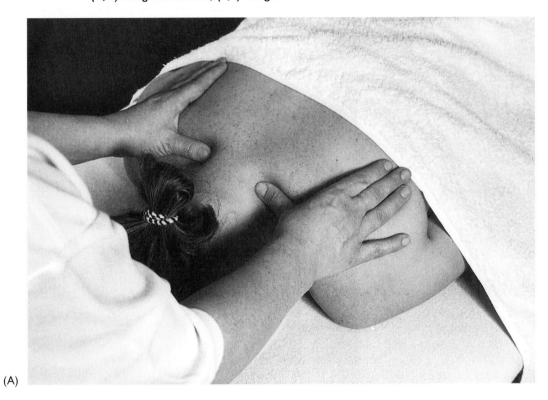

(A)

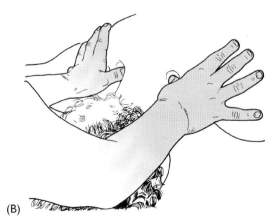

(B)

(Figure cont'd)

(Figure 9.6 cont'd)

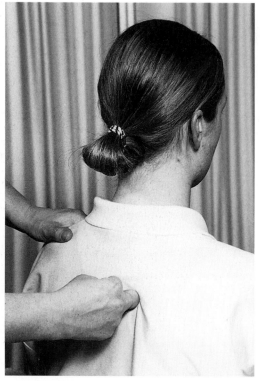

(C)

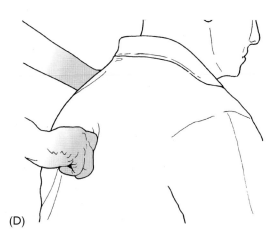

(D)

(Figure cont'd)

(Figure 9.6 cont'd)

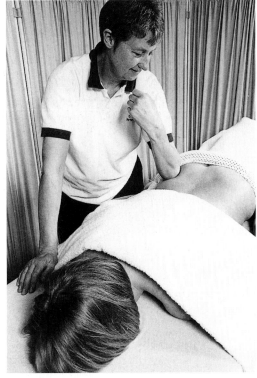

(E)

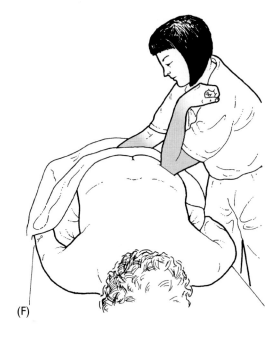

(F)

Lateral View (Fig. 9.7)

GV 20

Location: On the median line of the head, bisected by a line joining the highest points of the ears.
Indication: Psychologically effective point, general sedative and harmonizing effect, good for weakness of memory, headaches. Not to be used if the patient is hypertensive.

GB 20

Location: In a depression inferior to the occiput, between the origins of sterno-cleidomastoid and trapezius.
Indication: Common cold, occipital headaches, torticollis, vertigo.

GB 21

Location: On the highest point of the shoulder, over the angle of the first rib.
Indication: Pain in shoulders and upper back, stiff neck.

GB 25

Location: At the tip of the lower border of the 12th rib.
Indication: Intercostal neuralgia.

GB 30

Location: In a depression lateral to the greater trochanter.
Indication: Low back pain, hip pain, sciatica.

GB 31

Location: On the lateral border of the thigh, where the tip of the second finger touches when standing.
Indication: Aches and pains in the legs.

GB 34

Location: In the depression anterior and inferior to the head of the fibula.
Indication: An influential point for muscles and tendons anywhere in the body; also ankle pain, knee pain, mental disorders.

GB 39

Location: 3 cun above the tip of the lateral malleolus, between the posterior border of the fibula and the peroneus longus and brevis tendons.
Indication: Cervical spondylitis, torticollis, Achilles tendinitis, sprained ankle.

FIGURE 9.7   *Location of commonly used acupoints.*

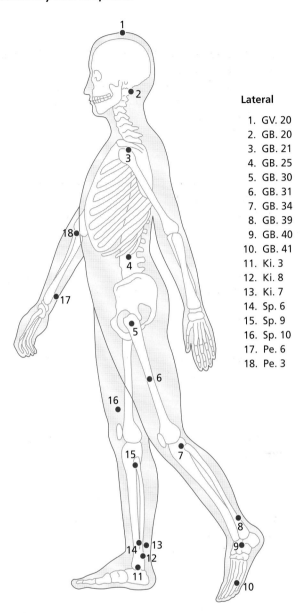

Lateral

1. GV. 20
2. GB. 20
3. GB. 21
4. GB. 25
5. GB. 30
6. GB. 31
7. GB. 34
8. GB. 39
9. GB. 40
10. GB. 41
11. Ki. 3
12. Ki. 8
13. Ki. 7
14. Sp. 6
15. Sp. 9
16. Sp. 10
17. Pe. 6
18. Pe. 3

GB 40

Location: In the depression inferior to the lateral malleolus posterior to extensor digitorum tendon.
Indication: Pain in the legs, arthritis, soft tissue problems around the ankle.

GB 41

Location: In the depression distal to the base of the fourth and fifth metatarsals.
Indication: Pain in the hand and wrist, headaches.

Ki 3

Location: Midway between the Achilles tendon and the tip of the medial malleolus.
Indication: Bladder and menstrual problems.

Ki 7

Location: 2 cun above the tip of the medial malleolus on the anterior border of the Achilles tendon.
Indication: Mental depression, night sweats, cystitis.

Ki 8

Location: 0.5 cun anterior to Ki 7 on the posterior border of the tibia.
Indication: Mental depression, urinary bladder disorders.

Sp 6

Location: 3 cun above the medial malleolus, slightly posterior to the border of the tibia.
Indication: Pain in the ankles, pain related to menstruation, nocturia, mental depression, insomnia, chronic fatigue syndrome.

Sp 9

Location: In the depression inferior to the medial condyle on the posterior border of the tibia.
Indication: Local problems at the knee joint, irregular menses, enuresis.

Sp 10

Location: At the highest point of vastus medialis, 2 cun proximal to the upper border of the patella.
Indication: Mental disorders, menstrual pain, itching skin, urogenital disorders.

P 6

Location: 2 cun proximal to the transverse crease of the wrist, between the tendons of flexor carpi radialis and palmaris longus.
Indication: Gastric problems, nausea, anxiety.

P 3

Location: Middle of elbow crease on medial side of biceps brachii tendon.
Indication: Palpitations, angina pain, mental disorders.

Posterior View (Fig. 9.8)

GV 14

Location: Between the spinous processes of C7 and T1.
Indication: Headaches, cervical spondylosis, torticollis, mental disorder, depression.

GV 4

Location: Between the spinous processes of L2 and L3.
Indication: Tinnitus, low back pain, sciatica.

BI 10

Location: 1.3 cun lateral to the midline at the C1/C2 vertebral joint.
Indication: Nasal obstruction, headache, cervical spondylosis.

BI 11

Location: 1.5 cun lateral to the lower border of the spinous process of T1.
Indication: Shoulder pain, neck pain.

BI 15

Location: 1.5 cun lateral to the lower border of the spinous process of T5.
Indication: Chronic chest disorders, angina pain, mental disorders.

BI 20

Location: 1.5 cun lateral to the lower border of the spinous process of T11.
Indication: Abdominal pain.

BI 22

Location: 1.5 cun lateral to the lower border of the spinous process of L1.
Indication: Low back pain, general fatigue.

BI 23

Location: 1.5 cun lateral to the lower border of the spinous process of L2.
Indication: Decreased energy, low back pain, sciatica.

BI 25

Location: 1.5 cun lateral to the lower border of the spinous process of L4.
Indication: Low back pain, sciatica, constipation.

FIGURE 9.8

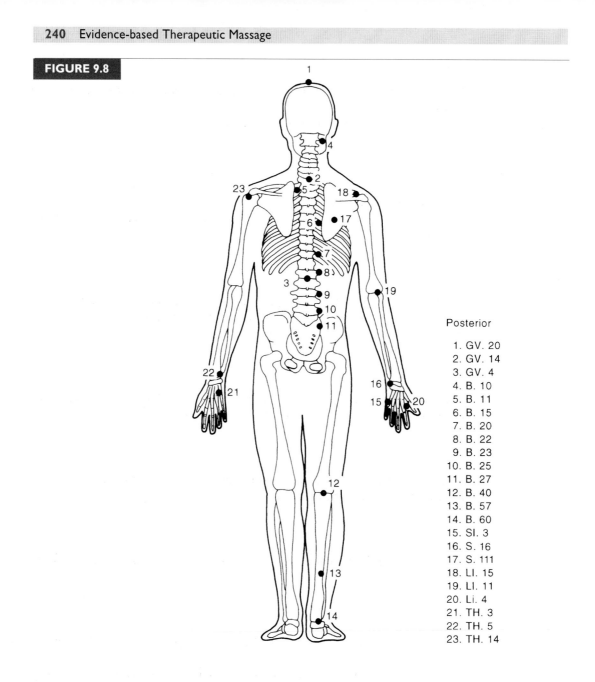

Posterior

1. GV. 20
2. GV. 14
3. GV. 4
4. B. 10
5. B. 11
6. B. 15
7. B. 20
8. B. 22
9. B. 23
10. B. 25
11. B. 27
12. B. 40
13. B. 57
14. B. 60
15. SI. 3
16. S. 16
17. S. 111
18. LI. 15
19. LI. 11
20. Li. 4
21. TH. 3
22. TH. 5
23. TH. 14

Bl 27

Location: On a level with the first sacral foramen, 1.5 cun lateral to the midline.
Indication: Low back pain, sciatica, intestinal disorders.

Bl 40

Location: At the midpoint of the transverse popliteal crease.
Indication: Sciatica, low back pain.

BI 57

Location: On the midline of the calf at the musculotendinous junction of gastrocnemius.
Indication: Sciatica, muscle spasm in the legs.

BI 60

Location: At the midpoint of a horizontal line connecting the highest point of the medial malleolus and the Achilles tendon.
Indication: Local pain, sciatica, low back pain, cervical spondylitis, Achilles tendinitis.

SI 3

Location: With the hand making a fist, this point is on the transverse crease just proximal to the head of the fifth metacarpophalangeal joint.
Indication: Tinnitus, headaches, torticollis.

SI 6

Location: In the depression on the radial side of the styloid process of the ulna.
Indication: Painful or stiff joints in the arm or neck.

SI 11

Location: In a depression at the centre of the infrascapular fossa.
Indication: Shoulder and upper back pain.

LI 15

Location: With the arm abducted the point is located at the anterior–inferior border of the acromioclavicular joint.

LI 11

Location: With the elbow flexed to 90 degrees, the point is at the lateral end of the transverse cubital crease.
Indication: Immune enhancing point, local elbow pain, depression, general fatigue.

LI 4

Location: At the highest point of adductor pollicis with the thumb adducted.
Indication: Toothache, face pain, headache.

TH 3

Location: On the dorsum of the hand between the fourth and fifth metacarpals and proximal to the metacarpophalangeal joints.
Indication: Ear disorders, pain in the hands, mental disorder.

TH 5

Location: 2 cun proximal to the dorsal wrist crease, between the ulna and radius.
Indication: Pain in the arm and hand, torticollis, headache.

TH 14

Location: With the arm abducted to 90 degrees, the point is in the depression dorsal to the greater tubercle of the humerus.
Indication: Shoulder joint pains, arm pain.

Anterior View (Fig. 9.9)

LI 20

Location: Between the nasolabial groove and the nasal ala.
Indication: Trigeminal neuralgia, tension of the facial muscles, toothache.

CV 12

Location: On the midline, midway between the inferior border of the xiphoid process and the umbilicus.
Indication: Nausea, vomiting, diarrhoea, abdominal distension.

CV 7

Location: 1 cun below the umbilicus.
Indication: Irregular menstruation.

CV 6

Location: On the midline, 1.5 cun below the umbilicus.
Indication: Together with Sp 6 and St 36 is a general tonification point for chronic fatigue, depression.

CV 4

Location: On the midline 3 cun below the umbilicus.
Indication: Dysmenorrhoea, cystitis, enuresis, depression.

St 34

Location: 3 cun superior to the superolateral border of the patella.
Indication: Knee pain, abdominal pain.

St 36

Location: 0.5 cun lateral to the tibial tubercle and 3 cun inferior to the tibial plateau.
Indication: General pain relief, depression.

FIGURE 9.9

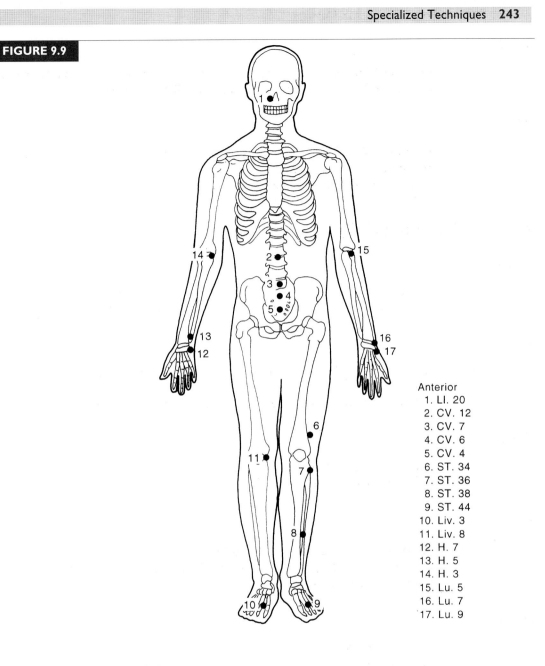

Anterior
1. LI. 20
2. CV. 12
3. CV. 7
4. CV. 6
5. CV. 4
6. ST. 34
7. ST. 36
8. ST. 38
9. ST. 44
10. Liv. 3
11. Liv. 8
12. H. 7
13. H. 5
14. H. 3
15. Lu. 5
16. Lu. 7
17. Lu. 9

St 44

Location: 0.5 cun proximal to the web between the second and third metatarsals.
Indication: Headache, toothache, abdominal pain.

Liv 3

Location: 2 cun proximal to the web between the first and second metatarsals.
Indication: Headache, eye disorders, mental disorders.

Liv 8

Location: In a depression at the medial end of the transverse popliteal crease.
Indication: Disorders of the knee joint, leg pain, dysmenorrhoea.

H 7

Location: On the transverse wrist crease, in the depression on the radial side of flexor carpi ulnaris.
Indication: Stress, anxiety, insomnia, irritability.

H 5

Location: 1 cun proximal to H 7, on the radial side of flexor carpi ulnaris.
Indication: Wrist pain, insomnia, mental disorder.

H 3

Location: With the elbow flexed, midway between the end of the cubital crease and the medial epicondyle of the humerus.
Indication: Tennis elbow, anxiety, irritability.

Lu 5

Location: On the cubital crease lateral to the tendon of biceps.
Indication: Tennis elbow, sore throat, lung disorder.

Lu 7

Location: 1.5 cun proximal to the transverse wrist crease on the radial border.
Indication: Common cold, headache, respiratory disorders, pain or tension in the muscles of the neck.

Lu 9

Location: On the radial end of the anterior wrist crease, lateral to the radial artery.
Indication: Useful for reviving a person who has fainted, influential in circulatory disorders such as arteriosclerosis and intermittent claudication.

TECHNIQUE: REFLEXTHERAPY

Purpose

Reflextherapy is also an example of an ancient therapy which originated in the East. It is known variously as reflextherapy, reflexology or zone therapy. Reflexologists believe that each area of the body is represented by zones on the feet and that the feet can be used as a diagnostic tool to uncover imbalances.

FIGURE 9.10 *Reflextherapy zones of the feet.*

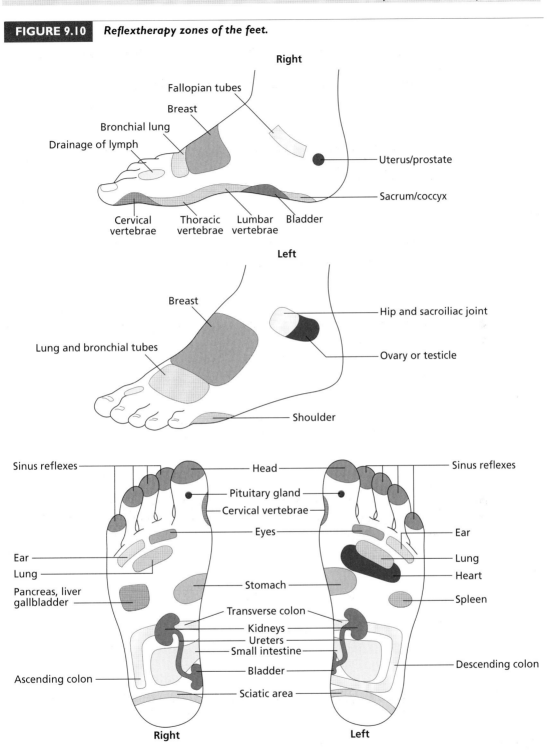

The therapist treats the relevant area to produce a reflex response in the connected somatic area (see Fig. 9.10).

Two recent studies have examined reflexology as a diagnostic tool. Baerheim et al (1998) engaged three reflexologists to find the clinical problems of 76 patients by examination of the soles of the feet. Inter-rater agreement, measured by weighted Kappa, was significantly better than chance for six parts of the body but was too low to be of clinical significance. White et al (2000) investigated whether reflexology charts could be used as a valid method of diagnosis. Two reflexologists examined 18 patients with six specified clinical conditions. The therapists were blinded to the conditions and rated the probability that each of the six conditions were present. Inter-rater reliability scores were very low, providing no evidence of agreement between examiners. The researchers concluded that this method of diagnosis was very poor at distinguishing between the presence or absence of medical conditions. Blood flow has been examined in two further studies. Using Doppler sonography, blood flow changes in the right kidney were measured in a placebo controlled double blind, randomized study. One group of 15 adults were given reflexology on the zone of the right kidney, the control group had reflexology on other foot zones. There was a significant difference between groups with the kidney group showing an increase in renal blood flow (Sudmeier et al 1999). Support is given to the findings by Mur et al (2001). Here the treatment group ($n = 16$) received foot massage on the intestinal zone, while the placebo group ($n = 16$) had foot massage on unrelated zones. Blood flow velocity in the superior mesenteric artery and a resistive index as a parameter of vascular resistance were calculated. During treatment there was a significant reduction in the resistive index for the treatment group, suggesting an increase in blood flow in the superior mesenteric artery and the subordinate vascular system.

Reflexology has been found to significantly decrease premenstrual symptoms (Oleson & Flocco 1993) and to decrease anxiety in patients with breast or lung cancer who were on a medical oncology unit. In the latter study, the patients with breast cancer also experienced a significant reduction in pain. Degan et al (2000) found that of 40 patients with pain associated with a lumbar–sacral disc herniation, 62% reported a reduction in pain after three sessions of reflexology. This supports the earlier work of Kovacs et al (1993) with patients who had low back pain. After reflextherapy they showed significant improvement in pain scores.

Two contrasting studies have examined the role of reflexology in bronchial asthma. Brygge et al (2001) gave 10 weeks of either active or placebo reflextherapy to two groups of 20 with bronchial asthma in a blind, controlled trial. Objective lung function tests did not change for either group, beta$_2$ inhalation and quality of life scores improved in both groups with no significant difference between them. This is at odds with a study by Hui-Xian (1994) in which it was reported that all 45 children with bronchial asthma showed improvements in symptoms after reflexology. These two studies clearly demonstrate the value of controlling for placebo. Frankel (1997) examined the effect of reflexology on baroreceptor reflex sensitivity (BRS), blood pressure and sinus arrythmia. There were two experimental groups, one receiving reflexology and the other foot massage, plus a control group. Both experimental groups showed a decrease in BRS and an increase of over 30% in frequency of sinus arrythmia compared to the control. This may indicate that simple foot massage could be as effective as reflexology in certain conditions but further research is needed. A recent German paper has raised the issue that reflexology is not always beneficial. The researchers investigated the possible usefulness of foot reflexology on recovery after a surgical intervention. A total of 130 patients who had undergone abdominal surgery for gynaecological reasons were given reflexology. The authors concluded that reflexology is not recommended for acute, abdominal post-surgical situations in gynaecology because it can trigger abdominal pain (Kesselring 1999).

Features

The zones of the feet are usually pressed gently with the thumb or fingers of the therapist. Some writers advocate deeper pressure with a knuckle if this is thought appropriate.

Position

Reflexologists generally position their clients in a specially developed chair which is comfortable for the client and for the therapist. Alternatively, a treatment couch can be used. The client is in a supine-lying or semi-recumbent sitting position.

Procedure

The treatment is usually begun with a bilateral foot massage leading to treatment of specific zones. Many therapists treat all the zones of the foot in one session. Others concentrate on specific zones to achieve the desired therapeutic effect.

TECHNIQUE: THAI MASSAGE

Purpose

Thai medicine is rooted in Buddhism and the philosophical belief that everything is made of the four elements: earth, water, wind and fire. The causes of all disease can be linked to the three aspects of the body: bile, wind and phlegm. Thai massage aims to influence the wind present by liberating it where it has become stagnant and redistributing it (Gold 1998).

Features

Points along the energy lines are treated by circular pressure from the practitioner's thumb, foot, palm or finger. Stretches are then applied to liberate the wind from joints. Compression is applied to the femoral and axillary arteries to temporarily restrict blood flow, and abdominal massage is an important feature.

Position

A variety of positions are adopted, mostly on a mat on the floor. This approach requires considerable physical flexibility on the part of the therapist. Further detail is beyond the scope of this book.

Procedure

Pressures and stretches are intermingled, using a variety of interactive positions. The stretches can be strong, but the therapist should be sensitive to end-range discomfort and work within it.

TECHNIQUE: TUI NA

Purpose

Tui na is part of Traditional Chinese medicine and is generally used to treat musculoskeletal disorders. It influences the flow of *Qi* (life energy), to enable it to flow freely around the body. This improves physical, emotional and spiritual well-being (Mercati 1997).

Features

Tui means 'push' and *na* means 'grasp'. The basic techniques include pressing (using the palm, thumb or elbow), squeezing, kneading, rubbing, stroking, vibration, thumb rocking, plucking, percussion, shaking, rotation, push/pull (with a joint manipulative element) and stretching.

Position

This is a strong approach. The patient will be sitting and lying and the therapist will work around her/him in an active, dynamic way.

Procedure

The tissues and Qi points of the body are worked in regional sections, using a combination of the techniques.

REFERENCES

Baerheim A, Algroy R, Skogedol K R et al 1998 Feet a diagnostic tool? Tidsskrift for Den Norske Laegeeforrening 118(5): 753–755

Benor D J 1993 Healing research, vol 1. Helix Deddington. Cited in: Charman R A (ed) 2000 Complemenary therapies for physical therapists. Butterworth-Heinemann, Oxford

Benor D J 1994 Healing research, vol 2. Deddington: Helix. Cited in: Charman R A (ed) 2000 Complementary therapies for physical therapists. Butterworth-Heinemann, Oxford

Brygge T, Heinig J H, Collins P et al 2001 Reflexology and bronchial asthma. Respiratory Medicine 95(3): 173–179

Chapman C R, Chen A C, Bonica J J 1977 Effects of intrasegmental electrical acupuncture on dental pain: evaluation by threshold estimation and sensory decision theory. Pain 3(3): 213–227

Degan M, Fabris F, Vanin F et al 2000 The effectiveness of foot reflextherapy on chronic pain associated with a herniated disc. Professioni Infermieristiche 53(2): 80–87

Dundee J W, Chestnut W N, Ghally R G, Lynas A G A 1986 Traditional Chinese acupuncture: a potentially useful antiemitic? British Medical Journal 293: 583–584

Frankel B S 1997 The effect of reflexology on baroreceptor reflex sensitivity blood pressure and sinus arrythmia. Complementary Therapies in Medicine 5(2): 80–84

Gold R 1998 Thai massage: a traditional medical technique. Churchill Livingstone, Edinburgh

Haase H 1962 Bindegewebsmassage Wirkungsphysiologische grundlagen und methodik. Zschr Artzl Fortbild 62(13): 134–136

Hui-Xian 1994 A clincial analysis of foot reflex massage for the treatment of 45 cases with infant bronchial asthma. AOR Research Reports, 4th edn. AOR, Henfield

Kaptchuk T J 1983 Chinese medicine: the web that has no weaver. Rider, London

Kesselring A 1999 Foot reflexology massage: a clinical study. Forschende Komplementarmedizin 6(Suppl. 1): 38–40

Kovacs F M, Abraira V, Lopez-Abente G, Pozo F 1993 Neuro-reflextherapy of non specified low back pain. AOR Research Reports, 4th edn. AOR, Henfield

Lavier J 1977 Chinese micro-massage. Thorsons, Wellingborough

Mercati M 1997 Tui na. Gaia Books, London

Mur E, Schmidseder J, Egger I et al 2001 Influence of reflex zone therapy of the feet on intestinal blood flow measured by color doppler sonography. Forschende Komplementarmedizin 8(2): 86–89

Oleson T, Flocco W 1993 Randomized controlled study of premenstrual symptoms treated with ear hand and foot reflexology. Obstetrics and Gynecology 82(6): 906–911

Oschman J L 2000a Energy medicine – the new paradigm. In: Charman R A Complementary therapies for physiotherapists. Butterworth-Heinemann, Oxford

Oschman J L 2000b Energy medicine: the scientific basis. Churchill Livingstone, Edinburgh

Seto A, Kusaka C, Nakazato S et al 1992 Detection of extraordinary large biomagnetic field strength from human hand. Acupuncture Electrotherapeutics Research Int Journal 17: 75–94. Cited in: Oschman J L 2000 Energy medicine: the scientific basis. Churchill Livingstone, Edinburgh

Sudmeier I, Bodner G, Egger I et al 1999 Changes of renal blood flow during organ-associated foot reflexology measured by color Doppler sonography. Forschende Komplementarmedizin 6(3): 129–134

White A R, Williamson J, Hart A, Ernst E 2000 A blinded investigation into the accuracy of reflexology charts. Complementary Therapies in Medicine 8(3): 149

Wittlinger H, Wittlinger G 1982 Textbook of Dr Vodder's manual lymphatic drainage, vol 1. Basic course, 3rd edn. Haut Verlag, Heidelberg

Zimmerman J 1990 Laying-on-of-hands healing and therapeutic touch: a testable theory. BEMI Currents Journal of the Bio-Electro-Magnetics Institute 2: 8–17. Cited in: Oschman J L 2000 Energy medicine: the scientific basis. Churchill Livingstone, Edinburgh

3

Section 3
Clinical Uses of Massage

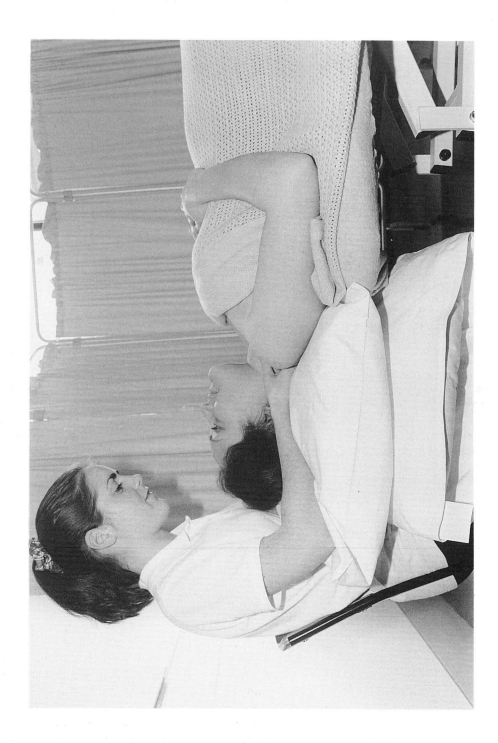

10 Sedative Massage

STRESS

The autonomic nervous system (ANS) was discussed in Chapter 3 in connection with the reflex effects of massage. That discussion is extended here, applied specifically to stress and autonomic arousal. The relevant function of the ANS to sedative massage is that when an individual experiences severe fear, pain or has a strong emotional reaction, the hypothalamus is stimulated to transmit impulses to the spinal cord which cause a sympathetic discharge, resulting in the alarm response, or general adaptation syndrome (Seyle 1982). This is the protective mechanism which prepares an animal or human for 'flight or fight', to ensure that, whichever of these actions is chosen, the animal is physiologically prepared for vigorous activity. The changes include an increase in blood levels of glucose, cortisol, adrenaline (epinephrine) and noradrenaline (norepinephrine), and an increase in blood pressure, blood flow to skeletal muscles, muscle tone and heart rate (Figs 10.1 and 10.2).

In Chapter 3 the concept of a stressor was briefly examined in relation to various types of touch and other stimulation via the sense organs. A stressor acts to arouse the sympathetic branch of the ANS; massage is frequently used to achieve the opposite effect, the aim being to provoke a decrease of activity in the sympathetic branch and an increase of activity in the parasympathetic branch of the ANS, thus returning the body to a normal balance.

Arousal is the result of an individual's personal response to any stimulus perceived as a threat. *Clinical stress* may occur if the arousal persists and the individual develops feelings of being unable to cope; thus, stress can be viewed as a form of chronic arousal. Prolonged stress may result in raised levels of cortisol, which can have further harmful effects, such as decreased immunity and hypertension. Unremitting stress is undesirable for the human organism. To maintain health there must be a reversal of the arousal and a return to a normal baseline state of homoeostasis.

FIGURE 10.1   *Current concepts of the stress syndrome. Reproduced, with permission, from Thibodeau & Patton (1999).*

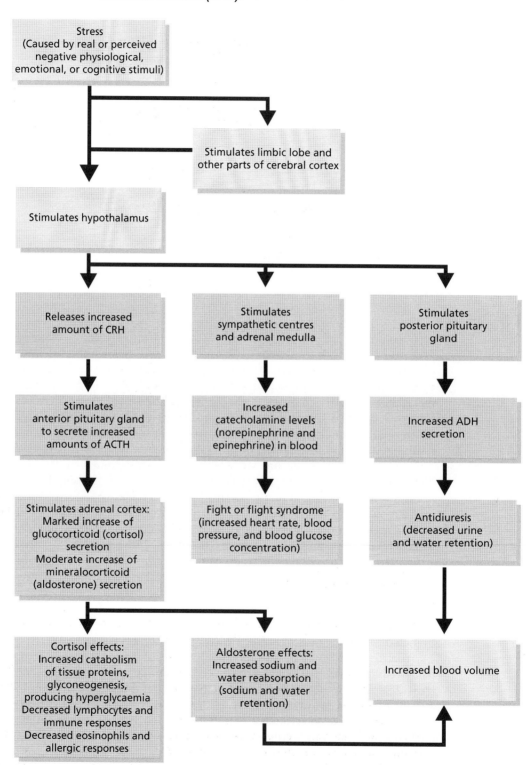

FIGURE 10.2   *Seyle's hypothesis about activation of the stress mechanism Reproduced, with permission, from Thibodeau & Patton (1999).*

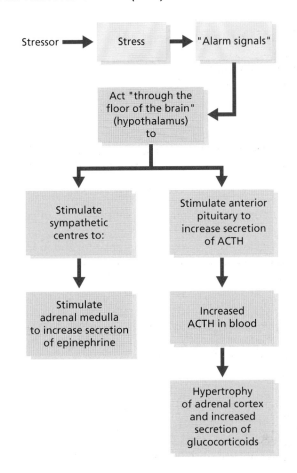

Some people with clinical stress initially require pharmacological intervention, but longer-term therapies focus principally on developing coping strategies which may be in the form of:

- cognitive approaches
- behavioural methods
- body awareness techniques.

Therapists who work in mental health care find that massage is a useful component when teaching body awareness techniques; this is often the first stage of physical treatment which attempts to reverse the musculoskeletal aspects of stress, such as muscle tension. Massage is not used in isolation but as an integral part of the rehabilitation programme; it may enhance relaxation and also promote integration of the physical senses.

Outside the orthodox health care setting, people often seek massage for 'stress', which has become a common term used to describe feelings of fatigue, tension and general weariness brought on by, for example, overwork, lack of sleep and worry. This condition is clearly to be differentiated from clinical stress, but massage is an appropriate prophylaxis if used in conjunction with exercise and other activities which promote physical and mental well-being.

ANXIETY AND DEPRESSION

Feeling anxious or depressed is a normal response to harrowing life events such as bereavement, loss of a job or financial difficulties. In healthy people these feelings reduce as the person adapts to the situation, uses coping strategies, and returns to a state of mental well-being. Anxiety and depression become mental disorders when the feelings are prolonged and constant.

In *anxiety* states people may experience irrational fears concerning everyday activities or the carrying out of normal routine tasks. They may exhibit physical symptoms which are consistent with increased sympathetic nervous system activity, such as muscle tension, palpitations, sweating and insomnia. Training in relaxation should be a component of anxiety management for these patients, and for many individuals massage will be a valuable prelude to this. Most patients with anxiety states have forgotten how it feels to be physically relaxed and massage is valuable in preparing these people for subsequent self-relaxation techniques.

A *depressed* patient will express profound sadness and social withdrawal; other symptoms may include impaired concentration, loss of interest in life, emotional lability, eating disorders, fatigue, irritability, insomnia, early morning waking and suicidal thoughts. Treatment is often long term and complex. Antidepressant medication is commonly prescribed together with occupational, physical and psychotherapy. Initially a patient with depression may be more comfortable with a passive type of treatment. Some depressed patients will also have symptoms of anxiety and for these people a sedative massage is appropriate but, to reduce the risk of therapy dependence developing, the therapist may encourage the individual to learn self-massage or self-acupressure. Dependence is less likely to result if it is explained that any passive treatment administered by the therapist is a preliminary to the patient being taught how to massage him- or herself or to start active exercises. This explanation will also help to prevent any feelings of rejection when the massage treatment comes to an end.

Many patients with chronic stress, anxiety or depression will also exhibit dysfunctional posture and movement patterns. This reflects the effect of the psyche on physical function and exemplifies non-verbal communication of the emotions of an individual. These dysfunctions signal the need for body awareness training, the object of which is to create the conditions necessary for a patient to begin to integrate sensory information, thus becoming more aware of posture and movement. For these patients massage may be the chosen treatment to reduce muscle tone and to facilitate physical activities. It may also be of benefit by prompting the patient to connect with pleasant physical sensations, thereby promoting a positive body image and, ultimately, helping to restore self-esteem.

Massage may be the only regular experience of caring touch for a large proportion of the population. Sedative massage is used frequently as a treatment by therapists, particularly nurses, for those who are tactually deprived. This client group is largely found among elderly people who are being cared for within institutions, the terminally ill and the chronically sick. The importance of massage to these groups is that, in its absence, they may experience not only tactual deprivation but also sensory deprivation, as the opportunities for normal sensory input are not currently a feature of many hospitals and other residential care environments. The massage session also provides an opportunity to establish an effective therapeutic relationship by enhancing the rapport between patient and therapist.

GROUP THERAPY

This approach to treatment works well with groups of clients who are survivors of abuse, provided an experienced therapist supervises and counselling is available should the need arise. Mutual support groups for carers may also benefit from learning how to give relaxation massage to each other; carers are often tense and so benefit from relaxation techniques and caring touch.

Massage can be used as a means of promoting trust and cohesion within the group. Hand or foot massage should be demonstrated by the therapist and, under her supervision, massage can be given and received by group members. Even individuals who initially are tactually defensive may be drawn into this activity when they recognize the benefit that other members derive from the massage. Members of such a group tend to become enthusiastic learners. Inevitably the activity leads to questions from individuals about the benefit of massage, which presents an opportunity for the therapist to discuss topics of health education.

OTHER USES OF RELAXATION MASSAGE

A further area for the use of sedative massage is as a prophylaxis against musculoskeletal dysfunction secondary to occupational stresses. Many workers sit, stand or move in ways that engender pathologically increased tone in some muscle groups. A classic example is the computer operator who frequently has increased tone in the upper back and neck muscles, as a result of prolonged static contraction of these muscle groups. The condition may go undetected until the therapist begins to massage the involved muscles, which are often painful. Once an employee is alerted to the potential problems he/she should be advised on how to work with ergonomic efficiency, to take regular breaks and to maintain good posture. Intervention at an early stage may help to avoid chronic muscle tension, muscle imbalance, adverse neural tension and postural dysfunction. Relaxation massage may serve a similar purpose for amateur athletes, many of whom, despite having a high level of body awareness, tend to dismiss warning signs and attempt to work through muscle pain.

Although we have discussed in this section specific groups of people who are likely to benefit from massage as a relaxation therapy, there is no intention to suggest that the therapy should be confined to those with specific medical disorders. A large section of society choose to have massage for the pleasurable experience and the positive psychological feelings of health it can give. Many people are now taking responsibility in promoting their own health and engaging in illness prevention. They are turning to various complementary therapies which they believe give them some control over their own health care. A growing fitness and leisure industry promotes activities that encourage an increasing number of people to become actively involved in maintaining a healthy lifestyle. Receiving regular massage is often a part of that endeavour.

THE RESEARCH

Several studies have explored the link between massage, autonomic effects and/or perceived levels of anxiety (Table 10.1). While some of the studies have shown significant changes of indices of autonomic activity, self-reported anxiety, or both, others present conflicting results, making interpretation of the studies as a whole difficult. Many of the studies have methodological and statistical limitations, and demonstrate potential internal bias. There are differences in sample sizes, populations, types of massage employed, time scales and number of massages. Some are pilot studies carried out to ascertain the relevance of massage to a particular profession working with a certain client group, and as such the results cannot be generalized. Despite these deficiencies it is possible to draw some inferences from the studies viewed as a whole. It is clear, for example, that studies which used a population who were residing in potentially stressful circumstances or with disease states (as opposed to a normal population) show results that appear to be more consistent, even when a widely different methodology was employed.

Two of the studies, those of Fakouri & Jones (1987) and Meek (1993), show consistent results, suggesting a decrease in autonomic arousal. However, the one measurement that shows consistent results across the studies in which it was employed is that of the State–Trait Anxiety Inventory, suggesting that this is a more predictable indicator of anxiety than the more traditionally used physiological measurements of autonomic arousal. The importance of the studies, taken as a whole, is that there appears to be no clear link between autonomic arousal and self-reported anxiety. The assumption that there is a correlation between autonomic arousal and perceived anxiety needs to be reappraised, since, in the light of these studies, the link appears to be tenuous.

The results suggest that the hypotheses of future studies of this genre would be better tested by the employment of psychological measurements. A paradigm shift may be necessary to ensure that what is being tested is *clinical effectiveness*, which is defined as 'the scientifically proven usefulness of a treatment in alleviating symptoms or combating disease' (Ernst & Fialka 1994). Research in this area has traditionally focused on physiological effects, rather than clinical effectiveness. As it is widely accepted, in the present context, that massage is used as a coping mechanism and not a cure, physiological measures will not translate as showing clinical effectiveness. It is evident that randomized longitudinal field studies are needed which are capable of measuring self-reported anxiety and any consequent changes in behaviour and function.

FORMS OF SEDATIVE MASSAGE

A *full body massage* will usually take from 45 to 90 minutes, depending on the time available, the variety of strokes used and regions of the body that may

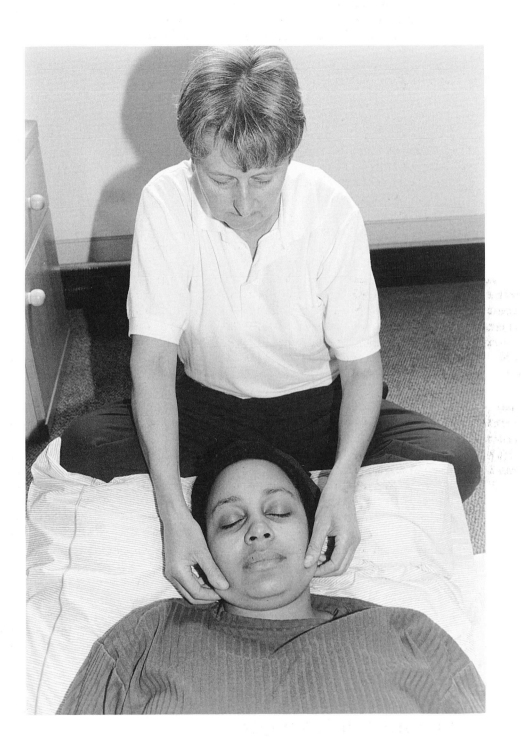

TABLE 10.1	Table of studies which have examined the link between massage and ANS sympathetic activity and anxiety

Reference	Subjects and controls	Intervention, length and no.	Results for massage groups
Barr & Taslitz (1970)	$n = 10$; F; healthy; 19–21 yrs; own control	'Conventional' back massage, 'frictions' on sacrum; 20 min × 3	SBP & DBP; ↓; delayed effects: SBP↑; DBP↑; HR↑; GSR↓; BT↑; PD↑; RR↓
Longworth (1982)	$n = 32$; F; healthy; 19–52 yrs; own control	SSBM; 9 min × 1	STAI↓; HR↑; EMG↓; delayed effects: SBP↑; GSR↑
Bauer & Dracup (1987)	$n = 25$; 18 M, 7 F; 37–76 yrs; acute myocardial infarction; no control	SSBM; 6 min × 1	No changes in physiological indicators; subjective reports of relaxation
Fakouri & Jones (1987)	$n = 18$; 4 M, 14 F; 56–96 yrs; in nursing care; no control	SSBM; 3 min × 3	SBP↓; DBP↓; delayed effects: HR↓; ST↓; subjective reports of relaxation
Field et al. (1993)	$n = 72$; 40 M, 32 F; 7–18 yrs; adjustment disorder and depression; massage group + control group	SSBM; 30 min × 5	Depressed subjects: STAI↓; urine cortisol↓; urine noradrenaline (norepinephrine)↓ Both subjects: POMS↓; observed behavioural arousal↓
Meek (1993)	$n = 30$; 16 M, 14 F; 50–90 yrs; terminally ill; no control	SSBM; 3 min × 2	HR↓; SBP↓; DBP↓; ST↑
Fraser & Ross Kerr (1993)	$n = 21$; 4 M, 17 F; 60+ yrs; in residential care; massage group +2 controls	SSBM; 5 min × 4	SBP↓; STAI↓; delayed effects: EMG↓; HR↑; DBP no change Subjective reports of relaxation
Ferrell-Tory & Glick (1993)	$n = 9$; M; 23–77 yrs; patients with cancer pain; no control	Effleurage and petrissage to back and feet, myofascial trigger point therapy for 30 min, then SSBM 3 min × 2	Pain (VAS)↓; relaxation (VAS)↓; STAI↓; HR↓; RR↓; SBP↓; DBP↑
Groer et al. (1994)	$n = 32$; 10 M, 22 F; 44–77 yrs; healthy; massage group + control group	Nursing back rub, 10 min × 1	STAI↓; s-IgA↓
Field et al. (1998)	$n = 28$; debridement of burns patients; control	Stroking to six body regions, 20 min × 7	STAI↓; BOS improved; saliva cortisol↓; HR↓; POMS↓
Hernandez-Reif et al. (2000)	$n = 30$; hypertensive adults; control	Massage therapy, 30 min × 10	DBP↓; urinary cortisol↓; salivary cortisol↓; reports of anxiety, depression, hostility↓
Kim et al. (2001)	$n = 59$; cataract surgery patients; control	Hand massage	Anxiety (VAS)↓; SBP↓; DBP↓; HR↓; adrenaline (epinephrine)↓; noradrenaline (norepinephrine)↓

Trends have been included as well as results with statistical significance.

Key: M: male; F: female; SSBM: slow-stroke back massage; SBP: systolic blood pressure; DBP: diastolic blood pressure; HR: heart rate; RR: respiratory rate; ST: skin temperature; GSR: galvanic skin resistance; EMG: electromyograph; STAI: State–Trait Anxiety Inventory; POMS: Profile of Mood States; VAS: visual analogue scale; s-IgA: salivary secretory immunoglobin A; BOS: behaviour observation scale; PD: pupil diameter; BT: body temperature.

require extra attention. When increased muscular tone is found, the therapist may spend more time working in this region until a decrease in tone is achieved. Alternatively, it can occasionally be advantageous to continue with the full body massage and then return to troublesome areas, which may then be found to have reduced in tone. It is unlikely that very ill patients would tolerate a full body massage. With the very ill it is advisable to concentrate on one area, such as the back, the neck and shoulders, or the face. In addition, many therapists working in a health care environment are so constrained by time that a full body massage is not possible. It is suggested that a *3-minute slow-stroke back massage* may prove effective in these circumstances (Fakouri & Jones 1987, Meek 1993, Labyak & Metzger 1997). If possible, the patient should lie prone. The therapist, using both hands, should use reciprocal strokes bilaterally over the posterior rami from the occiput to the sacrum in slow and rhythmical movements.

The starting point for the full body massage can be variable and is best decided upon by the preferences of the client and therapist. At the first massage the client may prefer to start in the prone position with the therapist beginning work on the back; for anyone who is anxious or ill at ease, this is the least threatening position.

When giving a relaxation massage the strokes should be light but firm, care being taken not to be so light as to stimulate rather than sedate. The therapist must be calm and avoid giving the impression that she is in a hurry – if the therapist is not feeling relaxed, then neither will the patient. Appropriate music may be played if the patient finds it soothing.

The lubricant may be applied by superficial stroking of the body region to be massaged; for a sedative massage it is acceptable to use slightly more than the normal quantity of oil as traction of the skin is unnecessary and undesirable. Essential oils may be used for their therapeutic properties and to enhance the pleasurable qualities of the massage (see Ch. 7).

Presented below is a suggested sequence for a full body sedative massage in the absence of complicating factors. The depth of pressure should be light to moderate and the strokes should be made slowly and rhythmically.

Full body sedative massage

Positioning of the patient

■ Lying prone on a treatment couch, pillows underneath the abdomen and ankles

Sequence of massage and manipulations
Begin all the regions by stroking:

■ The back: effleurage, light palmar and finger kneading, effleurage, transverse stroking, effleurage
■ The back of the legs: effleurage, light kneading, effleurage

The patient turns to supine, pillows under the head and knees:

■ The front of the legs: effleurage, light kneading, effleurage
■ The arms: effleurage, light kneading, effleurage
■ The abdomen: effleurage, transverse stroking, effleurage
■ The chest, shoulders and neck: effleurage, light finger kneading, effleurage
■ The face: effleurage, light finger kneading, plucking, effleurage

REFERENCES

Barr J S, Taslitz N 1970 The influence of back massage on autonomic functions. Physical Therapy 50(12): 1679–1691

Bauer W C, Dracup K A 1987 Physiological effects of back massage in patients with acute myocardial infarction. Focus on Critical Care 14(6): 42–46

Ernst E, Fialka V 1994 The clinical effectiveness of massage therapy: a critical review. Forsch Komplementarmed 1(5): 226–232

Fakouri C, Jones P 1987 Relaxation treatment: slow stroke back rub. Journal of Gerontological Nursing 13(2): 32–35

Ferrell-Tory A T, Glick O J 1993 The use of therapeutic massage as a nursing intervention to modify anxiety and the perception of cancer pain. Cancer Nursing 16(2): 93–101

Field T, Morrow C, Valdeon C et al 1993 Massage reduces anxiety in child and adolescent psychiatric patients. International Journal of Alternative and Complementary Medicine (July): 125–131

Field T, Peck M, Krugman S et al 1998 Burn injuries benefit from massage therapy. Journal of Burn Care and Rehabilitation 19(3): 241–244

Fraser J, Kerr J R 1993 Psychophysiological effects of back massage on elderly institutionalized patients. Journal of Advanced Nursing 18: 238–245

Groer M, Mozingo J, Droppleman P 1994 Measures of salivary secretory immunoglobin A and state anxiety after a nursing back rub. Applied Nursing Research 7(1): 2–6

Hernandez-Reif M, Field T, Krasnegor J et al 2000 High blood pressure and associated symptoms were reduced by massage therapy. Journal of Bodywork and Movement Therapies 4(1): 31–38

Kim M S, Cho K S, Woo H, Kim J H 2001 Effects of hand massage on anxiety in cataract surgery using local anesthesia. Journal of Cataract and Refractive Surgery 27(6): 884–890

Labyak S E, Metzger B L 1997 The effects of effleurage backrub on the physiological components of relaxation: a meta-analysis. Nursing Research 46(1): 59–62

Longworth J C D 1982 Psychophysiological effects of slow stroke back massage in normo-tensive females. Advances in Nursing Science 6: 44–61

Meek S S 1993 Effects of slow stroke back massage on relaxation in hospice clients. Journal of Nursing Scholarship 25(1): 17–21

Seyle H 1982 History and present status of the stress concept. In: Goldberger L, Breznitz S (eds) Handbook of stress: theoretical and clinical aspects. Macmillan, New York

Thibodeau G A, Patton K T 1999 Anatomy and physiology, 4th edn. Mosby, St Louis

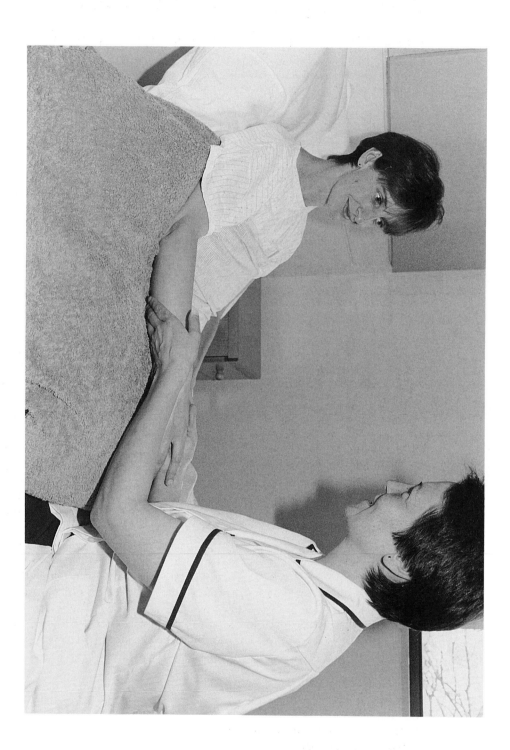

11 Massage for People with Long-term and Terminal Illness

Long-term conditions present specific problems and therefore require that health care workers take an appropriate approach. Patterns of progression may differ and these conditions may be chronic but stable, or may deteriorate, as, for example, in motor neurone disease. Alternatively they may exacerbate and remit, as with multiple sclerosis, for example. In terminal illnesses, progress may be either slow or rapid from the time of diagnosis.

Common to all these conditions is distress, fear, stress, unavoidable symptoms and a severe disruption of lifestyle. In all cases, health care workers should emphasize the maintenance of quality of life (QoL) for these patients, reducing stress and supporting the patients by equipping them with coping strategies. If cure is not an option, then acceptance and learning how to cope and maintain independence are the challenges facing patients and their carers. Carers are an integral part of the process and helping the patient to maintain close supportive relationships is important.

Although the difficulties and emotional trauma must not be minimized in any way (these diagnoses are clearly devastating and the trauma not fully appreciated by anyone without personal experience), care should be directed towards assisting patients and those close to them through this time in shared experience, rather than feeling they are under an impossible burden. Thus, goals are not focused on cure or passive receipt of care but on patient-led strategies and therapies which respect and involve their personally identified unit of significant others.

Massage can be used to:

● reduce pain
● reduce oedema
● reduce musculoskeletal symptoms
● reduce muscle tone
● desensitize hypersensitive skin
● reduce stress

- reduce anxiety
- alleviate constipation
- help prevent pressure sores
- improve body image
- enhance coping strategies
- promote relaxation and well-being
- facilitate communication and intimacy.

Massage may therefore be an obvious choice as a useful and often powerful tool when working with this client group, as it can help in the ways listed above. It should be stressed, however, that the problems faced by this client group are complex – massage by itself cannot achieve these effects but it can make an important contribution to all of them.

MASSAGE FOR PEOPLE WITH CANCER

Patients with cancer often endure a long period of anxiety and uncertainty as they wait for diagnosis, medical test results, unpleasant drug treatments, sometimes disfiguring surgery and new prognoses. Their physical fight against the disease may be accompanied by emotions such as denial, fear, anxiety, sorrow and loss. They may have to let go of work, leisure pursuits and loved ones at the same time as they endure pain and sometimes disablement. A stress management programme incorporating health education, muscle relaxation and massage has been found to be helpful in reducing stress in people with cancer (Lin et al 1998).

Modern medicine can sometimes cure cancer and can offer considerable relief from symptoms. This section relates more specifically to the terminally ill patient who may be at home, in hospital or in a hospice. Massage has been found to be beneficial in reducing perceptions of distress, fatigue, nausea and state anxiety in cancer patients undergoing autologous bone marrow transplant (Ahles et al 1999). A randomized controlled clinical trial, which was conducted within a hospice, examined the effects of massage on cancer pain intensity, prescribed intramuscular morphine equivalent doses (IMMEQ), hospital admissions and QoL. Pain intensity was significantly reduced after the massage and current QoL scores were significantly higher in the massage group. IMMEQ doses were comparable in the massage and control group, as were hospital admissions (Wilkie et al 2000). These two studies underscore the benefit of massage in both hospital and hospice environments with patients at different stages of disease.

Relationships with carers are crucial at this stage, as they offer love, support and intimacy to the patient. It is important, then, that therapeutic intervention helps to strengthen relationships rather than disrupt them. Touch can be a strong need of the cancer sufferer, who may have lowered self-esteem, particularly if disfiguring surgery has been necessary. Touch may also be important for carers, as something they can give to the patient, 'something to offer' that is positive and therapeutic, enabling them to take an active role rather than one of passive observation which can lead to feelings of helplessness and uselessness. If a carer wishes to learn massage a good starting point would be for the therapist to instruct him/her in how to give a foot massage. There is evidence that a 10-minute foot massage (5 minutes each foot) can have a significant effect on perceptions of pain, nausea and relaxation (Stephenson et al 2000). A further study has examined the effects of foot reflexology on anxiety and pain in patients with breast or lung cancer who were on a medical/oncology ward. All the patients treated with massage experienced a significant decrease in anxiety and patients with breast cancer showed a significant decrease in pain (Stephenson et al 2000).

Touch can also help to restore intimacy, which may be lost due to fear of hurting the patient, or because of separation through periods of medical treatment. The therapist must work with those close to the patient, and must sometimes relinquish her role and pass it on to the carer. Carers may also be stressed and in need of massage themselves, in which case 'time out' should be encouraged. Another option is reciprocal massage, between patient and carer, which may facilitate communication and intimacy. It can be a non-strenuous but fulfilling form of sensuality. It may restore the early experiences in a relationship – exploration, physical awareness and gentle, sensitive responses to each other's needs. Scented oils and music may enhance the experience. The advice and support of the therapist may facilitate this activity. The relaxation effects of massage can also aid in reducing sleep disturbance (Richards 1998).

McCaffery & Wolf (1992) suggest that massage is especially helpful when the patient is confined to bed (either because of specific treatment or the terminal stage) and lies supine much of the time, as it improves circulation to the skin and reduces skin breakdown. This can enhance nursing strategies to reduce pressure sores such as turning and positioning regimens. Care should be taken if the skin has become reddened, as this can indicate that there is tissue breakdown underneath the skin, and manipulation of skin may worsen the situation.

Modifications usually make a treatment possible and it is always worth pursuing, as a study with female cancer patients showed that massage gave them 'meaningful relief from suffering' (Billhult & Dahlberg 2001).

Patients should be respected as individuals and encouraged to direct the best time for the massage and how long it should last, and to decide whether the massage should be conducted in silence or whether it offers a welcome opportunity for talking, either general discussion or expression of feelings. The areas to be massaged may be modified by the presence of any open lesions. The hands and feet may be good options if accessibility to other parts of the body is limited by surgical wounds, drips or drains. These areas are often acceptable to the individual who does not welcome further personal intimacy. The addition of an essential oil to the lubricant may enhance the effects of massage. Wilkinson et al (1999) found that the addition of Roman chamomile essential oil to a carrier oil enhanced the therapeutic effects of reduced anxiety and improved overall QoL.

Is Massage a Safe Intervention for People with Cancer?

Early writers on massage placed little emphasis on cancer as a contraindication to massage. It was not listed by Goodall-Copestake (1926) or Tidy (1932), although this omission could indicate the scant attention the disease received generally in physiotherapy texts. Hollis (1987) gives tumour as a contraindication and Tappan (1988) lists melanoma, as this type of cancer metastasizes easily through lymphatic and blood vessels. In its traditional use, within ortho-dox medical care, massage has previously been regarded as being contraindi-cated for patients with active malignant disease.

Physiotherapists, by taking a detailed medical history and having access to patients' medical records, have avoided techniques that might increase local metabolic rate or blood flow in the vicinity of active disease. This statement needs some clarification, as massage has been used to reduce local symptoms, or to aid relaxation in the terminally ill patient, when emphasis is on comfort rather than cure. Massage has also proved useful, for example, in spinal cancer which has produced uncomfortable sensory changes such as hyperaesthesia. This can be sufficiently severe to make touch uncomfortable to the point where washing becomes distressing. Gentle rhythmical stroking can prove useful to desensitize the skin, and the use of warm water to massage the skin gently (via gentle movements in a hydrotherapy pool, for example) may be helpful. Heavier stroking can be used as a counterirritant, acting through the pain gate to reduce pain. Also, after radical mastectomy for example, patients can be given or taught oedema massage for the arm following removal of the lymph glands. Effleurage was formerly the main treatment of choice; it has now largely been superseded by the more superficially applied manual lymphatic drainage. Traditionally, however, massage has been taboo in the earlier active stages of the disease, but acceptable at the later and terminal stages.

Of course, patients with cancer have the right to treatment of other injuries and physical problems unrelated to the cancer. They also have the right to support for symptoms of stress, and help with coping mechanisms. Thus, as long as the tissues are not actively manipulated over any active disease site, an increase in lymphatic and venous flow is avoided in patients with melanoma or Hodgkin's disease and the lymph nodes are not directly stimulated mechani-cally, then massage can be a useful adjunct to other therapies. Stationary and light pressure techniques are probably the safest (holding, therapeutic touch, acupressure, for example); the more superficial techniques – as used in gentle stroking, whole body sedative massage or through an oily medium – would be the next treatment of choice from a safety viewpoint. It is unlikely that these techniques would be physiologically more stimulating than everyday activities such as walking or housework. Hadfield (2001) used aromatherpy massage in patients with a primary malignant brain tumour who were attending their first follow-up appointment after radiotherapy. There was a statistically significant reduction in four physical parameters of the autonomic nervous system (ANS) which suggested a relaxation response.

In relation to drug therapy, it has been suggested that massage may increase the rate at which chemotherapeutic agents flow around the body when admin-istered into the bloodstream, that it increases the rate at which drugs enter the bloodstream when administered by other means, and that the dosage should be reduced accordingly (McNamara 1994). However, this has not yet been sub-stantiated experimentally. Also, it has been suggested that massage increases the rate at which chemotherapy and its toxins will be lost from the body, although it should be recognized that we have insufficient experimental evi-dence to support these suppositions. Of course, as in all conditions, techniques and approaches should be modified to match the stage of disease.

Another pertinent study was undertaken by McNamara (1994). She sent out questionnaires to 24 volunteer massage practitioners and asked for their views and knowledge on the use of massage for people with cancer. The main findings in relation to dangers and contraindications were that practitioners had often been taught or had read that massage was contraindicated in the earlier stages of the disease but not in the terminal stages. There was obviously some concern about the lack of research evidence to support or refute this suggestion, but massage was generally being offered to people with cancer.

An *absolute contraindication* for massage is undiagnosed cancer. It is important that the massage therapist is alert to the possibility and that any patient experiencing symptoms which may relate to a serious condition should be urged to seek advice from a doctor immediately. Look for:

- intractable pain – no relief on rest, significantly disturbed sleep (this may indicate inflammatory or malignant disease)
- feeling of being generally unwell
- change in temperature
- inflammation and heat in the absence of trauma
- unexplained weight change
- any lump bigger than 5 cm, especially if it is a recurrence of a previous lump or is deeper than fascia or is increasing in size (Grimer & Dalloway 1995).

Within the physiotherapy profession there has been a long tradition of concern about the safety of massage for patients with cancer. Its unwritten nature leaves an apparent controversy in this area, which has prompted research in the subject (McNamara 1994). The consensus is that massage is *not* acceptable if:

- the cancer is metastasizing
- the cancer is active
- the massage is in the region of a contained tumour
- cancer is undiagnosed
- the therapist is not sensitive to any fragile areas of bone.

Generally speaking, massage is considered quite appropriate for use in the terminal stages of the disease.

If a therapist is unsure of any of these factors and is unable to receive specific guidance from the patient's doctor, then she should err on the side of caution.

If in doubt, *stationary holding* or *therapeutic touch techniques* can be used as there is no evidence to suggest that these are unsafe under any circumstances.

Gentle stroking, a *back rub*, *foot massage* or *whole body massage* are techniques of choice for relaxation.

Heavier *stroking* or *classical Swedish massage techniques* can be used to influence the pain gate or to have a counterirritant effect to relieve pain.

The reflex techniques of *acupressure* may be preferred, to promote relaxation or for their balancing effect to strengthen immunity and improve general health.

Massage should be modified to match the medical condition and desires of the individual patient, and the type of massage and structure of the sessions negotiated beforehand. Essential oils may be found to be pleasant, or they may worsen nausea. If tolerated, specific oils can be chosen, such as rosemary, applied as a shampoo to the head or as a massage oil, to stimulate hair growth following chemotherapy. If applied in excess, however, it may cause convulsions and fitting, so the therapist should be cautious. Massage may be preferred for a whole hour or may be tolerated only for short periods of time.

Tyler and colleagues (1990) demonstrated that the 1-minute back rub (a traditional nursing procedure) showed no statistically significant worsening of mixed venous oxygen saturation and heart rate levels when applied to 173 patients in receipt of critical care. This suggests that massage is safe even in critically ill patients, though the considerable variability shown reinforces the principle of close monitoring of physiological responses in this client group. Dunn et al (1995) also found that massage and aromatherapy with lavender oil did not adversely affect vital signs in patients being nursed on an intensive care unit. Stress or coping measures were not altered to statistically significant levels post-massage, or aromatherapy, or rest; but aromatherapy significantly improved mood and decreased anxiety levels.

Oedema in Oncology

A specific use of massage is in the treatment of oedema. Hydrostatic oedema may result from the pressure of a malignant growth, whereas lymphoedema may be caused by the removal of lymph glands during cancer surgery or their obliteration by radiotherapy or tumour mass, and may occur in Kaposi's sarcoma, associated with human immunodeficiency virus (HIV)/acquired immune deficiency syndrome (AIDS). This oedema is protein rich and must therefore be removed by the lymphatic system.

To summarize, the principles of treating *hydrostatic oedema* are to clear proximal areas first; thence to direct strokes from distal to proximal; increase pressure in the tissue spaces; and supplement massage by elevation of the limb, compression and circulatory exercises. The principles of *lymphoedema* treatment are that: massage is light in order that lymph vessels, which are placed superficially in the tissues, are stimulated; healthy glands are stimulated first, before clearing trunkal areas; swelling is then drained into these cleared areas before being moved towards healthy glands; and massage is accompanied by compression bandages, exercises and benzopyrone therapy for maximum effect. Manual lymphatic drainage (MLD) is the technique of choice for lymphoedema. The selection of strokes includes stationary circles, light effleurage, pump technique, scoop technique and rotary technique, which can be applied with a little oil. The effectiveness of this regimen in the treatment of lymphoedema has been demonstrated by Bunce et al (1994), who studied 25 women referred for post-mastectomy lymphoedema treatment. Massage (Foldi MLD), pneumatic compression, compression bandaging and exercises were undertaken for 3 hours daily, 5 days per week for 4 weeks. The length of time since mastectomy was found not to affect the results. After the intensive phase of treatment, there was a mean reduction in excess volume of the affected limb of 40%. At 12 months, the affected limbs were no more than 5% larger than the unaffected limbs. The results in this well-designed study were statistically significant.

MASSAGE FOR LYMPHOSTATIC OEDEMA

Lymphoedema is swelling due to an abnormality in the lymphatic system, often occurring in one limb. It is classified according to cause:

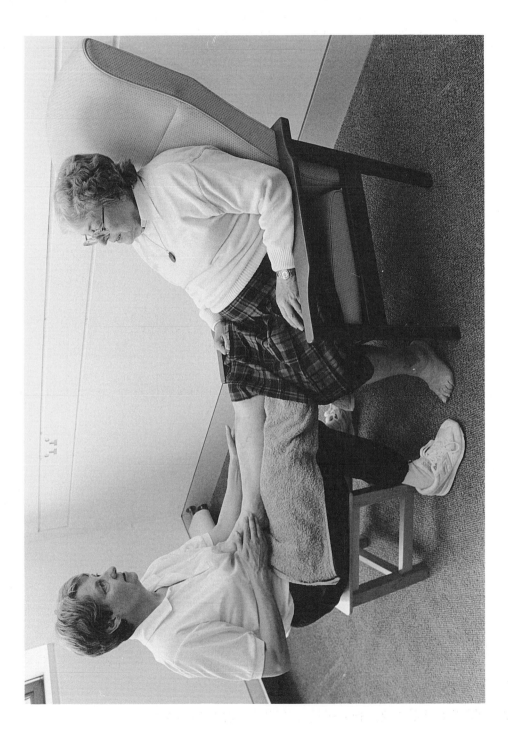

Primary Lymphoedema

Dysplasia
    Aplastic: no vessels
    Hypoplastic: few vessels
    Hyperplastic: incompetent valves (Kinmonth 1982).
Congenital dysplasia: occurs at birth (Turner's syndrome, Nonne–Milroy–Meige disease).
Lymphoedema praecox: develops in late puberty.
Lymphoedema tarda: apparent later in life.

Secondary Lymphoedema

Parasitic lymphoedema is caused by filarial parasites, transmitted through mosquito bites. The parasites block the lymphatics causing massive oedema and large skin vesicles, when it is often called elephantiasis.

Iatrogenic lymphoedema results from surgical removal or radiotherapeutic destruction of the glands in the treatment of cancer.

Additionally, *obliterative lymphangitis* can occur secondary to deep vein thrombosis, *trauma* can damage vessels or glands, and *kinetic insufficiency* can occur in paralysis.

Lymphoedema is also classified according to severity (Foldi 1994, Casley-Smith & Casley-Smith 1992):

Grade 1: Pitting oedema which reduces on elevation.
Grade 2: No pitting or reduction on elevation; fibrosclerosis which may feel hard; skin changes.
Grade 3: Elephantiasis.

Traditional techniques for the removal of excess tissue fluid, such as deep massage, electrical stimulation under pressure, compression devices and muscle pump exercises, have been used with variable results in this condition. The current treatment of choice is a regimen termed complex physical therapy (CPT) or complex decongestive physical therapy (CDP), which is time-consuming and therefore costly, but which achieves excellent results. An integral part of the regimen is the specialized massage technique of manual lymphatic drainage (MLD), which was originally developed by Vodder (1936) and has since been modified by Leduc (Leduc et al 1981) and Foldi (1994) (see also Ch. 9).

MLD is thought to be preferable to other forms of massage in the treatment of lymphoedema as it is based on the anatomy and physiology of the lymphatic system and deeper forms of massage are thought to damage the lymphatics. Rapid massage at a pressure of 70–100 mmHg has been found to create artificial cracks in lymphatic vessel walls, loosen subcutaneous tissue, form large tissue channels and release lipid droplets (Eliska & Eliskova 1995). The massage in this study, however, was particularly vigorous.

Manual Lymphatic Drainage

Aims

To stimulate lymphatic drainage (Fig. 11.1) and to clear proximal lympho-tomes (adjacent areas of the trunk); to promote movement of lymph across

The lymphatics in fluid balance. Reproduced, with permission, from Thibodeau & Patton (1999).

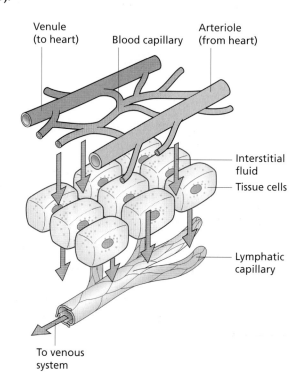

lymphatic watersheds; to open up superficial collateral lymphatic vessels; to facilitate lymph removal by opening up the flaps in the vessel walls; and to stretch and assist in the reabsorption of fibrous tissue.

Principles

Lymphatic oedema cannot be removed via the bloodstream as it is protein-filled. The plasma proteins are too large to be reabsorbed through blood vessels, so must be removed via lymph channels. If the lymphatic system is poor, the proteins will increase the colloid osmotic pressure in the tissue spaces, drawing fluid out of the bloodstream. This results in massive oedema. Fibrin is formed which traps the swelling, and the cells are separated from their source of nutrition. The skin becomes hard and altered in quality. Compressive techniques do not open the flaps in the walls of lymphatic vessels, to allow fluid in. Massage should therefore gently move the skin, opening the flaps in the superficial vessels and have a pumping effect on the deeper vessels. It should also bypass the damaged vessels and facilitate removal across the lymphatic watersheds. Massage should be given for 1 hour daily. It should not be undertaken in the presence of untreated acute infection (cellulitis) and reddening of the skin must be avoided, as histamine is thought to increase oedema (Kurz 1989, 1990).

Media

A small amount of oil should be used, but not enough to cause a gliding over the skin.

Strokes

- stationary circles
- light effleurage
- pump technique
- scoop technique
- rotary technique.

Treatment should start in the left supraclavicular space, to drain the ductus thoracicus followed by clearance of the adjacent lymph gland area (axilla or groin) (Kurz 1989, 1990). If the lymph glands are removed or damaged, the strokes should sweep across to the glands on the opposite aspect of the body. For example, if the oedema is in the arm and the axillary glands have been removed during mastectomy, the massage should continue to the opposite axilla. In severe cases it may be necessary to clear the opposite side of the trunk and adjacent quadrants on the opposite side of the trunk before moving towards the affected limb. Once the starting point has been decided, the areas of treatment must progress by clearing proximal areas before distal. The massage cannot continue across a scar: it should progress on the opposite aspect of the body.

Self-care

The patient should be advised that MLD is only one component of a complex programme of treatment. Treatment is much more effective if the patient conscientiously follows the regimen of prescribed benzopyrones (a form of vitamin P which causes resorption of the tissue proteins), pressure garments, measured to a precise fit and worn 24 hours a day, and skin care. Mechanical pumps may occasionally be used in secondary lymphoedema under supervision, but should be used judiciously. If used in primary oedema, they merely shunt the swelling to a proximal area, for example the genital region. They can also result in the formation of a fibrous band around the top of the limb, which reduces the effectiveness of other treatments.

When severe, the fluid can sometimes be felt to ripple in the tissues under the therapist's hand. Aching within the trunk, for example over the thoracic spine area, often reduces as the swelling reduces.

Progress can be monitored by measuring the girth along a limb, every 10 cm, with a tape measure. The volume of the limb is then calculated by dividing the limb into four, then adding the volumes of each segment using the formula for a cylinder (volume = π (circumference/2π) $2 h$, where circumference is the mean of adjacent circumferences and h is 100 mm).

Effectiveness of Massage in Oedema

Some time-consuming techniques have been described here. Just how effective is massage in oedema? Ladd et al (1952) examined the effects of massage on lymph flow. They cannulated the lymph channel in the neck of 17 dogs and collected lymph in a test tube during an experimental procedure. The nearest limb of each dog was put through a routine of massage, passive movement and electrical stimulation interspersed with 10 minutes' rest, the whole cycle being repeated between two and four times and rotated in order between dogs. The massage was a modified Hoffa-type routine of stroking, effleurage, petrissage and Hoffa frictions, and it was found to raise lymph flow to significant levels above those found in the other techniques. Passive movements worked better than electrical stimulation. Of further interest was the finding that, in one dog which shivered, lymph flow was as good as when massaged. This mirrors the findings of Wakim and co-workers (1949) that blood flow is increased more by active movement than passive movement or massage, suggesting that in normal healthy individuals massage is not required to improve certain physiological parameters. This does not, of course, negate its use for psychological or musculoskeletal benefits.

In 1990, a study was conducted in which Mortimer et al measured skin lymph flow by an isotope clearance technique in anaesthetized pigs. It was found that the flow rate varied naturally between pigs and between parts of the body, and that subdermal flow was faster than deep flow. Local massage, described as 'Gentle, local massage using a hand-held massager' increased flow rates to highly significant levels statistically. These results are interesting, because they suggest that local mechanical manipulation of the tissues will increase the lymphatic flow. It can be postulated that this is due to a mechanical movement of the tissues opening the flaps in the lymphatic vessel walls, to allow passage of the proteinous fluid. Further evidence was provided by Ikomi & Schmid-Schonbein in 1996. They measured the effects of passive leg movement and massage on lymph flow rates in a dog and found that both movement and massage increased the rate of lymph flow. The rate was dependent on the frequency of tissue movement and the amplitude of skin displacement. These results were independent of heart function, indicating that expansion and compression of the lymphatics provide a mechanism for the pumping of lymph.

There is much interest in the specific effectiveness of MLD. One such study was undertaken by Kurz (1989, 1990) who gave MLD (Vodder method) to 29 patients suffering from lymphoedema due to varying causes. The results were compared with those of 10 healthy controls. It was found that three to four times the quantity of urine was excreted after the massage. The subjects underwent controlled food and drink intake before the study and full urine analysis was conducted after the massage phase. The significant findings were that urine levels of 17-OH-cortisone and serotonin decreased, whereas those of adrenaline (epinephrine) increased by 50% and histamine by 129%. The authors found the results elucidating in that cortisone is sodium retaining and oedema producing, so its elimination will have obvious effects on oedema. The reduction in serotonin levels demonstrates destruction of this oedema-producing hormone. The researchers thought that the increases in adrenaline (epinephrine) and noradrenaline (norepinephrine) were due to the fact that they were stimulated to increase the circulation, and that the presence of large quantities of histamine indicates that this might contribute to the oedema formation as it creates and sustains tissue fluid. They consider that this research substantiates Kuhnke's (1975) claims that MLD causes reabsorption of oedema, contraction of vascular muscle (as shown in the catecholamine levels), and decompression of nociceptors (as evidenced by the reduction in the concentration of serotonin and other metabolites). This research, however, did not have an experimental and control group equal in size and the explanation for the meaning behind the urine analysis is speculative.

Zanolla et al (1984) studied 60 patients, aged between 37 and 80 years, and divided them into three groups. No difference was found between the groups in terms of sex, age and disease status. MLD was compared with uniform pneumatic pressure and differentiated pneumatic pressure and the circumference of the arm was measured in seven places before and after treatment. MLD produced the best results, and uniform pneumatic pressure also showed a significant improvement over differentiated pressure. The results for the differentiated pressure and control device were not significant. Unfortunately, the groups were not large enough for between-group comparison of effectiveness. What was interesting, however, was that the massage was very effective, although it was applied for only 1 hour three times weekly for 1 month, whereas the mechanical treatments were applied for 6 hours daily over 1 week. Not only has intermittent mechanical pressure been found clinically to worsen the problem in some cases, it was not shown to be particularly effective in this research. These findings suggests that MLD is the treatment of choice for lymphoedema but the use of pressure garments (which mimic the uniform pressure applied in this study) can considerably enhance the treatment. A complex approach of MLD, pressure garments, exercises and skin care is advocated as the treatment approach of choice by lymphoedema specialists (Casley-Smith & Casley-Smith 1994, Foldi 1994) and is recommended in the UK Department of Health guidelines for managing the treatment of post breast cancer lymphoedema (Kirshbaum 1996).

The effectiveness of using a combined approach has been documented by Casley-Smith & Casley-Smith (1992), who described their results of treating 78 patients with oedema following mastectomy with CPT (including the Foldi method of MLD). In the first 4 weeks of treatment, the mean reduction of swelling in grade I lymphoedema was 103% of its initial volume and the mean volume reduction in grade II lymphoedema was 60%, both sets of results being highly significant. A smaller but significant drop in volume was maintained over the following year. Examining each separate leg, mean losses of fluid were 1.1 litres for grade I, 1.3 litres for grade II and 3.7 litres in elephantiasis. Ko et al (1998) found similarly good results with a reduction in per cent volume and reduced infection rate following CPT in this large study. These positive results have been substantiated by Wozniewski et al (2001) who found that the milder the lymphoedema, the better the results of CPT.

MLD may be more effective than a simplified version often taught to patients for self-massage (simple lymphatic drainage, SLD), as suggested by the results of a small pilot study conducted by Sitzia et al (2001). In addition, aromatherapy with lavender oil can be included in a CPT programme to enhance the comfort, relaxation and self-esteem of women who have had breast cancer (Kirshbaum 1996).

Conclusion

Oedema is present in many of the patients who consult or are referred for physical therapy. It must be controlled immediately it occurs, because chronic oedema can cause fibrosis, adhesions, resultant loss of joint movement and pain. The excess fluid itself causes pain as pressure is exerted on nociceptors; it further prevents cells from being bathed in fresh, newly nourished tissue fluid, thereby reducing normal cellular metabolism. Metabolic circulation may be reduced, together with metabolites, and protein remains in the tissues. Prevention, containment and removal of swelling is the essential hierarchy of care for the tissues, regardless of cause, and massage can be a cornerstone of effective treatment, with skilful application of MLD being essential in the treatment of lymphoedema.

MASSAGE IN HIV/AIDS

The issues already discussed may apply to individuals who have HIV or AIDS, who may also experience particular problems which warrant further discussion. As with all seriously ill patients, patients with HIV or AIDS may have skin highly sensitive to touch, and the type of massage used must be chosen with care. Slow stroking may appear to be less desirable but may work to desensitize the skin, if the patient is able to tolerate this approach and to persevere with a technique that may initially have been uncomfortable. Some patients have Kaposi's sarcoma, which appears as brown, reddish or purple lesions which can be several inches across. Of course, any open lesions should be avoided and closed lesions massaged lightly.

Hygiene is very important: many people with AIDS suffer from skin rashes and these should be diagnosed accurately before massage. Fungal infections, for example *Candida albicans*, may be highly contagious. Direct contact with herpes must also be avoided. Hand or foot massage may be appropriate if skin problems are widespread, or sensitive acupressure massage can be given through clothing or bedcovers. Depending on the general medical condition of the patient with AIDS, there may be coughing, vomiting or diarrhoea. No one should be excluded from treatment should they desire it, but massage may have to be interrupted to assist with other needs. When helping with bodily fluids or to change soiled clothing or bedding, gloves should be worn and hands washed thoroughly before recommencing treatment. The therapist should be fully aware of the unit's infection control policy and an appropriate standard of hygiene must be maintained at all times.

The therapist may treat individuals with this diagnosis at an early stage when they may want to boost their immune systems and acquire relaxation and coping skills. Alternatively, she may treat people at the opposite extreme, in the later stages of terminal illness. In the latter situation, the therapist must be prepared to deal with the presenting symptoms, which may be neurological, respiratory or involve the eyesight. Lang (1993) found, in a retrospective study of community physiotherapy with 10 people with AIDS, that pain was often musculoskeletal in origin.

There is some evidence that massage can decrease stress and increase natural immunity. Ironson et al (1996) studied 29 gay men, of whom 20 were HIV positive, and their responses to daily massage over 1 month. The subjects had a significant increase in natural killer cell number and cytotoxicity, and soluble CD8; a significant decrease was found in anxiety and urinary cortisol levels. The massage was designed specifically to be relaxing; it included elements of Swedish, Trager, polarity, acupressure and craniosacral therapy. Interpretation of the term 'massage' was, therefore, very loose and it would be difficult to replicate, either clinically or in a subsequent study. However, the results are supported by later research with adolescents who were HIV positive (Diego et al 2001). Massage twice a week for 12 weeks was compared with a group who received progressive muscle relaxation. It was reported that the immune changes in the massage group included increased natural killer cell number (CD56); in addition, the HIV disease progression markers CD4/CD ratio and CD4 number showed improvement. This study contrasted with that of Birk et al (2000), who found massage did not enhance immune measures. The study by Birk et al was a randomized prospective controlled trial of adults with HIV infection; massage alone was compared with massage in combination with either exercise or stress management–biofeedback treatment and a control group receiving a standard treatment intervention. No significant changes were found in any enumerative immune measure and the conclusion was that massage administered once a week to HIV infected people does not enhance immune measures. However, all these studies add support to the supposition that massage reduces feelings of stress, anxiety and depression and this can affect natural immunity. There are clear implications, therefore, for the treatment of people with immune-related conditions.

Essential oils may be beneficial for any of these clients, but allergies should be considered as immunity is compromised. As with all clients, but more so with this group, the therapist should ask what the patient's body needs are at each treatment session; a preordained programme may be inappropriate with a fluctuating medical condition and a patient who may feel very ill or be in acute pain. Treatment may be further restricted by drips and drains. Working with this client group can be demanding both professionally and emotionally. It is important to encourage and allow expression of feelings and emotions. It is better for the therapist to attempt to advise and to give clients what they desire in support of their personal strategy, rather than trying to achieve great things. If you work with the client on equal terms, leaving self aside, then you can remain strong, conserving emotional energy for personal, non-professional life, and so work with this client group can be long term rather than transient.

KEY POINTS

- ◆ Goals of care should not focus on cure or passive receipt of care, but should support and reinforce patient-led strategies.
- ◆ Massage may be preferred for short periods of time.
- ◆ Be flexible if the condition is fluctuating.
- ◆ Abdominal massage may alleviate constipation.
- ◆ Massage can reduce oedema, and manual lymphatic drainage is effective in lymphoedema.
- ◆ Be prepared to hand over your role to a carer.
- ◆ Ensure your intervention enriches, rather than disrupts, relationships.
- ◆ Massage can reduce pain and muscle tone, and promote relaxation and well-being.

REFERENCES

Ahles T A, Tope D M, Pinkson B et al 1999 Massage therapy for patients undergoing autologous bone marrow transplantation. Journal of Pain and Symptom Management 18(3): 157–163

Billhult A, Dahlberg K 2001 A meaningful relief from suffering: experiences of massage in cancer care. Cancer Nursing 24(3): 180–184

Birk T J, McGrady A, MacArthur R D, Khuder S 2000 The effects of massage therapy alone and in combination with other complementary therapies on immune system measures and quality of life in human immunodeficiency virus. Journal of Alternative and Complementary Medicine 6(5): 405–414

Bunce I H, Mirolo B R, Hennessy J M et al 1994 Post-mastectomy lymphoedema treatment and measurement. Medical Journal of Australia 161: 125–128

Casley-Smith J R, Casley-Smith J R 1992 Modern treatment of lymphoedema. I. Complex physical therapy: the first 200 Australian limbs. Australian Journal of Dermatology 33: 61–68

Casley-Smith J R, Casley-Smith J R 1994 Information about lymphoedema for patients. Lymphoedema Association of Australia, Adelaide

Diego M A, Field T, Hernandez-Reif M et al 2001 HIV adolescents show improved immune function following massage therapy. International Journal of Neuroscience 106(1–2): 35–45

Dunn C, Sleep J, Collet D 1995 Sensing and improvement: an experimental study to evaluate use of aromatherapy massage and periods of rest in an intensive care unit. Journal of Advanced Nursing 21(1): 34–40

Eliska O, Eliskova M 1995 Are peripheral lymphatics damaged by high pressure manual massage? Lymphology 28(1): 21–30

Foldi M 1994 Treatment of lymphedema [editorial]. Lymphology 27: 1–5

Goodall-Copestake B M 1926 The theory and practice of massage. Lewis, London

Grimer R J, Dalloway J 1995 Tumour recognition – signs and symptoms [letter]. Physiotherapy 81(7): 413

Hadfield N 2001 The role of aromatherapy massage in reducing anxiety in patients with malignant brain tumours. International Journal Of Palliative Nursing 7(6): 279–285

Hollis M 1987 Massage for therapists. Blackwell, Oxford

Ikomi F, Schmid-Schonbein G W 1996 Lymph pump mechanics in the rabbit hind leg. American Journal of Physiology 271(1/2): H173–183

Ironson G, Field T, Scafidi F et al 1996 Massage therapy is associated with enhancement of the immune system's cytotoxic capacity. International Journal of Neuroscience 84(1–4): 205–217

Kinmonth J B 1982 The lymphatics: surgery, lymphography and diseases of the chyle and lymph systems. Edward Arnold, London

Kirshbaum M 1996 Using massage in the relief of lymphoedema. Professional Nurse 11(4): 230–232

Ko D S, Lerner R, Klose G, Cosimi AB 1998 Effective treatment of lymphedema of the extremities. Archives of Surgery 133(4): 452–458

Kuhnke E 1975 Die physiologischen grundlagen der mannuellen lymphdrainage. Physiotherapie 66: 12

Kurz I 1989 Textbook of Dr Vodder's manual lymphatic drainage. Vol. 2. Therapy. Haug, Heidelberg

Kurz I 1990 Textbook of Dr Vodder's manual lymphatic drainage. Vol. 3. Treatment. Haug, Heidelberg

Ladd M P, Kottke F J, Blanchard R S 1952 Studies of the effect of massage on the flow of lymph from the foreleg of the dog. Archives of Physical Medicine 33(10): 604–612

Lang C 1993 Community physiotherapy for people with HIV/AIDS. Physiotherapy 79(3): 163–167

Leduc A, Caplan I, Lievens P 1981 Traitment physique de l'oedeme du bras. Paris

Lin M L, Tsang Y M, Hwang S L 1998 Efficacy of a stress management program for patients with hepatocellular carcinoma receiving transcatheter arterial embolization. Journal of the Formosan Medical Association 97(2): 113–117

McCaffery M, Wolf M 1992 Pain relief using cutaneous modalities positioning and movement. Hospital Journal 8(1–2): 121–153

McNamara P 1994 Massage for people with cancer. Wandsworth Cancer Support Centre, London

Mortimer P S, Simmonds R, Rezvani M et al 1990 The measurement of skin lymph flow by isotope clearance – reliability, reproducibility, injection dynamics and the effect of massage. Journal of Investigative Dermatology 95(6): 677–682

Richards K C 1998 Effect of a back massage and relaxation intervention on sleep in critically ill patients. American Journal of Critical Care 7(4): 288–299

Sitzia J, Sobrido L, Harlow W 2001 Manual lymphatic drainage compared with simple lymphatic drainage in the treatment of post-mastectomy lymphoedema. Physiotherapy 88(2): 99–107

Stephenson N L, Weinrich S P, Tavakoli A S 2000 The effects of foot reflexology on anxiety and pain in patients with breast and lung cancer. Oncology Nursing Forum 27(1): 67–72

Tappan F M 1988 Healing massage techniques. Appleton and Lange, Norwalk, CT

Thibodeau G A, Patton K T 1999 Anatomy and physiology, 4th edn. Mosby, St Louis

Tidy N M 1932 Massage and remedial exercises. John Wright, London

Tyler D O, Winslow E H, Clark A P, White K M 1990 Effects of a one minute back rub on mixed venous saturation and heart rate in critically ill patients. Heart and Lung 19(5): 562–565

Vodder E 1936 Le drainage lymphatique: une nouvelle methode therapeutique santé pour tous. Cited in: Wittlinger H, Wittlinger G 1982 Textbook of Dr Vodder's manual lymphatic drainage. Haut, Heidelberg, vol. 1

Wakim K G, Martin G M, Terrier J C et al 1949 Effects of massage on the circulation in normal and paralyzed extremities. Archives of Physical Medicine 30: 135–144

Wilkie D J, Kampbell J, Cutshall S et al 2000 Effects of massage on pain intensity analgesics and quality of life in patients with cancer pain: a pilot study of a randomized clinical trial conducted within a hospice care delivery. Hospice Journal 15(3): 31–53

Wilkinson S, Aldridge J, Salmon I et al 1999 An evaluation of aromatherapy massage in palliative care. Palliative Medicine 13(5): 409–417

Wozniewski M, Jasinski R, Pilch U, Dabrowska G 2001 Complex physical therapy for lymphoedema of the limbs. Physiotherapy 87(5): 252–256

Zanolla R, Monzeglio C, Balzarini A, Martino G 1984 Evaluation of the results of three different methods of postmastectomy lymphedema treatment. Journal of Surgical Oncology 26: 210–213

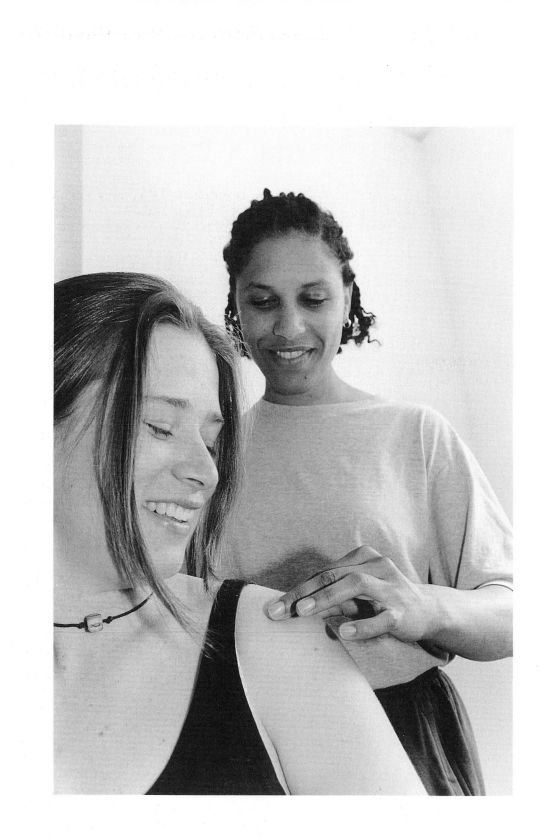

12 Neuromusculoskeletal Disorders

Massage has a particular role in the traditional treatment of musculoskeletal disorders. Its popularity as a core therapeutic intervention within this clinical area of orthodox medicine has varied over time, from being a primary intervention to becoming almost totally disregarded as a useful technique. As physical therapy evolved, Swedish massage was an essential element in the treatment of back and neck pain until techniques with a perceived higher status such as electrotherapy and manipulative therapy became predominant. Consequently the use of massage waned in state-run health care in some countries but it remained an important feature of sports medicine and osteopathy.

One of the problems was that massage was generally assumed to be a symptomatic treatment. Therapists generally believe that, where possible, the cause of symptoms should be identified and eliminated, as treatment that is purely symptomatic is less satisfactory and not cost-effective. Certainly, many patients' problems stem from mechanical, degenerative and inflammatory problems of the joints themselves and massage cannot be said to effect a cure of such problems. However, massage *can* influence the soft tissue problems that occur either in isolation or in association with joint dysfunction.

As structures in the body are neuronally interconnected, a joint cannot undergo changes that alter its normal movement pattern without the surrounding muscles and their connective tissues responding in some way. These secondary changes often become symptomatic. The reflex effect of joint manipulation will prevent development of, and may ease, some of these alterations but is unlikely to reverse long-standing or complex changes.

It is through an *integrated* approach that acute dysfunction of the musculoskeletal system is best treated, ensuring that causative factors are identified and where possible eliminated, and that reflex soft tissue adaptation is corrected, providing total relief of symptoms and preventing recurrence. It should also be recognized that this scenario may occur in reverse, whereby soft tissue problems arising from excess muscle tension can produce postural change and muscle imbalance, thus precipitating joint problems (Marks 1993).

In this chapter, we explore the different soft tissue injuries and responses to bone and joint dysfunction. We also discuss how massage is an essential component of effective musculoskeletal therapy, by examining the total musculoskeletal system in the context of the whole person.

THE MUSCULOSKELETAL SYSTEM

The (neuro) musculoskeletal system comprises the bones of the skeleton, the joints at which movement occurs, the muscles that move them and the nerves that stimulate the muscles. The central nervous system (CNS) must also be included as it is the coordinator of all activity, for example that which occurs in the autonomic nerves to control the blood vessels essential for tissue nutrition, and that in the brain and spinal cord which controls the protective and coordinated movement patterns occurring in response to sensations arising from the periphery.

The skeletal and muscular systems are interconnected through joints and connective tissue. Dysfunction in one part will ultimately affect adjacent parts and may also have a broader effect through postural or gait adaptations. There are many factors that contribute to the original causative factor of musculoskeletal problems and, in some cases, one can lead to another. Those considered here are:

- mechanical
- postural
- occupational
- traumatic
- surgical
- disease.

They are dealt with as: mechanical and postural (including occupational factors, discussed in more detail in Ch. 14); disease; and trauma and surgical factors.

MECHANICAL AND POSTURAL FACTORS

The majority of patients with musculoskeletal problems who seek medical help have back or neck problems. Spinal problems and rheumatological conditions are thought to be much more common in the West than in countries where individuals lead a more active lifestyle. It is widely believed, therefore, that inactivity and resulting postural stresses, or sedentary or repetitive occupational stresses, are responsible for many of the symptoms. Generally, the human body must adjust in accordance with the person's lifestyle. Individuals with physical limitations experience this in reverse: aspects of their lifestyle and behaviour may be dictated by their bodies to a greater extent. Lifestyle requires a particular excursion of joints and stretch of soft tissues which are unique to the individual, and specific activities will put physical structures through a wider range of movement more frequently. In an inactive person or someone whose job involves sitting, repetitive movements or inappropriate physical loading, plastic adaptation of a mechanical or postural nature must occur to accommodate this particular lifestyle.

The postural changes may be as a result of habit, for instance many hours over several years spent slumped in easy chairs, or sitting with rounded shoulders and a poking chin at a keyboard until, gradually, less muscular effort is made to maintain an upright posture against gravity (Figs 12.1, 12.2). The postural (antigravity) muscles have a tendency to shorten (Janda 1983) and become structurally tight, and their antagonists tend to become reflexly inhibited and weakened. This produces postural changes and instability. A typical pattern is one of weakened, lengthened abdominal muscles and weak glutei. The hip flexors and

| FIGURE 12.1 | *Poor sitting posture.* |

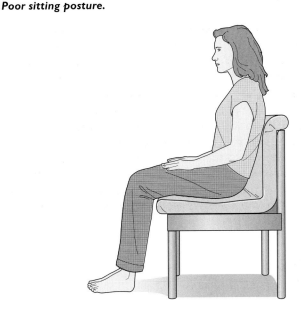

| FIGURE 12.2 | *Use of a lumbar roll to correct poor posture.* |

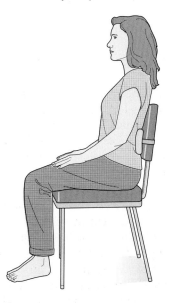

the back extensors become short and tight. This was identified by Janda as the 'crossed pattern'; it is accompanied by tight hamstring muscles, thought to be an attempt to stabilize the pelvis. The situation becomes more complicated where there are many short muscles together. The erector spinae, for example, although seen as one muscle mass running along either side of the spinal column, consists of three groups of muscles (iliocostalis, longissimus and spinalis), each of which has a subgroup in each area of the spine. The fibres of erector spinae run in several different directions over different distances. It is important that these muscles act in coordination, but imbalance can occur within the group. According to Janda, antagonist muscles tend to react in a way that is opposite to their agonist, either weakening or shortening, resulting in a muscular imbalance around a joint and eventually throughout the body.

The muscles adapt to their shortening, probably losing sarcomeres (Williams & Goldspink 1978), and their connective tissue loses length and flexibility. As the reflex weakening of the antagonist occurs, these postural changes become self-perpetuating. They can be exacerbated, or indeed caused, by body language, whereby tall people may develop rounded shoulders, shy people a protective flexed posture in which the pectoral muscles become tight and the thoracic spine flexed and stiff, the chronically depressed a poking chin in which the extensor muscles of the neck become short (for further discussion see Kurtz & Prestera 1984). The normal mechanical stresses which the tissues experience through everyday functional activities are correspondingly altered and may be magnified as some (spinal) joints may now be held at an extreme of their range. The increased stress on the connective tissue causes remodelling and the fibres become laid down along the new lines of stress, so they actually change structure to accommodate the postures. Usual patterns of movement may start to strain this altered tissue. For example, sporting activities, or sudden explosive movements, such as running for a bus which places dynamic stretch on tissue, may strain or partially tear connective tissue. Adhesions or excess fibrous tissue may be laid down in response and attempts to correct the posture to a 'normal' one, or attempts at exercising to strengthen weakened antagonists, will produce pain. This is because 'normal' stress which protects joints has now become 'abnormal' as far as the collagenous tissues are concerned. Applying normal stress will in fact weaken the tissues as the fibres now lie in the direction of the abnormal stress and are therefore ill-equipped to resist normal stress. The obvious result of these attempts to correct the situation will be pain. This scenario was recognized by McKenzie (1981) in his postural syndrome (see box). He recommends fully stretching ligaments and surrounding tissue following injury.

Muscle imbalance leads to altered biomechanical stresses in joints which may precipitate cartilaginous degeneration and stiff or hypermobile joints (Marks 1993). Often, in the spine, one segment becomes damaged or degenerative as the

---

Postural syndrome

Characterized by pain that:

- is alleviated by rest or lying down or by altering position
- is fairly localized (low back pain not referring lower than the knee, or neck pain no lower than the elbow)
- improves on movement
- is accompanied by no history of trauma

stress it experiences is altered from that which the joint was designed to withstand. The accompanying inflammation causes fibrosis and stiffening so an adjacent joint becomes hypermobile and painful in an attempt to maintain normal functional movement. A common example of this is where stiffness of thoracic vertebral joints 1–4 causes pain at cervical 5–6, as is typical in cervical spondylosis, recognized by the forming of a 'ledge' between C6 and C7 and a so-called 'dowager's' or 'buffalo' hump. Adaptation takes place in ligaments and muscles to guard the painful area, and symptoms can be produced from these soft tissues. The loading on muscles may produce spasm, fibrosis and the development of myofascial trigger spots (Travell & Simons 1992), and further postural adaptation may result.

It eventually becomes difficult to understand which changes occurred first – habitual posture, joint dysfunction or occupational stress – and a complete treatment regimen must address all aspects: correcting poor posture and poor ergonomic habits, freeing joints and their surrounding tissues, and settling soft tissue symptoms. Treatment that addresses only some facets of the problem will have only limited success. Weintraube (1986) states that treating only secondary soft tissue changes will remove compensatory mechanisms and may worsen symptoms. He suggests that, in chronic conditions, the joints should be treated first to balance the joint and soft tissue changes.

Some persistent spinal problems fall into the category of a complex chronic back pain model. As the symptoms follow a pattern of quiescence and flare-up, the patient gradually adapts her/his lifestyle. Attempts to increase activity, whether by beginning exercise programmes to increase fitness or changing work or leisure patterns, will create pain as a result of the adaptations already described. This increased irritability of symptoms may cause irritability of mood, which affects relationships with partners, family and friends. Depression or anxiety – whether transient or long term – can become a feature. The increased muscle tone experienced in either of these conditions can exacerbate musculoskeletal symptoms. An altered sleep pattern will perpetuate the problem as sleeplessness due to pain will worsen depression, while 'tossing and turning' due to psychological factors will worsen physical pain and stiffness. Drugs to relieve insomnia, pain or psychological symptoms may cause side-effects such as constipation, which, accompanied by a reduction in physical activity, contributes to the general loss of well-being. Chronic pain can become more complex in that behavioural patterns of the sufferer generally within relationships can become inextricably bound up with the whole syndrome and the disability can be a focus for dependence or caring within a relationship. This scenario can be further complicated when the patient tends to respond emotionally to pain. Further discussion of this is outside the scope of this book, but a full understanding is essential for anyone working in this field. Touch and massage can contribute to a multifactorial, holistic treatment programme for these patients but should be used as *enabling* techniques, to support patients in sharing in the responsibility for their own recovery, rather than to perpetuate passivity. This is particularly important for patients in whom the psychological factors outweigh the physical factors in chronic pain 'syndrome'.

A recent and rigorously controlled study which compared massage, acupuncture and self-care education for chronic low back pain had surprising results. Patients in each of the treatment groups received therapy which was appropriate to their condition, thus following normal clinical practice. Treatments lasted 10 weeks, the patients being assessed at week 4 and week 10.

The massage group scored significantly better than the other groups throughout the trial. A follow-up at 1 year later showed massage and self-care scored almost equally. Acupuncture did not even achieve a significant placebo effect (Cherkin et al 2001).

Where *muscle damage* has occurred as a result of long-term postural stresses or trauma, inflammation will occur at the site of the lesion, which may be at a muscle-connective tissue interface, and fibrous scarring will result. If this is ignored, it will become shortened and adherent, with symptoms persisting even when the active inflammatory processes have resolved. In acute problems, muscle *contraction* causes pain, although a minor lesion in a strong patient may require hard muscle work to reproduce symptoms. Widthways expansion may be allowed during contraction, so contracting the muscle may not cause pain. However, *stretching* the muscle longitudinally may be painful. Thus, exercises to strengthen opposite muscle groups may be ineffective if reciprocal lengthening is not possible, and stretching (both active and through massage) should be an integral part of the rehabilitation of injured muscles. The damage may result in inhibition within a different part of the muscle group, or in altered patterns of recruitment, where the precise coordinated sequential fibre contraction is disturbed. For example, the multifidus is a segmental muscle (Macintosh & Bogduk 1986) and altered preferential recruitment may occur (Norris 1995). A similar situation occurs at the knee where the vastus lateralis may be recruited before the vastus medialis oblique if the latter is inhibited, for example following knee trauma (Gerrard 1989).

The aims of massage in muscle damage should be to: contain inflammation and promote repair; increase nutrition to the area; reduce swelling and inflammatory byproducts; gradually increase mechanical stresses on the immature collagen; ensure strength and mobility at tissue interfaces; facilitate full excursion of the tissue in all directions; and prevent soft tissue contracture. These will reduce pain and promote normal function.

Massage can help alleviate secondary muscle *spasm*. This tends to be due to an acute problem. It is generally thought that muscle tone increases in response to pain as a splinting, protective mechanism. A spasm cycle becomes established in which the spasm is self-perpetuating. Eventually, the circulatory compromise caused by the excess tone may lead to muscle wasting. Shortening of connective tissue occurs and the muscle decreases in length. This mirrors the history of muscle 'tension' which is often found in shoulder girdle and neck muscles as a physical response to stress.

Massage can interrupt the cycle of:

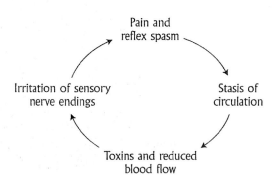

These events can be replaced by a therapeutic cycle, created by massage, whereby an interruption of this pathophsiological cycle will break the chain of ongoing events. However, this theory has more recently come under scrutiny as pain and tenderness in muscles has not been found to correlate to increased muscle tone. In fact, pain tends to inhibit rather than facilitate muscle contraction (Mense et al 2001). Other theories vary from hyperactive muscle spindle activity (Hubbard 1996) to spontanous electrical activity at the motor endplate (Bohr 1995). These theories are supported by some contradictory physiological evidence but tend to focus on specific aspects of the clinical picture such as the presence of myofascial trigger points (see below) and not the whole clinical picture, and ignore the effects felt in the *total* muscle following massage.

Myofascial Trigger Points

Myofascial trigger points (MTPs) were identified by Travell & Simons (1992). They can occur due to any factor (postural, mechanical, metabolic, nutritional, etc.) which alters the local circulation to a few muscle fibres. MTPs are narrow bands of fibres within a muscle which have been held in excess tone or spasm for some time. Eventually, the fibres become ischaemic and fibrous (Fig. 12.3). They are identified by palpation and by a particular pattern of symptoms (see Travell & Simons (1992) for charts of referred pain patterns, and Fig. 12.4).

Symptoms of Myofascial Trigger Points

- Pressure reproduces the pain, including the exact recognizable pattern of referral.

FIGURE 12.3 *Trigger point complex.* **ATrP = Active Trigger Point.**

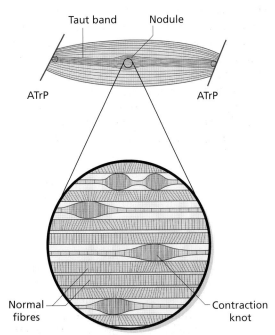

FIGURE 12.4 *Myofascial trigger points and usual areas of referred pain.*

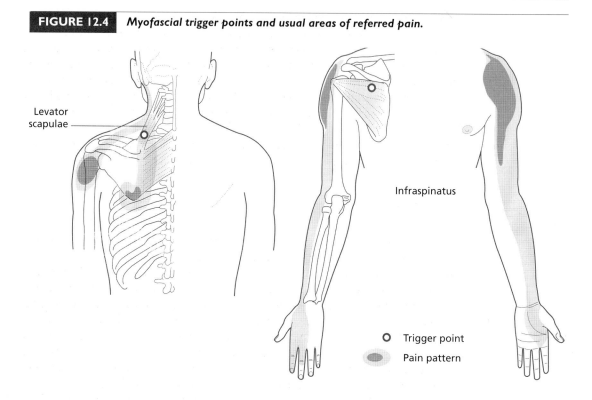

Levator scapulae

Infraspinatus

O Trigger point

● Pain pattern

- A distinct tight band can be felt.
- When the finger slides over the band, a distinctive clear twitch response occurs.
- An active MTP might be described as 'exquisitely tender'.

Treatment

Successful treatment of MTPs has two distinct stages:

1. The first is deactivation – pain relief and reducing the tonicity of the fibres involved.
2. The second is stretching.

Deactivation may be by injection, dry needling, Cyriax frictions, ultrasound, direct pressure or a 'milking' massage technique. The most effective manual therapy methods of MTP deactivation are direct pressure or massage. The pressure must be accurately applied directly on the MTP (which may be perhaps 2 mm in length) at 90 degrees to the fibres, and held for approximately 20 seconds (Travell & Simons 1992). A thumb, elbow, tennis ball or mushroom-shaped wooden implement (Prudden 1984) can be used for either treatment by a therapist or self-treatment. The 'milking' massage technique is a deep stroking performed by the fingertips along the length of the affected fibres. It usually elicits a vivid local erythema.

These techniques all produce relief but must be followed by full-range passive stretching to restore full resting length to the muscles. The initial deactivation will offer only short-term relief. Travell & Simons (1992) recommend the use of vasocoolant spraying prior to stretch but many therapists now use muscle energy techniques whereby the muscle is contracted against static resistance (approximate guidelines are: 5 seconds at 20% of maximum strength if acute, 10 seconds at 30% of strength if chronic, to vary according to patient need and response) before stretching. This utilizes postisometric relaxation of the muscle to allow passive stretch, so there must be a slight pause after contraction and before stretching. Even where the MTPs are chronic, three to five repetitions are often sufficient to produce a full range of stretch and this restored length and function with its accompanying reduction in pain can be maintained by active stretching exercises. Once full range has been achieved, the MTP becomes silent, but predisposing factors must be addressed to prevent recurrence.

DISEASE FACTORS

Arthritis, both inflammatory and degenerative, is often met by the physical therapist and can be a primary cause of many of the secondary soft tissue problems outlined above. The inflammatory type is commonly rheumatoid arthritis or ankylosing spondylitis but many less common syndromes exist, such as infective arthritis and Sjögren's syndrome. Inflammatory arthritis has a systemic component which produces symptoms of fatigue and listlessness when the condition is active. The joints undergo severe inflammatory changes which result in ligament erosion and joint deformity with instability. Degenerative arthritis (osteoarthrosis or spondylosis) is a response to biomechanical, genetic and metabolic factors, and leads to joint deformity with stiffness.

Massage in inflammatory arthritis must be undertaken with great care. The skin is often fragile and must not be overstretched. Bruising may occur easily and joints must be fully supported in a comfortable position. Local massage is contraindicated in an active stage of the disease and general massage is contraindicated where the disease is active systemically. At other times, gentle massage can be therapeutic. Massage in degenerative arthritis is often of considerable value in relieving the secondary soft tissue problems; for example, neck massage in an exacerbation of cervical spondylosis can be beneficial. Care must be taken to ensure the underlying joints are resting in a neutral well-supported position during the massage.

TRAUMA AND SURGERY

Muscle strains and ligament sprains can be minor, involving just a few fibres, or can be severe where the structure undergoes complete rupture. Details of the healing process have been given in previous chapters but, to summarize, the main problems created by soft tissue trauma are oedema and fibrous scarring within the structure. Oedema leads to fibrosis and adhesions, and should be controlled. Pain is caused by the pressure exerted by the tissue fluid and is worsened when movement stretches the damaged tissue.

These problems also occur after surgery (to repair a ruptured muscle or ligament or to fixate a fracture internally, for example). Post-surgical oedema and scarring literally stick tissue layers together, both underneath the scar and in the area of repair. This can seriously compromise joint movement.

Fractures in bones that are not weight-bearing, or which can be fairly readily immobilized externally, may still be treated by the plaster cast method.

This splintage will be left *in situ* until union has occurred, which can take as long as 6 weeks for a Colles' fracture. This immobilization may leave weakening and contracture of the connective tissues. Adhesions may render the joint almost immobile initially. Therapy is required to promote movement, and graded muscle strengthening and massage can play an important part in the early stages, replenishing tissue fluid, restoring pliability to the tissues, stretching adhesions and possibly promoting resorption and remodelling of the fibrous tissue. It is especially valuable, over any type of scar, to stretch and mobilize the new skin and restore mobility at tissue interfaces.

Appropriate stress applied correctly during healing can increase the final length of a scar (Hardy 1989). Scars often turn pale when exercise first puts them on a stretch but eventually they become a healthy colour, reflecting the colour of the surrounding skin. Swelling, which is often trapped in pockets near the scar, eventually dissipates with massage and the scar lifts from the underlying tissue, becoming pliable.

Active exercises will produce these effects to a certain extent, but individual patients often require help in the form of massage. It can be particularly valuable following joint replacements, especially if the patient has been inactive for some time and post-surgical rehabilitation progresses slowly. Massage will promote functional recovery following internal fixation of fractures which have necessitated extensive scarring, for example where the iliotibial tract is involved.

Scar Massage

- Effleurage to increase circulation.
- Static pressure to reduce pockets of swelling.
- Finger and thumb kneading to mobilize the scar and surrounding tissue.
- Skin rolling to restore mobility to tissue interfaces.
- Wringing the scar to stretch and promote collagenous remodelling.
- Cyriax frictions to loosen adhesions.

We will now examine various sections of the body and discuss the specific application of these concepts and principles to each section.

HEADACHES AND NECK PAIN

Many clients suffer from headaches. The types of headache that have relevance to the massage therapist are tension headaches and those of cervical origin. One of the somatic responses to stress is increased tone in shoulder girdle muscles. Subtle changes in body language and posture may occur, the shoulders being held high and the upper back held stiff and straight. This can lead to muscle fatigue, when the muscles ache and feel tired because of metabolic insufficiency and toxin build-up. On palpation, there is increased tone, 'stringy' areas where several muscle fibres are held in increased tension, sometimes surrounded by shortened connective tissue. This is often felt like a rope in the paravertebral muscles. The affected muscles may be extremely tender or may have tender spots in them, or active MTPs. Muscles particularly at risk are those in the cervicothoracic region. Trapezius, supraspinatus, levator scapulae, rhomboids and the scalenes are commonly involved. A painful spot midway between the acromial process (acromion) and T1 is commonly present in the trapezius muscle, and a point in supraspinatus, just above the mid-point of the spine of scapula, can often be found. Most sufferers of tension headaches and neck pain also have tenderness and thickening at the insertion of trapezius on the nuchal line of the occiput, and tenderness and fibrosis at the insertion of levator scapulae (at the superior angle of the scapula), with the borders of this muscle sometimes clearly palpable along its length. The scalenes are often extremely uncomfortable on palpation, the palpation eliciting a toothache-like pain and feeling 'stringy' and tight to the therapist.

Massage often enables the patient to adopt a better neck posture; retraction of a poking chin, for example, may become possible after massage. Range of movement is often increased to a surprising degree following massage, and functional activities such as driving and sleeping become easier. Even migraines can reduce in frequency following a combination of massage, muscle energy technique and postural correction. Massage has been found, when used in combination with relaxation therapy, to be more effective than acupuncture in terms of pain frequency and severity, duration of migraines and severity and number of migraine days (Wylie et al 1997). This approach can be particularly useful where the underlying joints are irritable and do not readily tolerate mobilizing and manipulative techniques, or where manipulation is contraindicated. Hernandez-Reif et al (1998) found that 30 minutes of massage, performed twice-weekly, over 5 weeks, reduced pain, anxiety, frequency of headaches, and also increased serotonin levels and improved sleep patterns in the massage group compared with the control group. Nine out of the 26 patients had migraine headaches. This was a scientifically designed study but it does not differentiate between the effects of massage itself and the effects of touch. A similar study comparing massage with a touch-based placebo would give more information about specific therapeutic effects of massage. Wylie et al (1997) found that both acupuncture and massage and relaxation significantly improved pain ratings in patients suffering from chronic headache, but that massage had a greater effect than acupuncture. More detailed examination of the cervical spine is often possible following massage as tenderness is reduced and movement increased. Underlying joint problems can be treated more satisfactorily due to reduced tenderness and guarding spasm.

Grimsby & Grimsby (1993) compared joint manipulation with massage and passive stretching in the cervical spine of 14 patients with C3 dysfunction. Both groups showed increased angle of movement following treatment, but muscle tone, as measured by electromyography, reduced following manipulation and increased in the massage and stretching group in five of seven subjects. Unfortunately the effects of massage were not studied separately, a small sample was used and each patient had the left scalenes stretched, regardless of the symptoms. Stretching did not involve postisometric techniques, which have been shown to be the most effective method of stretching (Entyre & Abraham 1986). While this study is thought provoking, its results are inconclusive because of the small sample size and provide insufficient justification for the choice of stretching technique.

Nilsson et al (1997) found that deep friction massage and laser therapy, given to the lower cervical and thoracic region including all MTPs, was less effective for the treatment of cervicogenic headache than therapeutic exercise or manipulation. This is not surprising as clinical reasoning would suggest that treatment targeting spinal joints would be more effective than a treatment which targeted the soft tissues where headaches are derived from the cervical spine. The researchers had used frictions as a control treatment as it was so unlikely to be effective.

BACK PAIN

Back pain is an increasingly serious problem in the UK, accounting for 14–15 million consultations annually with general practitioners (Clinical Standards Advisory Group 1994). Back problems range from those of traumatic origin, where a single incident results in identifiable damage, to the spontaneous episodes of self-resolving back pain, which can be thought of as 'normal occurrences'.

In the acute stage, back pain is accompanied by spasm and soft tissue pain. Muscle imbalance is commonly seen, for example a shortened quadratus lumborum can produce a 'shortened leg' or a scoliosis. The paraspinal muscles can be very tender in acute spasm. In more chronic conditions, the lumbar fascia can become tight, especially where periods of immobility have occurred. Tenderness and thickening may be present around the margins of the lumbar fascia, at the points of attachment along the lower costal margin, at the junction with the abdominal fascia, along the iliac crest and sacrum and supraspinal ligaments. MTPs may be present, particularly in the buttock muscles. A 'piriformis syndrome' can exist where an MTP in this muscle involves branches of the sciatic nerve (which may pass directly below or through this muscle), referring pain down the leg. Nodules are often palpated around and below the iliac crests. Grieve (1990) suggests that these are fat herniations through the fascial layer. They appear to become painful when they are adhered to the surrounding tissue, or inflamed. Massage increases circulation and mobilizes them, often rendering them painless.

Massage in *acute* back pain should aim to:

- promote local and general relaxation
- increase circulation
- reduce oedema
- reduce muscle spasm.

Massage in *chronic* back pain should aim to:

- reduce muscle spasm
- stretch shortened tissues
- mobilize adhesions and tissue interfaces
- relieve symptoms of stress.

The strokes and massage routine will therefore be varied accordingly.

The number of treatments required by these patients can often be reduced if manual therapy is augmented by massage. Manual therapy must, however, be followed by an active rehabilitation programme. Research has shown that active functional rehabilitation is effective in the treatment of back pain (Frost & Klaber Moffet 1992); thus manual techniques are to be used as enabling techniques, to facilitate dynamic self-rehabilitation.

UPPER LIMB PROBLEMS (Box 12.1)

In many upper limb problems, the whole arm and posture must be examined and included in the treatment. Many work-related upper limb disorders involve adverse neural tension which occurs in the neck region due to poor postural habits. In conditions such as tennis elbow and carpal tunnel syndrome the neck must be assessed and, if massage is incorporated into the treatment, areas such as the scapula region, where 'grating' may be felt by the patient, and nodules underneath or along the vertebral border of scapula should be included.

Li Zumo (1984) reported on 235 patients with frozen shoulder who were treated by manipulation and massage, for at least four sessions each: 146 of the 205 patients in the group having massage and exercises had complete recovery, whereas only three patients improved in the group having manipulation, exercises and hand massage. The samples were uneven in size and subjective measures were used. However, all 205 patients in the massage group showed 'satisfactory' results and a significant difference was demonstrated between the two groups.

Scapula release is often important in the treatment of patients with shoulder problems; Cyriax friction techniques are useful in the treatment of rotator cuff tendinitis, tennis or golfer's elbow, and de Quervain's syndrome. Massage of the upper limb, especially the flexors of the forearm, can offer relief to chronic carpal tunnel syndrome sufferers, particularly following release surgery; however, where neural tension or poor posture (increasing pressure in the anterior triangle of neck) precipitates the symptoms, then massage is merely palliative and the cause should preferentially be addressed. Care must be taken where the condition exists in pregnancy. It is thought to be due to increased fluid retention and thus any increase in pressure in the wrist induced by massage will be detrimental.

Massage is particularly valuable following hand injuries. Swelling is often trapped in the fascial spaces of the hand and massage will aid its reabsorption. A combination of massage and string wrapping has been found to be effective for swollen fingers (Flowers 1988). Scarring in the hand, which inevitably follows trauma or surgery, can have serious consequences. A small loss of excursion of soft tissue, following scarring or immobilization, can have

BOX 12.1	*Common upper limb disorders*
Shoulder:	Supraspinatus tendinitis
	Rotator cuff lesions
	Bicipital tendinitis
	Subacromial bursitis
Elbow:	Tennis elbow
	Golfer's elbow
	Ligament sprain
Wrist and hand:	Tendinitis/tenosynovitis
	De Quervain's syndrome
	Ligament sprain
	Carpal tunnel syndrome

significant functional implications in a hand, which depends on full movement of many small joints for essential functions such as power grip and pinch grip. Scar massage with lanolin-type creams is therefore usually an important part of a hand rehabilitation programme, particularly in conditions such as Dupuytren's contracture, in which scarring tends to be thick and dense. Massage is also important following splintage, to mobilize the tissues and facilitate active exercises.

THE LOWER LIMB (Box 12.2)

Particular issues in the lower limb include swelling around the ankle, which occurs following local injuries such as sprains or is caused by gravitational movement of more proximal oedema. Firm strokes with the thumb or fingertips can be applied in the tissue spaces on either side of the malleoli and Achilles tendon. These are known as Bisgaard strokes. Friction techniques are useful in chronic sprains of the ankle, coronary ligaments of the knee, and muscle tears. Deep techniques along the iliotibial tract can promote stretch in cases of trochanteric bursitis or where post-surgical scarring is present. In addition, circulatory massage is often beneficial in a wide range of individuals, and leg massage is helpful to the sportsperson.

BOX 12.2	*Common lower limb disorders*
Hip and thigh:	Iliotibial band syndrome
	Trochanteric bursitis
	Piriformis syndrome
	Muscle tears
Knee and lower leg:	Ligament sprain
	Compartment syndrome
	Tendinitis
	Bursitis
	Meniscal tears
	Patellofemoral dysfunction
Foot and ankle:	Tendinitis/tenosynovitis
	Ligament sprain
	Stress fractures

KEY POINTS

♦ The best approach to the treatment of acute musculoskeletal problems involves treating the cause and correcting reflex soft tissue adaptation.

♦ Soft tissue changes, either primary or secondary, can be symptomatic and may be helped by massage.

♦ Touch and massage can contribute to the management of patients with chronic pain but must enable the patient to change aspects of lifestyle.

♦ Massage should not inadvertently perpetuate passivity in a patient with a chronic condition: it should facilitate dynamic self-rehabilitation.

♦ Massage should be used in muscle trauma to: promote reduced pain and improved local nutrition; reduce swelling and inflammatory by-products; promote remodelling; prevent scar contraction.

♦ The cycle of muscle spasm can be interrupted by a therapeutic cycle initiated by massage.

♦ Scar massage can reduce local swelling, mobilize, stretch and promote remodelling of the scar.

♦ In acute back pain, massage can reduce pain, spasm, oedema, increase circulation and promote relaxation.

♦ In chronic back pain, massage can reduce spasm, stretch and mobilize shortened tissues and reduce stress.

REFERENCES.

Bohr T W 1995 Fibromyalgia syndrome and myofascial pain syndrome: do they exist? Neurology Clinics 13(2): 365–384

Cherkin D C, Eisenberg D, Sherman D et al 2001 Randomized trial comparing traditional Chinese medical acupuncture, therapeutic massage, and self-care education for chronic low back pain.

Clinical Standards Advisory Group 1994 Report of a CSAG committee on back pain. HMSO, London

Entyre B R, Abraham L D 1986 Gains in range of ankle dorsiflexion using three popular stretching techniques. American Journal of Physical Medicine 65: 189

Flowers K R 1988 String wrapping versus massage for reducing digital volume. Physical Therapy 68(1): 57–59

Frost H, Klaber Moffet J 1992 Physiotherapy management of chronic low back pain. Physiotherapy 78(10): 751–755

Gerrard B 1989 The patello-femoral pain syndrome: a clinical trial of the

McConnell programme. Australian Journal of Physiotherapy 35: 74–80

Grieve G P 1990 Episacroiliac lipoma. Physiotherapy 76(6): 308–310

Grimsby D, Grimsby K 1993 Electromyographic and range of motion evaluation to compare the results of two treatment approaches: soft tissue massage versus a segmental manipulation of the cervical spine. Nederlands Tijdshcrift Voor Manuele Therapie 12(1): 2–7

Hardy M A 1989 The biology of scar formation. Physical Therapy 69(12): 22–32

Hernandez-Reif M, Field T, Dieter J, Swerdlow Diego M 1998 Migraine headaches are reduced by massage therapy. International Journal of Neuroscience 96: 1–11

Hubbard D R 1996 Chronic and recurrent muscle pain: pathophysiology and treatment and review of pharmacological studies. Journal of Musculoskeletal Pain 4(1/2): 124–142

Janda V 1983 On the concept of postural muscles and posture in man. Australian Journal of Physiotherapy 29(3): 83–84

Kurtz R, Prestera H 1984 The body reveals. Harper and Row, New York

Li Zumo 1984 Two hundred and thirty-five cases of frozen shoulder treated by manipulation and massage. Journal of Traditional Chinese Medicine 4(3): 213–215

Macintosh J E, Bogduk N 1986 The biomechanics of the lumbar multifidus. Clinical Biomechanics 1: 205–213

McKenzie R A 1981 The lumbar: spine mechanical diagnosis and therapy. Spinal Publications, Waikanae, New Zealand

Marks R 1993 Muscles as a pathogenic factor in osteoarthritis. Physiotherapy Canada 45(4): 251–259

Mense S, Simons D G, Russell I J 2001 Muscle pain: understanding its nature, diagnosis and treatment. Lippincott/Williams and Wilkins, Philadelphia, PA

Nilsson N, Christansen H W, Hertvigsen J 1997 The effect of spinal manipulation in the treatment of cervicogenic headache. Journal of Manipulative and Physiological Therapeutics 20(5): 326–330

Norris C M 1995 Spinal stabilisation: 3. Stabilisation mechanisms of the lumbar spine. Physiotherapy 81(2): 72–79

Prudden B 1984 Myotherapy: Bonnie Prudden's complete guide to pain-free living. Doubleday, New York

Travell J G, Simons D G 1992 Myofascial pain and dysfunction: the trigger point manual, vol. 2. Williams and Wilkins, Baltimore, MD

Weintraube A 1986 Lumbar soft tissue mobilisation. In: Grieve G (ed) Modern manual therapy of the vertebral column. Churchill Livingstone, London

Williams P E, Goldspink G 1978 Changes in sarcomere length and physiological properties in immobilised muscle. Journal of Anatomy 127: 459–468

Wylie K R, Jackson C, Crawford P M 1997 Does psychological testing help to predict the response to acupuncture or massage/relaxation therapy in patients presenting to a general neurology clinic with headache? Journal of Traditional Chinese Medicine 17(2): 130–139

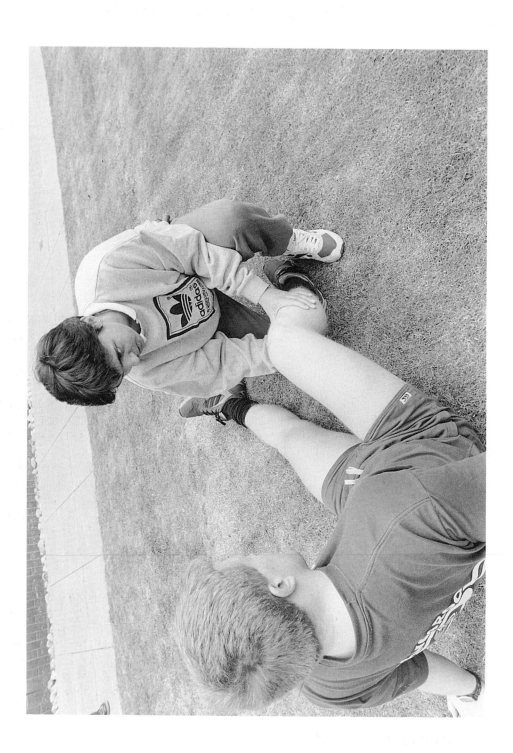

13 Massage in Sport

Massage is widely used in the training of athletes and in the treatment of sports injuries, being an essential component of sports rehabilitation. It is used to enhance athletic performance, to assist recovery from sport and exercise, to assist training, to facilitate the healing and remodelling of damaged tissues and to promote local and general relaxation.

When assisting the body to prepare for sport, the specific needs of the sportsperson should be identified and addressed. This applies whether the individual is a reluctant or enthusiastic amateur or a highly motivated, finely turned, world-class athlete. Training and rehabilitation, in which massage may play a part, should be at the optimum level for the type and class of sport played by the individual. Massage needs to be adapted to the specific situation, for example an amateur sports player may neglect training, warming up and stretching, and massage would play an important role in maintaining tissue pliability to prevent injury. A well-motivated top-class athlete, on the other hand, might have a tendency to overtrain, so recovery from fatigue is an essential component of training and massage could play a central role in this.

The effects of massage have already been discussed in this book. In this chapter we concentrate on specific effects of particular relevance to sport, and discuss their application in this specialized field. To apply massage to this client group, it is necessary to have an understanding of the effects of exercise on the soft tissues and the symptoms that exercise may produce. It is also essential for knowledge of the pathophysiology of soft tissue stress, healing and repair to guide clinical decision-making, or therapeutic massage may result in damage to tissues and, consequently, to reduced performance.

HEALING AND REPAIR

For sport to be safe, the body must adapt to the extra stresses placed upon it. These can be the dynamic stresses of power, agility, coordination and concentration. The body also has to cope with activity at the extremes of joint movement and muscle length, heavy demands in terms of endurance and strength, and physical contact with team-mates or opponents. Any one, or a combination, of these factors may be needed in a particular sport.

For the body to be able to meet these demands, it must have freely moving joints which have a full range of movement in all available directions. It also needs good muscle strength and strong and pliable connective tissue. The cardiovascular requirements are of peripheral importance to this discussion and, although their importance should be acknowledged, they are not expanded on here.

Excess or repetitive stresses or overwork applied to musculoskeletal structures result in a higher incidence of minor strains and sprains than would be found in an individual who does not participate regularly in sport. These events may occur in the muscles and connective tissue of any sportsperson. In addition, there may be specific injury – muscle and ligament tears, for example. In either case, contractile tissue or pliable connective tissue is replaced by scar tissue. This can bind the interfaces of adjacent tissues as well as interfaces within the same tissue such as between fibre bundles. Adhesions can occur within tissues such as joint capsules, and these adhesions ultimately become part of the tissue itself. However, as they are of non-specialized collagen and of different fibre orientation, their presence can result in a loss of length, pliability, widthways stretching and movement between fibres and fibre bundles. If they are left, any activity which takes a structure to its normal physiological limit will re-strain it, owing to its extensibility being slightly reduced, and this will begin the process over again. Thus, continuous stress or overuse will lead to a cycle of:

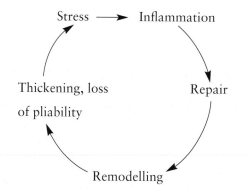

The purpose of massage in these circumstances is to stretch and mobilize the adhesions and to restore the level of mobility to as near normal as possible. Massage will also assist remodelling and promote absorption of the scar, encouraging connective tissue to be laid down in a more appropriate way. This will enable the tissue to withstand the stresses placed upon it, thus ensuring its strength. Adhesions, therefore, are not 'broken down' as such, as is commonly assumed. This would seriously compromise the structure by causing a breakdown of the capsule or ligament itself, setting up a whole new cycle of inflammation, healing and repair. A more natural part of the healing and remodelling process is influenced rather than the massage introducing a new trauma to the tissues (Fig. 13.1).

FIGURE 13.1   *Phases of wound healing.*

Phases of Wound Healing

Phase	Onset	Peak	Duration	Pathophysiology	Wound Strength	Management
Traumatic inflammation	0	12 hours	24–48 hours	Vascular response: bleeding, oedema Cellular (phagocytosis) response: leucocytes, macrophages	Negligible	Rest Elevation Ice
Proliferation of fibroblasts	12 hours	2–5 days	10 days	Fibroblasts proliferate, migrate and bridge wound edges by 5 days	Some	Rest Elevation
Collagen (fibroplasia)	5 days	3 months	6 months	Collagen fibrils: initially weak random fibrils, later strong flexible fibres depending on the stress placed upon them	Rapid rise	Splintage of the repaired tissue Exercise
Remodelling	1 month	→	2 years or more	Collagenase removes excess collagen, fibroblasts contract, and there is vascular and wound shrinkage	Continued gradual rise	Exercise and return of function

Adapted from The Hand Fundamentals of Therapy, p. 2, by Boscheinen-Morrin *et al.* (1992). Butterworth-Heinemann, Oxford.

FATIGUE

In periods of increased training, the body may not be allowed to recover fully between sessions and this results in reduced performance. Overtraining can be recognized by local symptoms of muscle and joint inflammation and discomfort, and also by the general effects of sleeplessness and restlessness. This is accompanied by an increased susceptibility to injury. Massage can be useful in reducing muscle tone and tension, reducing muscular discomfort and promoting a local and general relaxation; it has also been shown to increase recovery from fatigue in the quadriceps (Ask et al 1987). Research by Balke and co-workers (1989) showed that manual and mechanical massage aids the resolution of post-exercise fatigue more effectively than rest. Seven subjects performed a gradual exercise test on a treadmill and then had 15–20 minutes of rest, manual or mechanical massage of the legs. The Thumper percussive massager was used for the mechanical massage. The same procedure was followed twice: once when the exercise taken was predominantly cardiovascular and once when it involved strength and endurance of the leg muscles. Recovery from fatigue, indicated by the level of repeat performance, was shown in both massage groups. Unfortunately, details of statistical analysis were not given so further evaluation of this research is not possible. The authors suggest that the results indicate that mechanical self-massage should be used more widely, rather than just reliance on a therapist.

MUSCLE SORENESS (Fig. 13.2)

Massage is often sought by the sportsperson to reduce post-exercise muscle soreness. Research has suggested that the type of soreness needs to be identified and the massage adapted accordingly. There are two types of exercise-related muscle soreness, one which arises during the exercise, which is usually referred to as 'muscle stiffness', and the second occurring after a delay. The latter is known as delayed-onset muscle soreness (DOMS).

Pain during exercise is familiar to us all. It can occur quickly when walking up an unaccustomed steep hill, for example. With exposure to the task, the muscles become capable of performing more of the activity before the onset of pain. It is widely accepted that this type of pain is due to metabolic insufficiency: the muscle outperforms its metabolic supply and an algesic substance is thought to be released from the muscle itself. Energy demands are met by phosphate levels, which are maintained through oxidative metabolism in Krebs' cycle (Lamb et al 1984). If the blood supply cannot meet these demands for oxygen, glycolysis can assist, though less efficiently, and lactic acid will be

---

FIGURE 13.2   *Structure of a muscle organ. Reproduced, with permission, from Thibodeau & Patton (1999).*

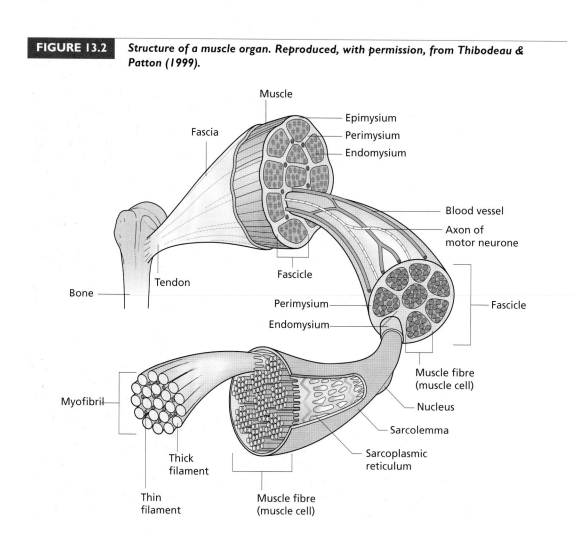

formed. This has previously been assumed to be the primary algesic substance in exercised muscles. A muscle in top condition will have a well-functioning capillary bed which ensures that the muscle is well perfused with oxygenated blood; the algesic substance (i.e. the by-product of metabolism whose production exceeds its removal by the bloodstream) will be slow to appear and will be removed quickly. However, in a deconditioned muscle, the algesic substance will be produced faster than it can be removed in the bloodstream and therefore the muscle may become much more painful. It has been widely thought that lactate is responsible for the pain, but it is now believed that the algesic substance is more likely to be potassium, which stimulates pain fibres (Jones & Round 1990). It has been shown that massage does, in fact, influence lactate levels (Bale & James 1991), which are indicative of metabolic processes, but the common assumption that this is of significance to muscle soreness no longer holds. Bale & James (1991) examined nine male athletes who were required to run for 2.5 minutes on a treadmill at 12–13.5 miles per hour. Following a 3-minute rest period, they had passive rest, massage or a warm-down run. The warm-down and massage groups showed statistically significant drops in blood lactate levels following treatment. The massage group also showed drops in perceived stiffness scores. The small sample size undermines the strength of this research, which also showed no increased flexibility in any of the groups. The reduction in perceived stiffness in the massage group is interesting and could be due to the mobilizing effects of massage on connective tissue, a flushing of the tissues with new, replenished tissue fluid or thixotrophy effects. Martin et al (1998) found that, in a group of 10 male cyclists, active recovery produced a significant reduction in blood lactate levels compared with sports massage and rest. These findings were substantiated by Monodero & Donne (2000) who found that active exercise was better than passive rest or massage in removing blood lactate at minutes 9 and 12. Combined recovery (active exercise and massage) was better at removing blood lactate at 15 minutes than passive or active recovery or massage. Combined recovery was also better in maintaining performance time. This study could help to explain some of the conflicting research results – perhaps a combined intervention approach is needed.

Hemmings et al (2000) found that massage significantly increased perceptions of recovery but did not significantly change blood lactate levels or glucose when compared with rest, after a first performance on a boxing ergometer. Massage did, however, significantly increase blood lactate concentration after a second ergometer performance.

Delayed-onset pain is felt a few hours after exercise and may persist for several days. It is often noted the morning after a period of increased training or excessive gardening. The pain is accompanied by tenderness and a feeling of stiffness which can be disabling. This occurs as a result of eccentric muscle work, otherwise known as isometric lengthening. This is the most common type of muscle work when weight-bearing: the foot is on the ground and the large leg muscles lengthen gradually while supporting the body-weight against gravity (as in the action of the quadriceps, when 'paying out' to control the movement of descending stairs, for example, or the action of biceps when the elbow is straightened to lower a weight held in the hand). Pain is associated with fatigue: if muscles are exercised to the point where they exhibit tremor, they are more likely to experience DOMS. It is thought that the pain may be due to connective tissue inflammation as research has found poor correlation between muscle damage and tenderness. Research has found evidence of myofibre disruption and collagen breakdown, thought to be due to an inflammatory response (Brown et al 1997). Vincent & Vincent (1997) found that, in weight lifters, soreness can be experienced without the high serum creatine kinase levels indicative of muscle damage. Training and massage delay the onset of the soreness, which suggests that compliance and/or strength of connective tissue increases. Clinically, massage appears to reduce the soreness, facilitating an earlier commencement of training. Research evidence, however, is inconclusive due to methodological flaws and lack of standardization across studies. Much of the research does suggest that massage may have a positive effect on DOMS, and Ernst (1998), following a review of the research, concludes that massage may be a positive treatment for DOMS. However, an earlier review by Tiidus (1997) led him to conclude that the paucity of evidence should lead to its use in athletic settings to be questioned. Armstrong (1990) has suggested that the events surrounding DOMS are acute inflammation, inflammatory pain, swelling, reduced range of movement, reduced force output, and reduced adherence and willingness to exercise. This is a phenomenon of considerable significance to any individual wishing to participate regularly in sport/exercise.

Pertinent research has been conducted by Smith et al (1994), examining the role of massage in DOMS. Untrained male subjects performed five sets of isokinetic eccentric contractions of the elbow flexors and extensors. The experimental group ($n = 7$) were given an 'athletic' massage for 30 minutes, 2 hours after exercising, while the control group ($n = 7$) rested. DOMS and creatine kinase levels were assessed before exercise and at 8, 24, 48, 72, 96 and 102 hours after exercise. Circulating neutrophils were assessed before, immediately after and at 30-minute intervals for 8 hours post-exercise. It was found that massage reduced DOMS and creatine kinase levels (showing skeletal muscle specificity) in the massage group and that massage also produced a prolonged increase in the level of circulating neutrophils. The explanation offered for this was that the DOMS was, indeed, due to inflammatory changes in the connective tissue. Neutrophils are essential for an inflammatory response to occur. Thus, if the neutrophils were dissipated in the bloodstream by massage, the inflammation would resolve and further inflammation be prevented, reducing the level and duration of DOMS. However, this promising research (there were only seven subjects in each group, which may be too small a number for conclusive inferences to be drawn from the statistical results) contradicts previous findings.

Molea et al (1987), Wenos and colleagues (1990), Weber et al (1994) and Hemmings (2000a) have shown massage to be ineffective in reducing DOMS. In these earlier studies, massage was conducted either immediately following, 24 or 48 hours after exercise. Smith et al (1994) were guided in their methodological decisions by the Soviet literature (Krilov et al 1985, Paikov 1985, Burovych et al 1989), which suggests that massage should be given 1–3 hours after exercise to enhance athletic performance. Soviet sports massage is well developed and Smith et al (1994) accepted their recommendations and chose 2 hours as the time required for an accumulation of neutrophils to occur. Massage before this point may increase circulation but would precede the specific time when grouped neutrophils could be dissipated into the bloodstream. This research therefore suggests that not only can massage reduce DOMS, but that its timing is crucial. Post-event massage should be conducted 2 hours after the event for best therapeutic benefit, although this research should be substantiated by a larger study as the small sample size weakens its statistical base.

Further research which may help to inform the use of soft tissue manipulation is that conducted by Wiktorsson-Möller et al (1983). This research has shown that, although stretch is better than massage and warm-up in increasing range of motion, massage of triceps surae increases the range of dorsiflexion both with the knee flexed and with it extended, suggesting this is due to passive manual elongation. It would be expected, from our understanding of connective tissue biomechanics, that stretch is superior to massage as prolonged longitudinal stretch (as produced by an active stretching exercise) straightens out the crimping in the collagen fibres in the toe region of the stress–strain curve, as discussed in Chapter 2. It is possible that the variation in fibre orientation within the triceps surae complex (soleus and the lateral and medial heads of gastrocnemius) means that the multidirectional stretching effect of massage is more effective than a unidirectional longitudinal stretching. It is probable that a combination of massage and active stretching would be the most effective approach. Research would elucidate this suggestion.

A more puzzling result was that massage alone was followed by a statistically significant reduction in muscle strength in the hamstrings and quadriceps of eight men, as measured by a Cybex II dynamometer. Again, it should be noted that many statisticians would dismiss statistical significance in so small a sample but an attempt should be made to understand the trend. Perhaps it could be due to a reduction in the resting tone of the muscle, establishing a lower starting point for the contraction. This was, unfortunately, not monitored in the study, and so must remain supposition.

Research into sports massage raises more questions than it answers. Is there a difference in result depending on whether deep tissue massage or more superficial massage is performed, through layers of slippery oil? How significant is the timing of the massage? Is a combined approach to post-exercise recovery better than the use of single modalities? Massage plays a big part in sports training and therapy. Many sports physiotherapists, however, believe that while clinical evidence shows that massage improves the pliability and general condition of the tissues (perhaps helping to prevent injury, improve the effects of healing and enhance performance if performed regularly), the effects of massage on enhancing recovery from exercise and reducing DOMS is doubtful. Massage is also believed to have an important psychological effect in a client group whose performance is strongly influenced by psychological factors. There is emerging evidence to support this (Hemmings 2000a, 2000b; Hemmings et al 2000).

An interesting study by Blackman et al (1998) found that while massage did not improve post-exercise anterior compartment pressures in seven athletes with suspected anterior chronic exertional compartment syndrome (ACECS), work performed in dorsiflexion to pain onset was improved following a course of massage. The authors concluded that intermittent massage and stretching may be useful in the treatment of ACECS.

To ensure that the massage is applied appropriately to the sportsperson, and also to the specific situation of training or rehabilitation, the therapist should ensure that her assessment of the client is comprehensive and includes details of the sport and training programme. An individualized plan should be drawn up in negotiation with the client. Consultation with other professionals such as the coach or doctor may be necessary to ensure that all approaches complement, rather than conflict, with each other. The type of massage should be based on rational therapeutic principles:

- *Is it a general conditioning or relaxing massage?* A general conditioning massage aims to promote faster recovery during training and two sessions should be added to the training schedule. All the strokes of classical massage can be used with pressure/trigger point stimulation.
- *Is it a post-travel massage, in which case stiffness, circulation and metabolic balance would be the main concerns?* Massage in this circumstance aims to increase circulation, tissue mobilization and well-being and all classical massage strokes can be used.
- *Is it a whole body treatment or is it aimed at a specific part of the body to assist in the treatment of a particular injury?* General all-body massage or selection of specific strokes to match individual treatment aims should be applied.
- *What stage of healing has the injury reached?* The timetable of healing should be used to inform clinical decisions.
- *At what time of day should it best occur and on what day?* Relative to the training programme or events diary.
- *Is it a pre-competition (warm-up) massage?* The aim here is to increase circulation and temperature, and increase tissue mobility. Classical massage strokes and pressure/trigger point stimulation should be given.
- *Is it an inter-competition (for soreness and cramp) massage?* This type of massage should promote recovery – identifying injuries, preventing soreness and having a psychological effect. The usual strokes should be constantly interspersed with effleurage to remove waste products liberated by the massage. If the massage is given before a warm-up, then stimulatory strokes should be added such as shaking and vibrations.
- *Or is it a post-competition massage?* Post-competition, the cardiovascular system must return to normal and removal of waste products, identifying injuries and preventing soreness are standard aims which accompany the positive psychological effects. Classical massage strokes should be used within the athlete's pain threshold, so without tapotement and with plenty of effleurage. Careful techniques such as light feathering with fingertips, to reduce cramp, may be added (Watt 1999).

It is thought that a vigorous massage may stress the body like a training session and therefore activity should be reduced slightly over the following 24–48 hours (Ylinen & Cash 1988). There is, however, dispute as to whether massage causes significant mechanical trauma to muscles. Arkko et al (1983) suggested that the rise in lactate dehydrogenase levels during their massage study (see Ch. 3) was due to mechanical trauma; however, these findings did not substantiate those of Danneskiold-Samsoe and colleagues (1982), who found no increased levels of lactate dehydrogenase. In this earlier study there were further findings which suggest that muscle damage did not occur (see Ch. 3 for a more detailed discussion). Obviously, massage can be conducted at different intensities to differing effect, and further research is essential for our understanding of the effects of massage and its safe application. Until this knowledge is available, the therapist should be fully aware of the possibility of massage-induced mechanical trauma and the detrimental effect this would have on fatigued muscle. It is wise to avoid massaging an athlete for the first time within 3 days of an event. Additionally, the media should be appropriate to the situation: for example, oils should not be used with ball players just before a game as it may make their hands slippery. It is worth noting that massage of the lower limbs does not affect an individual's oxygen consumption or cardiovascular function (Boone & Cooper 1995), so pre-event massage should not have an adverse effect on the athlete's cardiovascular performance during competition.

TREATMENT OF INJURY

Massage has a clearer role in the rehabilitation of sports injuries; however, it must be emphasized that there is *no* place for massage in the direct treatment of an *acute injury*; this should be clear to anyone who has sufficient under-standing of pathophysiological processes to qualify as a practitioner of thera-peutic sports massage. Inflammation is an important part of the healing process and should be *permitted, but contained* in rehabilitation. It is necessary to establish, from the history of injury and physical examination, which struc-ture is affected, and how. Examination should include a manual examination so that the therapist can feel whether there is any tightness or shortening, reduced pliability, stuck, immobile, or separated fibres, circulatory changes, swelling or pain. The treatment of choice in acute injury is:

Rest with controlled movement
Ice
Compression
Elevation.

A danger of massage being performed too early is that of increased inflamma-tion by provoked vasodilatation. It is also possible for clots to be dislodged and tiny emboli to occur. There is a further danger that myositis ossificans may be stimulated. Danchik et al (1993) reported a case in which a 20-year-old hockey player received a blow to the lateral aspect of the thigh. There was considerable swelling. At 4 hours following injury, radiography showed a huge mass develop-ing in the muscle. Immediate treatment after the injury had been vigorous massage, active stretching, heat with hot packs, analgesic cream and the applica-tion of an elastic bandage, before allowing a return to the field. According to the authors, any such mass normally reabsorbs with rest and would not normally be visible on radiography within 3–4 weeks of the injury. The appearance of a huge mass at 4 hours post-injury is clearly abnormal and was highly likely to have been stimulated by the massage. Such injuries are very common and it is widely agreed that ice is the first-aid measure of choice – massage is contraindicated. Inappropriate massage such as this would result in the athlete being prevented from participating in sport for a considerable length of time, while the myositis is reabsorbed with rest. This would clearly have serious implications for a top-class athlete. There is also the real risk of permanent damage.

It must be stressed that massage over recent injuries may dislodge the clot and cellular organization and initiate bleeding (Arnheim 1989). It could also disturb a haematoma, possibly dislodging emboli, and may lengthen the healing phase.

The Strokes

Like any other, a sports massage should be tailored to the individual client. However, experience has shown which strokes are of most use:

1. Effleurage should be chosen to increase drainage.
2. Petrissage must be included in order to release fluid from the tissues, increase fluid interchange, stretch and restore mobility at tissue interfaces and between individual fibres and fibre bundles, and stretch adhesions. The multidirectional stretch will be particularly pertinent to muscle with multidirectional fibres.
3. Cyriax cross-fibre frictions can be used to promote remodelling by encouraging resorption and reorientation of scar tissue.
4. Static pressures and deep kneading can reduce muscle tension.
5. Friction strokes produce a bow-string effect, reducing muscle tone.
6. Strumming (pushing the fibres sideways to produce a bowing effect, perpendicular to the direction of fibres) mobilizes muscle tissue widthways, across the full spread of the muscle.
7. Stretching techniques will mobilize local areas, for example the patella retinaculum or iliotibial tract.
8. Myofascial release can be given to stretch fascia; or connective tissue manipulation can be used for a more profound reflex autonomic effect.
9. J stroking (with fingertips, fingers applied perpendicularly to the muscle) can reduce tender spots.
10. Cross-hand stationary release techniques can be used to initiate a release in the tissues, felt as a palpable 'give' under and between the hands.
11. Neuromuscular technique can detect and treat particular trouble spots.
12. Travell's 'milking' technique can deactivate trigger spots. This must be followed by a full stretch of the affected muscle.
13. Medical vibrators and mechanical massagers can be used for a strong, less specific, effect.

A carefully selected combination of these techniques can be used to assist in preparation for sport, and recovery from it. It can also reduce pain, thereby increasing function and performance. If applied following the event (2 hours is probably the optimal time) it can reduce DOMS. Massage can be applied in a general way, as a whole body relaxation or conditioning massage to assist performance; it can be applied to the limb that will undergo the most stress; or it can be confined to one troubled or vulnerable area only, in which case 5 minutes may be sufficient.

COMMON SPORTING INJURIES

Strain

A strain is a partial or complete muscle or tendinous tear. Note that the vascular supply to the tendon is poor; therefore healing is slow and massage should be used to increase circulation. Minor strains involve muscle fibre damage but with the sheath remaining intact. More severe strains may involve partial or complete rupture of fibres and sheath. Tendon injuries are often caused by overuse, for example in repetitive actions. Where this occurs in the synovial tendon sheath it is termed tendovaginitis.

Sprain

A sprain is a partial or complete ligamentous tear caused by an overstretch injury. This commonly occurs in contact sports, for example where the player receives a blow to the outside of the lower leg when the foot is fixed on the ground. This causes an adduction stress at the knee joint and the ligament on the medial side of the knee may tear. The same mechanism occurs when a runner 'goes over' on an ankle, tearing the lateral ligament of the ankle.

Bursitis

Inflammation of the bursa can occur when the structure overlying it is constantly stretched or contracted. The repetitive friction can cause inflammation in the bursa. This situation is often due to poor biomechanics; for example, trochanteric bursitis near the hip may be due to abnormal biomechanics which cause an altered gait. Hammer (1993) has described two cases where Cyriax friction techniques were used successfully in the treatment of bursitis. Usually, injection with a mixture of local anaesthetic and steroid is advocated for bursitis (Ombregt et al 1995). Ombregt and co-workers (1995) have stated that Cyriax frictions are contraindicated in the treatment of bursitis; Hammer (1993), however, states that excellent results have been obtained with Cyriax frictions. It is suggested that, where the symptoms are chronic, frictions may initially worsen symptoms for two or three treatments, in which case the inflammation could be settled with ice. Therefore, the patient should be screened for chronic symptoms before choosing this technique. Hammer suggests that the direction of fibres in the underlying or overlying tendon should dictate the direction of friction strokes (across the fibres) but that circular strokes could be used for gluteus maximus. All tender areas should be included, as these denote the extent of the bursa. The use of Cyriax frictions in the treatment of this condition is thus controversial, and therapists are advised to proceed with caution.

Conclusion

In sport the injuries are mostly acute or severe versions of the injuries seen in those who do not participate. Specific rehabilitation is needed for each injury and each individual. It should take the athlete to levels of function appropriate to her/his lifestyle. The therapist must be prepared for the psychological considerations of competitive sport, and specialized skills are required for work with these highly motivated individuals who tend towards impatience and non-compliance where recovery from injury is involved. A multidisciplinary approach of mutual respect and support is essential for success in this field.

COMMON INJURIES IN POPULAR SPORTS

Athletics and Running

- ankle sprains
- plantar fasciitis
- shin splints
- Achilles tendon strain
- hamstring strain
- trochanteric bursitis
- supraspinatus tendonitis.

Rugby

- fractures and dislocations
- skin wounds.

Gymnastics and Dance

- ankle ligaments: chronic sprains with thickening
- scarring
- tenosynovitis of the ankle and foot
- leg injuries
- hyperflexion sprain of the back
- hyperextension injury (interspinous ligament nipped between spinous processes)
- kinking in the spine (due to one stiff segment)
- facet joint damage
- muscle imbalance
- ligament sprain of the neck.

Karate

- contact
- haematoma
- nerve injuries
- fractured knuckles.

Judo and Wrestling

- joint injuries
- fractures and dislocations.

KEY POINTS

- ◆ Massage can assist the warming-up process, facilitating increased flexibility.

- ◆ Massage can assist recovery from fatigue.

- ◆ Massage can promote healing and remodelling of soft tissues.

- ◆ Delayed-onset muscle soreness, blood lactate levels and perceived muscle stiffness can be reduced by massage.

- ◆ Post-event massage should be conducted 2 hours after the event for best therapeutic benefit.

- ◆ The multidirectional stretching effect of massage may be more effective than stretching exercises in a bi- or multipennate muscle, and stretching exercises more effective in a longitudinally oriented muscle.

- ◆ Massage should not be applied immediately following a soft tissue injury.

REFERENCES

Arkko P J, Pakarinen A J, Kari-Koskinen O 1983 Effects of whole body massage on serum protein electrolyte and hormone concentrations enzyme activities and haematological parameters. International Journal of Sports Medicine 4: 265–267

Armstrong R B 1990 Initial events in exercise-induced muscular soreness. Medical Science in Sport and Exercise 54: 429–435

Arnheim D D 1989 Modern principles of athletic training. Mosby, St Louis

Ask N, Oxelbeck U, Lundeberg T, Tesch P A 1987 Influence of massage on quadriceps function after exhaustive exercise. Medicine and Science in Sports and Exercise 19(53): 18

Bale P, James H 1991 Massage warmdown and rest as recuperative measures after short-term intense exercise. Physiotherapy in Sport 13(2): 4–7

Balke B, Anthony J, Wyatt F 1989 The effects of massage treatment on exercise fatigue. Clinical Sports Medicine 7: 189–196

Blackman P G, Simmons L R, Crossley K M 1998 Treatment of chronic exertional anterior compartment syndrome with massage: a pilot study. Clinical Journal of Sports Medicine 8(1): 14–17

Boone T, Cooper R 1995 The effect of massage on oxygen consumption at rest. American Journal of Chinese Medicine 23(1): 37–41

Brown S J, Child R B, Day S H, Donnely A E 1997 Indices of skeletal muscle damage and connective tissue breakdown following eccentric muscle contractions. European Journal of Applied Physiology 75(4): 369–374

Burovych A A, Samtsova I A, Manilov I A 1989 An investigation of the effects of individual variants of sports massage on muscle blood circulation. Soviet Sports Science Review 24: 197–200

Danchik J J, Yochum T R, Aspegren D D 1993 Myositis ossificans traumatica. Journal of Manipulative and Physiological Therapeutics 16(9): 605–614

Danneskiold-Samsoe B, Christiansen E, Lund B, Anderson R B 1982 Regional muscle tension and pain ('fibrositis'): effect of massage on myoglobin in plasma. Scandinavian Journal of Rehabilitation Medicine 15: 17–20

Ernst E 1998 Does post-exercise massage treatment reduce delayed onset muscle soreness? A systematic review. British Journal of Sports Medicine 32(3): 212–214

Hammer W I 1993 The use of friction massage in the management of chronic bursitis of the hip or shoulder. Journal of Manipulative and Physiological Therapeutics 16(2): 107–111

Hemmings B 2000a Sports massage and psychological regeneration. British

Journal of Therapy and Rehabilitation 7: 184–188

Hemmings B 2000b Psychological and immunological effects of massage after sport. British Journal of Therapy and Rehabilitation 7(12): 516–519

Hemmings B, Smith M, Graydon J, Dyson R 2000 Effects of massage on physiological restoration, perceived recovery and repeated sports performance. British Journal of Sports Medicine 34(2): 109–114

Jones D A, Round J M 1990 Skeletal muscle in health and disease. Manchester University Press, Manchester

Krilov V N, Talishev F M, Burovikh A N 1985 The use of restorative massage in the training of high level basketball players. Soviet Science Review 20: 7–9

Lamb J F, Ingram C G, Johnson I A, Pitman R M 1984 Essentials of physiology. Blackwell, Oxford

Martin N A, Zoeller R F, Robertson R J, Lephart S M 1998 The comparative effects of sports massage active recovery and rest in promoting blood lactate clearance after supramaximal leg exercise. Journal of Athletic Training 33(1): 30–35

Molea D, Mucek B, Blanken C, Burns R et al 1987 Evaluation of two manipulative techniques in the treatment of post exercise muscle soreness. Journal of the American Osteopathic Association 87(7): 477–483

Monodero J, Donne B 2000 Effect of recovery interventions on lactate removal and subsequent performance. International Journal of Sports Medicine 21(8): 593–597

Ombregt L, Bisschop P, ter Veer H J, Van de Velde T 1995 A system of orthopaedic medicine. W B Saunders, London

Paikov V B 1985 Means of restoration in the training of speed skaters. Soviet Sports Review 20: 7–12

Smith L L, Keating M N, Holbert D et al 1994 Effects of athletic massage on delayed onset muscle soreness, creatine kinase and neutrophil count: preliminary report. Journal of Orthopaedic and Sports Physical Therapy 19(2): 93–99

Thibodeau G A, Patton K T 1999 Anatomy and physiology, 4th edn. Mosby, St Louis

Tiidus P M 1997 Manual massage and recovery of muscle function following exercise: a literature review. Journal of Orthopaedic and Sports Physical Therapy 25(2): 107–112

Vincent H K, Vincent K R 1997 The effect of training status on the serum creatine kinase response soreness and muscle function following resistance exercise. International Journal of Sports Medicine 18(6): 431–437

Watt J 1999 Massage for sport. Crowood Press, Marlborough

Weber M D, Servedis F J, Woodall W R 1994 The effects of three modalities on delayed onset muscle soreness. Journal of Orthopaedic and Sports Physical Therapy 20: 236–242

Wenos J Z, Brilla L R, Morrison M D 1990 Effect of massage on delayed onset muscle soreness [abstract]. Medical Science in Sport and Exercise 22: S34

Wiktorsson-Möller M, Oberg B, Ekstrand J, Gillquist J 1983 Effects of warming up massage and stretching on range of motion and muscle strength in the lower extremity. American Journal of Sports Medicine 11(4): 249–252

Ylinen J, Cash M 1988 Sports massage. Stanley Paul, London

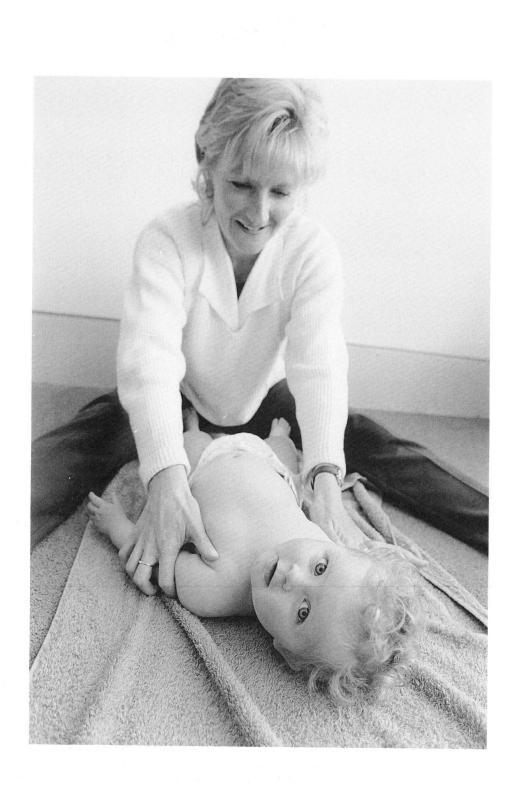

14 Client Groups

The possibilities for the clinical use of massage are extremely broad. In this chapter, we highlight its use with the client groups for which massage is most commonly used. It is hoped that this will encourage therapists creatively to widen the clinical application of massage.

MASSAGE FOR PEOPLE WITH NEUROLOGICAL DISORDERS

Patients with neurological conditions, just like any other individuals, may request massage to achieve a feeling of well-being. In mainstream health care, the use of massage with this client group is a controversial subject, as it is generally believed that restoration and maintenance of normal movement is the priority for use of patient–therapist contact time, to maximize natural neuroplastic changes and increase function. Massage should therefore be used selectively, to enhance the effects of other forms of physiotherapy. Where massage *is* used, for example in an attempt to reduce excess muscle tone, the type of spasticity must be understood because spastic reflexes are easily triggered by inappropriate handling. Examples of this are in flexor spasticity, when stroking the palm of the hand can stimulate the grasp reflex, or in extensor spasticity in the lower limb, when stroking the ball of the foot can trigger an extensor thrust response. As spasticity is due to loss of inhibitory control from the higher centres, reduction through peripheral stroking techniques is not of permanent value but can be used to evoke a temporary response, which enhances the effectiveness of subsequent movement techniques.

Slow stroking over the posterior primary rami region, based on the Rood approach, has been advocated by O'Sullivan (1988). Her suggested mechanism for the resulting reduction in muscle tone is activation of the inhibitory reticular system, which temporarily replaces the lost descending inhibition. In a study by Brouwer & Sousa de Andrade (1995), 10 patients with multiple sclerosis had measures taken of H-reflex amplitude, H-reflex amplitude during vibration and Achilles tendon jerk, in the triceps surae muscle. The measurements were taken before, immediately after and 30 minutes after stroking. The technique consisted of 3 minutes of continuous stroking from the occiput to the coccyx (with the patients lying prone), by the therapist's index and middle fingers on either side of the spinous processes. A significant reduction in H-reflex amplitude was found in the group with multiple sclerosis, particularly 30 minutes after the stroking ended. The study was well controlled except for use of baclofen (an antispastic drug), although analysis showed that subjects taking the drug demonstrated the same trend in results, albeit to a lesser degree. In addition, the subjects reported subjective feelings of relaxation. Farber (1982) suggests that 3–5 minutes should be the maximum length of time this type of massage is given to neurological patients, to avoid rebound effects of the autonomic nervous system (ANS) or skin irritation.

Sirotkina (1964) used massage on flaccid muscles in the hemiparetic arms of stroke patients, in an attempt to increase muscle tone. Electrical activity was shown to increase following massage. Massage has been shown to have a positive psychological effect on multiple sclerosis sufferers. Hernandez-Reif et al (1998) compared 'medical treatment' with massage and found that the massage group improved anxiety and depression scores after 10 45-minute massages over 5 weeks.

Massage can be used to mobilize and stretch shortened muscle groups, in conjunction with active exercise therapy techniques. This can be useful in the flexor muscles of the forearm. Soft tissue mobilizations (STMs) are commonly used, to stretch muscle and its surrounding tissues and to restore muscles in excess torsion back to their more usual position. The muscle belly is grasped within the therapist's palm and the muscle is lifted and rotated towards its normal position, repeated numerous times. This is done in conjunction with active exercise therapy, to help normalize muscle tone and increase the effectiveness of muscle activity.

MASSAGE IN RESPIRATORY DISORDERS

Massage is not in widespread use with this client group. Asthma and other conditions which cause breathlessness, however, can lead to feelings of panic and anxiety so it may be that massage has a use in assisting patients to manage these conditions. Connective tissue manipulation has been used to reduce bronchospasm. Beeken et al (1998) studied the effects of neuromuscular release massage therapy in five individuals. Four of the subjects had an increase in thoracic gas volume, peak flow, and forced vital capacity. The authors report significant improvements in heart rate, oxygen saturation and systolic blood pressure following 24 weekly treatments. These findings are of interest and may be worth repeating with a larger sample to explore whether the findings can be generalized to other individuals, and if massage was the only causative factor in the improved physiological measures. Massage was found to be superior to relaxation therapy in children with asthma (Field et al 1998a). The children were more relaxed after massage and over time experienced improvement in lung function. It is unclear whether the effects were psychological or physical, as again this research group did not control with another touch therapy. It also had poor reporting characteristics (Hondras et al 2001).

PAIN

Pain is an important symptom. Pain caused by cancer is experienced as 'negative' pain, possibly perceived to indicate a severity or worsening of the condition, therefore provoking fear and anxiety. This contrasts with 'positive' pain which can be endured more readily as it leads to reward, such as the pain of childbirth or athletic achievement. Massage can help an individual to cope with pain. Several approaches can be taken: whole body massage can be given to induce relaxation; local Swedish massage can be applied to close the pain 'gate' or to have a counterirritant effect. Reflex techniques such as acupressure can be used to promote relaxation and a feeling of general well-being or to improve specific organic functions.

Weinrich & Weinrich (1990) studied 28 patients with cancer, assigning them to two groups of 14 in matched pairs. The treatment group received 10 minutes of massage (performed by senior nursing students who had received less than 1 hour of massage training), while the control group was visited for 10 minutes. The back massage significantly reduced pain in men but not in women. This was short-term relief, as no significant differences remained after 1 hour. The levels of pain before the massage were, in fact, quite low, so significant falls would have been difficult to demonstrate in a sample of this size.

In a larger study, Marin et al (1991) studied the effect of massage on 116 patients who had had a thoracotomy. A visual analogue scale was used, as in the Weinrich study, and it was found that massage and physiotherapy reduced pain significantly. This is a French paper and unfortunately the English abstract does not give further details. Massage therapy was found to have superior effects to trancutaneous electrical nerve stimulation (TENS), a common treatment for chronic pain, and placebo TENS in fibromyalgia patients. The massage therapy group enjoyed improved sleep patterns and decreased pain, fatigue, anxiety, depression and cortisol levels following 10 30-minute massages over 5 weeks. The TENS group also improved across several parameters by the last treatment. The massage therapy was compared to modalities which were less intensive in terms of touch and direct individual contact, so the psychological effects of massage cannot be differentiated from any physiological effects in this study (Sunshine et al 1996). In a more recent study of the same client group, massage was found to have a positive effect on pain intensity, number of tender points in the neck and upper back region and functional status in fibromyalgia patients. Massage was added to a treatment regimen of heat and exercise and compared with heat, exercise and mobilizations. Neither approach was found to be superior but the sample sizes were small ($n = 7$) in this study which contained multiple variables (Aslan et al 2001). A randomized controlled trial undertaken by Hulme et al (1999) explored the effects of foot massage on patients' perceptions of day care following laparoscopic sterilization. The mean pain scores following surgery differed between the two groups (foot massage and analgesia compared with analgesia only), with the foot massage group reporting less pain over time, although this was not statistically significant. Field et al (2000) studied the effects of burn scar massage and found that twice weekly massage reduced the incidence of itching, pain and anxiety and improved mood. Unfortunately, the mechanical effects on the scar itself were not measured. Massage appears to be a promising intervention for pain relief but studies differentiating between the psychological and physiological effects would inform work with this client group.

PLASTIC SURGERY

Patients with cancer may be offered reconstructive ('plastic') surgery following disfiguring surgery. Massage following mastectomy is advocated by Field & Miller (1992) to reduce the thickening of the scar, facilitate revascularization and promote mobility and elasticity of the skin. These authors also describe massage of silicone breast implants to prevent capsular contracture, a common cause of disfigurement. These massage 'exercises' are recommended from 24 to 48 hours after operation and should then become a permanent routine for the patient. The implant under the skin is displaced superior and medially to counteract the effects of gravity. Laterally and inferiorally directed movements can be included, but are optional.

Bodian (1969) reported the efficacy of massage following ophthalmic plastic surgery to reduce thickening of scars and keloid formation and to prevent deformity caused by scar contracture. A technique was described whereby the skin of the eyelid is stretched to full excursion in a direction that is opposite to the tightening. This method, using approximately 20 excursions three times a day, was taught to the patient or parent 2 weeks or more after surgery. Reported results were softening and thinning of the eyelid, smoothing of the scar as underlying adhesions were released and reduction of keloid formation.

MASSAGE WITH OLDER PEOPLE

Within the client group termed the young old (65–74 years) and the old (over 75 years) (Rosenberg & Moore 1995), widely varying degrees of physical and mental health can be found. This is not a homogeneous group and, as far as health is concerned, there is no reason to assume they all have health or functional problems. It is noteworthy that about 80% of older people in the UK perceive their health and activity levels to be satisfactory (Partridge et al 1991). However, some of the changes associated with ageing can cause physical discomfort, loss of function and psychological change. Collectively these may lead to a loss of coping skills, which means that these elderly people will require varying levels of support to remain independent in their own home, or will require admission to long-term residential care. In both cases, the prime goals of care are to improve or maintain functional abilities for as long as possible and to enhance the quality of life (QoL). These aims are unlikely to prove successful in the long term if adequate attention is not given also to intellectual and emotional function. Thus, it is especially important to view a programme of care holistically and it may then be found that improvement in one function will often be followed quickly by improvement in others.

Some elderly and very old people are admitted to residential care because their support system has failed, for example when a carer has fallen ill. If the client does not deteriorate functionally then a return to semi-independent living will be possible once the support is reinstated. However, the majority of people in residential care are there because, even with a high level of support, they cannot function satisfactorily and safely in their own home. Many of these clients have multiple pathologies and other problems associated with old age. Physical discomfort, impaired function, social isolation, bereavement, decreased financial status and loss of home are also likely to have had a significant effect on people in this environment. While some clients display remarkable resilience in coping psychologically with these events, others suffer a consequent impairment in mental health.

Although depression is commonplace in the elderly (Gurland & Toner 1982), the therapist should guard against mistaking the symptoms of depression for dementia, which is an organic brain syndrome. A depressed person may appear confused and lack motivation but the condition may be helped by appropriate interventions. Highly developed interpersonal skills are required of the therapist to maximize the possibility of successful treatment. Empathy and an unconditional positive regard are prerequisites to developing a therapeutic relationship which may partially compensate for the social isolation and anxiety caused by a change in the client's environment.

Personal autonomy – the freedom to make one's own choices – is largely denied to elderly people in residential care. This frequently engenders a loss of self-esteem and sense of self, which is damaging to QoL and can also affect motivation. It is important, therefore, that clients should be empowered in such a way that they feel that they have some choices. This is pertinent to the therapist when considering massage with this group of clients. It should not be assumed that every elderly person will welcome touch or that it is necessarily appropriate. However, there is a body of opinion which supports the view that some institutionalized elderly and chronically sick people may be tactually deprived (Barnett 1972, Fakouri & Jones 1987). It has been reported that a group of elderly clients with anxiety and depression responded well to hand massage, experiencing feelings of relaxation and an improved sense of well-being (Cole 1992). Back massage with conversation has been shown to reduce anxiety in the elderly. Fraser & Kerr (1993) compared back massage with conversation to a conversation-only and a no-intervention group, in a population of institutionalized elderly clients. The results showed a significant difference in the mean anxiety score between the back massage and the no-intervention group; the results approached statistical significance between the back massage and the conversation-only group. Although the sample size was small ($n = 21$), which makes the validity of the statistics questionable, this study does lend some support to the use of massage as an intervention with anxious elderly clients in residential care.

The therapist should ensure that privacy is maintained throughout the massage and require the client to remove only the items of clothing that are essential to facilitate the treatment. Many elderly people are embarrassed to remove clothing in the presence of another and the therapist will be rewarded if she first takes time to establish a good rapport and remains sensitive to this issue. Care and attention need to be paid to the type of massage administered, particularly in relation to the soft tissues, which are not so resilient as those found in a younger age group. Extra lubricant should be used on dry skin to avoid stretching and uncomfortable friction; light techniques should be used in the presence of fragile blood vessels. The client may not be able to lie in the usual positions for massage: climbing on to a non-adjustable treatment couch may be impossible or unsafe, and for some elderly people the prone position will be uncomfortable. If a treatment couch is used the supine and side-lying positions may be more comfortable, but many clients will require the therapist to use ingenuity in achieving a position that is both effective for the massage and remains comfortable and ergonomically sound for client and therapist (Fig. 14.1). Massage to the upper and lower limbs can be administered with the client seated in a comfortable chair; back massage is facilitated when the client is seated on a stool of suitable height and supported anteriorly by

FIGURE 14.1 *Enabling massage in a seated position by use of a portable head rest.*

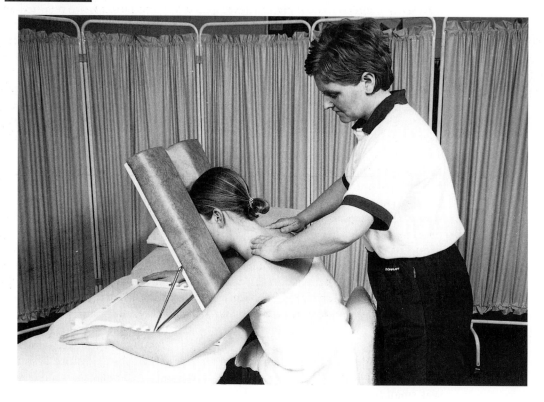

pillows placed on the couch or a table. If positioning is problematic, or if the client does not wish to remove clothing, then a hand massage may be acceptable. This is a useful alternative when privacy cannot be assured and can also be utilized as a component of a group programme to promote social interaction and shared enjoyment.

Dementia

This term denotes a global intellectual impairment associated with most areas of mental function and may be accompanied by decreased motor abilities. It is commonly the result of Alzheimer's disease, multiple cerebral infarcts, metabolic disorders or some degenerative diseases. Most dementias are chronic, with an unremitting deterioration in the condition. Occasionally a form of acute dementia is diagnosed which can be treated, for example in the case of vitamin B_{12} deficiency. The challenge facing health professionals, when caring for clients with dementia, is to provide an environment that offers opportunities for optimum QoL for each individual.

The therapist must be prepared to take much time in building a relationship of trust with the client and in acquiring the skills needed to communicate in the presence of intellectual and sensory deficits. Several studies support the view that the use of two sensory stimuli during communication are more effective than one, so that the addition of caring touch to a verbal approach may facilitate verbal or non-verbal responses (Kleinke 1977, Langland & Panicucci 1982). The utilization of touch may not have a universal application: in some patients with high agitation and severe cognitive impairment touch was found to be linked with an increase in aggressive behaviour (Cohen-Mansfield et al 1989). This work supports that of De Wever (1977), who found that nursing home clients often perceived discomfort when an arm was placed around their shoulder by a nurse. Thus, great care should be taken by the therapist to ensure that physical contact is not misinterpreted by the client: ensure that the client is able to observe your approach; attempt to maintain eye contact during communication; always explain what you require from the client; avoid making sudden movements which may startle the client; and, where possible, ensure that the client is in a familiar environment with minimal extraneous sensory distractions.

Massage of the hands may help to accustom the client to being touched, assist in building trust and promote relaxation. Poon (1991) found a 40% increase in self-reported relaxation scores after elderly clients with dementia were treated with hand massage. When the massage was combined with music, the scores increased to 60%. Hand massage may be taught to the family, carers and significant others of dementia sufferers; these are people who often feel helpless in the face of the unremitting nature of the disease and the difficulties in communicating with their loved one. Giving a massage may enable them to enjoy a form of caring touch once again.

KEY POINTS

◆ Many elderly people are healthy and do not have functional problems.

◆ Therapists who work with this client group need good interpersonal skills.

◆ Not all elderly people respond well to touch.

◆ Massage may help to reduce anxiety in some institutionalized elderly people.

◆ Client positioning for massage may need modifications.

MASSAGE IN OCCUPATIONAL HEALTH

There is currently a global trend for market economies to emphasize increased production at reduced cost. This inevitably leads to fewer workers working harder – at a faster rate and for longer hours. While work can have a positive effect on the individual – aiding the development of physical strength and flexibility, social skills, personal growth and providing financial security – it can also have a detrimental effect on well-being. Massage can be used to prevent and reduce psychosocial and musculoskeletal stress, but emphasis is currently placed on prevention of the latter. In Europe, attention has been focused on the prevention of musculoskeletal stress by the European Community Directive (1990) which resulted, in the UK, in the Manual Handling and Health and Safety Regulations of 1992. Broad health and safety issues are outside the scope of this book and require specialist knowledge from the fields of management, occupational psychology, ergonomics, engineering, and health and safety. To address the issues satisfactorily a workplace requires a detailed health and safety policy for which all the members of the workforce at all levels share responsibility. A comprehensive policy should ideally include health promotion in addition to addressing ill-health treatment and prevention. Massage has a particular role to play in the promotion of well-being and can also participate in treatment of musculoskeletal conditions.

It should be recognized that most of the issues that contribute to loss of well-being in the workplace are interrelated. This is apparent when examining the many factors that contribute to work-related musculoskeletal disorders:

- stress: work pressure, financial
- anxiety: job insecurity, workload
- relationships: inside and outside work
- environment: abnormal or fluctuating temperature, noise, dust, poor light, cluttered floor can all act as dangers or stressors
- unergonomic design of the workplace or task
- static loading on the musculoskeletal system
- repetitive tasks
- moving and handling of excess or awkward loads
- injury.

The most common musculoskeletal problems for which a physiotherapist is consulted are spinal pain and work-related upper limb disorders (WRULDs), otherwise known as cumulative trauma disorders. The latter includes the con-

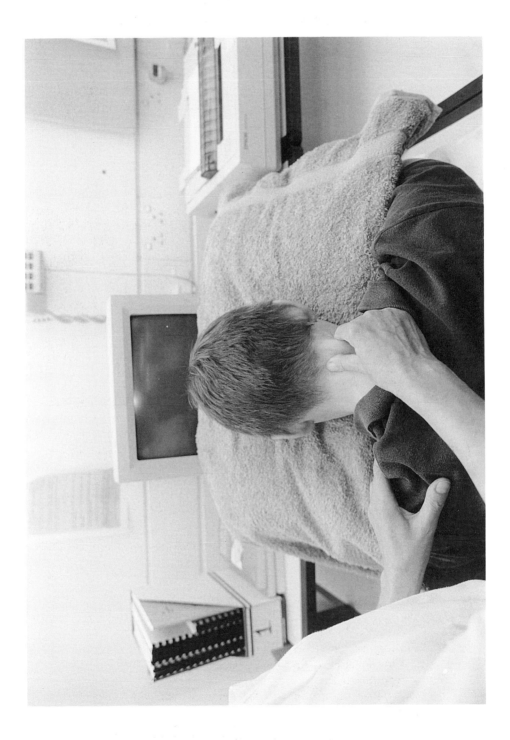

troversial repetitive strain injury (RSI). The mechanisms that produce the symptoms of RSI are poorly understood (Pheasant 1992) and therefore its recognition by the medical profession remains inconsistent. It is of interest that the symptomology can exist when repetitive strain is not a feature of the job.

Various terms are used throughout the world. WRULD is the most satisfactory as it covers upper limb symptoms that occur as a result of work, despite their cause. Risk factors appear to be actions that are repetitive, that load muscles statically or that load joints excessively or cumulatively, particularly when they are in a poor biomechanical position. Poor positioning is often seen in the small joints of the hands, wrists and trunk, and typically occurs in the lower back when lifting in a constrained space (for example, flexion with rotation).

Symptoms occur primarily in the soft tissues and may be diagnosed as carpal tunnel syndrome, tenosynovitis or tennis elbow, which are thought to be due to overuse (as in tennis elbow), repetitive friction between the tendon and its sheath (tenosynovitis), and fluid pressure build-up with resultant nerve pressure in a confined space (as in carpal tunnel syndrome). The latter is more likely in pregnancy when fluid retention can be a causative factor. However, in many work-related problems, while the symptoms may be local, the problem is often more complex. Symptoms and signs are often more diffuse, with discomfort felt at several sites. Thorough examination of the musculoskeletal system often reveals signs that are proximal to the site of discomfort. It is thought that this is often due to adverse neural tension (ANT) induced by postural factors, muscular tension or previous trauma, either instantaneous or cumulative. Therefore screening for ANT is essential in the treatment of WRULDs (Pheasant 1994). Massage can be used to reduce and prevent some of the contributing factors, and to reduce soft tissue symptoms.

Massage for Causative Factors

Static loading of muscle is known to contribute to WRULDs. This tends to occur in the shoulder girdle during tasks such as typing. Widespread use of word processors appears to have contributed to the increase of arm problems as modern machines require a fairly static action whereas traditional typewriters necessitated dynamic, varied movements of the whole arm – sliding the carriage, for example. As more office tasks such as filing are becoming electronic, an increasing amount of time is being spent at the visual display unit (VDU) and relatively static postures may be held for hours. Static muscle work leads to reduced circulation and anoxia in muscle with resultant pain, tenderness and thickening. Postural adjustment and muscle tension can lead to 'tension' headaches.

Massage can be beneficial in reducing the effects of static muscle work by increasing circulation to the muscles, reducing toxic accumulation and its resulting tenderness, and mobilizing connective tissue. This facilitates elongation of the neck muscles and trapezius, allowing postural correction such as head retraction, lowering of the shoulder girdle and restoration of normal spinal alignment. The muscles that require particular attention are trapezius (palpate for a thickened occipital attachment on the nuchal line), erector spinae in the neck and thoracic areas, levator scapulae (a thickened attachment at its insertion at the superior angle of scapula is common), the rhomboids, supraspinatus, infraspinatus and the scalenes.

Useful Strokes for Reducing Effects of Static Muscle Work

> Strokes which are useful are: *effleurage* to promote drainage and increase circulation, *petrissage* including *wringing* and *skin or muscle rolling* of the neck (and shoulder girdle if the patient is unclothed), and *finger kneading* especially at tendinous and aponeurotic insertions on to the scapula.

Massage can also be used to reduce some of the physiological effects of stress and, by promoting a feeling of well-being, may help to reduce stress itself. Relaxation massage can contribute to the promotion of good health, a point which is being addressed in some larger companies to assist workers in maintaining fitness and the flexibility necessary to carry out their work safely and efficiently, thus reducing sick leave costs. Aromatherapy may be the treatment of choice here due to the multisensory effects of massage with essential oils. The therapeutic properties of oils such as geranium and lavender can be utilized to promote relaxation. Field et al (1997a) found that a variety of relaxation therapies, including massage, were equally effective in decreasing anxiety, depression, fatigue and confusion scores in 100 hospital employees. The same research group found massage therapy to reduce anxiety, but also to enhance electroencephelogram patterns of alertness and speed and accuracy of mathematical computations (Field et al 1996a). This is interesting as it suggests that relaxation need not induce a drowsy state, but may instead produce alertness. Further work is needed to assess whether different types of massage or different body areas may influence the state of alertness. This study also demonstrates that improved psychological parameters improve work performance, as well as leading to improved well-being, therefore initiatives to improve the health of workers are likely to be cost-effective.

Massage in the Treatment of Work-Related Problems

In the treatment of musculoskeletal problems, it is important to consider the structures that may be implicated in the symptomology, even though they may seem to be symptomatically silent. Thus, in WRULDs, the neck, shoulder girdle and arm may require attention as well as the more distal areas of discomfort.

Strokes for Treatment of Work-Related Problems

> Locally, the strokes that may be useful are: *effleurage* to promote drainage; *petrissage*, *wringing*, and *skin and muscle rolling* to stretch and mobilize the tissues; *finger kneading* for stretching of deeper structures; and *Cyriax frictions* for chronic tendinitis.

Care must be taken of areas showing signs of acute inflammation, recognized by redness and heat. Local massage should be avoided if this is present, and massage confined to proximal areas.

Any interruption of typical muscle work patterns is beneficial and health promotion or rehabilitation initiatives are most likely to succeed if they have a good cost–benefit ratio for the client, whether an individual employee or company. This has led to the development of on-site services, pioneered in the USA, where workers are given massage through their clothing without leaving their workstation. Where possible, however, workers are best encouraged physically to leave their workstation as the change of position and the walk, however brief, will be therapeutic and biomechanically beneficial. Levoska & Keinanen-Kiukaanniemi (1993) found that muscle training was more effective than heat, massage and stretching in reducing symptoms of cervicobrachial disorders in 47 female office employees, although the incidence of headache was significantly less at 12 months' follow-up in the group receiving passive physiotherapy. This illustrates the need for a combined approach. However, seated massage through clothing can be helpful where privacy is not available (see Fig. 14.1). The portable chairs which have been specially designed for massage have facilitated massage that is performed with the client in a sitting position. For many years, physiotherapists have performed neck massage with the patient leaning forwards on to a pile of pillows; though effective, this can be cumbersome and is difficult to achieve in non-clinical situations. Massage chairs are often well designed and comfortable, and facilitate massage services in public areas.

Clothed massage, like any other, should be tailored to the needs of the individual client, but particularly useful are pressure techniques and modified classical massage type techniques. Care should be taken to ensure that massage over certain materials (for example lycra) does not irritate the skin. Katz et al (1999) conducted a small pilot study in which hospital nurses were given eight 15-minute workplace-based massage treatments. Pain intensity, tension, relaxation and the profile of mood states scores significantly improved after massage. This study suggests that workplace-based massage may be effective in reducing the effects of stress at work and is worth investigating further.

In summary, massage can be used to treat specific musculoskeletal problems such as WRULDs and low back pain in coordination with the other occupational health staff. Relaxation massage, preferably with essential oils, in a conducive environment can be used to reduce stress. The hands or neck and shoulders should be treated as a minimum, but whole body massage is preferable. Massage plays a small part in occupational health, which should include ergonomic design, education, postural correction and body awareness to reduce musculoskeletal strain. It is not satisfactory to put energy into reducing the negative effects of work without applying an equal amount of effort towards prevention. Massage should not be used to perpetuate bad working practices by reducing symptoms and appeasing the workers. It should contribute to the empowerment of employees, which will enable them to participate in improving their working practices and environment.

KEY POINTS

- ◆ Massage can help treat back pain and work-related upper limb disorders.
- ◆ Thorough assessment is necessary and postural factors should always be considered in this client group.
- ◆ Treatment, education and prevention should be undertaken together.
- ◆ Massage can be used to treat local problems such as neck pain or overuse injuries.
- ◆ Aromatherapy can induce relaxation, reduce stress and promote well-being.
- ◆ Seated, on-site massage can be a cost-effective way of promoting health among employees.

MASSAGE IN MENTAL HEALTH

This is an interesting and complex area of work for the therapist. People with mental disorders have a wide variation in symptoms and the approach to treatment is specific to the patient. Clients will typically display both cognitive and somatic signs and symptoms; cognitively there will be evidence of abnormal patterns of thought, and somatically various abnormal physical sensations may be reported. The therapist will be guided in her approach more by the symptoms experienced by the individual than by the diagnostic label that has been attached to that client.

Perhaps of primary importance when working with this group of clients is to ensure that informed consent to treatment has been obtained. People with mental illness may be particularly vulnerable to the power imbalance inherent in a therapist–client relationship and some will not possess the assertive powers needed to vocalize their feelings about treatment procedures. Others may have disordered thought processes which render them temporarily incapable of rational decision-making, including consent to treatment. In these cases the therapist may find it useful to discuss the proposed treatment methods with colleagues. For example, a client with mental illness and who has been sexually abused may experience flashbacks (a state of acute awareness of the traumatic event including the return of emotions felt at that time), which may be triggered by being touched. Consideration of the potential outcome of attempting massage with this client (information that may be offered by the clinical psychologist) may enable the therapist to adapt the treatment to avoid an unwanted effect.

The therapist should have a clear idea of the aims of massage so that there is unlikely to be any conflict with the objectives of the treatment plan as formulated by the multidisciplinary team. Massage should augment the therapeutic procedures that have been agreed by members of the multidisciplinary team. Occasionally massage may detract from the overall aims or may be thought to be an inappropriate intervention for a specific client. This is rare, however, and massage is usually a most versatile therapeutic tool in mental health care. It can, for example, be employed to sedate, to stimulate, to help develop a trusting therapeutic relationship and to decrease awareness of somatic symptoms.

It is likely that clients with a mental illness have the same incidence of musculoskeletal problems as the general population. If a client complains of symptoms, the therapist should assess in the usual manner and not assume that they are a somatized symptom of the mental illness. Occasionally certain prescribed medications may cause severe muscle spasm; the therapist may be the only person on the team to identify this and must therefore be aware of unusual signs of this nature. Therapists in private practice will occasionally be consulted by clients who ostensibly have purely physical symptoms but who may have an underlying mental health problem. Chronic physical illness is often accompanied by depression and anxiety. At some time during their life 25% of the population will experience a psychiatric illness (Rose 1995), and individuals often do not seek professional help for mental health problems. They may report only the physical symptoms of mental illness and so the underlying cause may be undetected. This clearly has implications for the degree of improvement that can be expected in the symptoms and for the outcome of treatment.

Many of the individuals in this client group will benefit from extra attention being paid to the environment in which the massage takes place. Privacy, quietness and freedom from interruption will ensure that conditions such as anxiety and paranoia are not likely to be exacerbated by procedures. The therapist should take the time to explain what she intends to do and ensure that the patient understands what the desired outcomes are. In this way it is possible to minimize any potential stress response, such as physiological arousal. It is important to formalize the massage treatment sessions to the extent that the patient knows when massage is going to be available and how many sessions are being offered, if these are to be limited. This will underscore the fact that massage is one element of the treatment plan and also decrease the likelihood of the client experiencing a sense of rejection when massage is discontinued. In this regard, care should also be taken not to promote therapist dependency. This can be avoided if the massage treatment is viewed by the client as part of a progressive rehabilitation programme. With patients who have chronic or recurring mental disorder, massage is more likely to be used as one of a number of strategies to promote coping abilities. In these cases it is better for the patient if timed appointments for treatment are made, rather than the sessions being viewed by the patient as being on demand or when the therapist can fit a massage into a busy schedule. Misunderstandings can easily arise which may detract from a valuable therapeutic relationship.

Many clients with mental illness enjoy hand massage. Even those with an aversion to touch (provided they consent), survivors of physical and sexual abuse, and others for whom general massage may be perceived as threatening or undesirable, usually respond well to hand massage. This form of massage is particularly useful in groups, where willing members can be taught to massage each other's hands, thus promoting interaction between members of the group (Valentine 1984). Although conversation is usually discouraged when massage is used for relaxation purposes, group massage sessions can create a helpful environment to encourage some light-hearted discussion, or give time for the therapist to teach health education and to dispel some unhelpful health beliefs. Most clients are interested in the process and become receptive to hearing explanations about the benefits of massage and other relevant health topics.

Teaching self-massage to clients provides them with a valuable tool of self-help and the therapist will occasionally be rewarded by the great enthusiasm with which some patients embrace this opportunity. By teaching a patient these techniques the therapist empowers the individual in a unique way. Clients with anxiety, depression and those who experience panic attacks are among those who will benefit from self-massage. One way to approach this is for the client to experience a therapist-administered head or hand massage and then be taught a modified form for self-treatment, which can be used as part of a relaxation programme. In addition, patients may be taught how to stimulate appropriate acupoints as an aid to composure or as part of their coping strategy against panic attacks.

A common assessment finding in many patients with mental disorder is that they have lost or distorted body image. Massage is valuable as a component of body awareness training, by stimulating sensory awareness of neglected areas. This presents a further opportunity for education, when body image can be related to the effect on emotions and attitude. It may aid clients who harm themselves by challenging feelings of self-loathing and helping to promote an enhanced self-image.

The therapist should always bear in mind that massage may provoke catharsis (the release of pent-up emotions); also, a trusting relationship between therapist and client may encourage emotive disclosure and the therapist must be competent to deal effectively with these situations when they occur. The release of emotions is often a prerequisite to the patient progressing towards wellness. If the therapist recognizes this she can provide a secure environment in which it may occur and an empathetic 'listening ear', which is often all that is required (Dennis 1995).

The Evidence

Ernst (1998), in his overview of complementary therapies for depression, concluded that, as far as massage is concerned, the evidence was promising but not compelling due to the fact that there were few studies which satisfied rigorous scientific standards. Nevertheless, there are some relatively small-scale randomized controlled trials which have shown massage to be beneficial for people with depression and post-traumatic stress disorder (PTSD).

Field et al (1996b) studied 60 children who were randomly selected from a pool of children who displayed classroom behaviour problems following Hurricane Andrew (these were symptoms previously reported for children considered to be suffering PTSD including numbness of responsiveness, increased arousal and conduct problems). The children were allocated to either a massage therapy group who received a 30-minute back massage 2 days per week for 4 weeks or a video attention control group who spent the same amount of time watching children's relaxing video tapes with a research assistant who provided physical contact. On the last day of the study the massage group showed significant decreases in anxiety and depression compared to pretreatment scores; there were also significant differences between the two groups.

In a different study Field et al (1996c) randomly assigned 32 depressed adolescent mothers to either a massage therapy or relaxation therapy group; the massage group received 30 minutes' massage on 2 days per week for 5 weeks; the relaxation therapy group spent the same amount of time doing yoga and progressive muscle relaxation. The profile of mood states scores significantly decreased from pre-treatment values in the massage therapy group over the trial and there was also a significant difference between groups. In addition, the massage therapy group showed a significant decrease in stress hormone levels (cortisol) over the period.

KEY POINTS

- ◆ The therapist should consult with other members of the multidisciplinary team.
- ◆ Massage should promote the objectives of the treatment plan.
- ◆ Physical symptoms need proper assessment.
- ◆ The client requires a full explanation of the treatment.
- ◆ Teaching self-massage is a way of empowering the client.
- ◆ The therapist should be prepared for emotive disclosure.

MASSAGE FOR PEOPLE WITH LEARNING DISABILITIES

Clients with learning disabilities have the same physiological and emotional needs as the rest of the population, but they often require support to learn 'living skills'. Massage can be used to fulfil some emotional needs such as the need for touch and intimacy and it can be used as a vehicle through which certain skills can be learned. Its incorporation into the lives of those with learning disabilities can be both valuable and pleasurable for the recipient and rewarding for the therapist, and it can be employed as an integral part of the therapeutic programme.

The learning of social skills is one of the keys by which an individual achieves 'normalization' or 'social role valorization' (Wolfsenberger 1983). However, this cannot be achieved without implications for all members of the learner's community. O'Brien (1987) has identified the widely accepted so-called Five Accomplishments which should be addressed by those providing services for people with learning disabilities in order that they might achieve a good QoL. The accomplishments are: community presence and participation, choice, competence and respect. Communication is an implicit skill required for the personal achievement of most of these goals and individuals may need help in developing their potential in this area, whether that potential involves speech, sign language or eye contact. Important stages in communication are trust, sharing and interaction, and these must be reinforced by reciprocity with others. Touch is a powerful route through which these can be developed and massage is advocated as an appropriate form.

Massage can also be used to assist the development of sensory awareness, augmenting the sophisticated multisensory workshops which include move-ment- or touch-generated light and sound systems, water beds, hammocks and tactile surfaces. They can be used to encourage interaction with the environment. Multisensory massage (Sanderson et al 1991), with objects of differing sensory quality such as brushes and cotton wool or with mechanical massagers, can desensitize psychological or physical touch intolerance and promote sensory differentiation. This physical interaction with another human being also requires trust and tolerance of sharing personal space. Sanderson and co-workers suggest that massage can be used with the eight steps identified by McInnes & Treffry (1982), through which a person with dual sensory impairment must progress before being comfortable with physical contact (Table 14.1). These are: resistance, toleration, passive cooperation, enjoyment, active cooperation, leading, imitation and initiation. They suggest that *passive massage* becomes *interactive massage* when the stage of active cooperation is reached. These stages are a useful guide to progression and goal attainment, but the support worker should be aware that, while they are a useful base for massage and other interventions, they can be regarded as oversimplistic as they are not necessarily linear and distinct (Chia 1995). More than one stage may be achieved at any one time and moves from interactive to passive stages do not necessarily imply regression, but may be dependent on factors such as mood and physical health (see Table 14.1). A study by Lindsay et al (1997) showed that hand massage/aromatherapy and active therapy (a bouncy castle) had a less positive effect on concentration than snoezelen and relaxation in eight subjects with profound learning disabilities. Rather than demonstrating that massage is not effective, it may indicate that massage must be skilfully applied and individualized according to McInnes and Treffry's interactive sequence if it is to be effective. Field et al (1997b) demonstrated that touch therapy can improve attentiveness and responsivity in autistic children.

Individuals who do not understand their environment or the intentions of others, or who are unable to identify or communicate their needs and feelings,

TABLE 14.1	The interactive sequence	
	Stage	**Interpretation and intervention**
Passive massage	1. Resists	Person may hide hands – switch to a form of touch which is more acceptable to the individual, e.g. stroking hair
	2. Tolerates	May be fleeting – aim to increase the time engaged on the activity
	3. Cooperates passively	Subtle change in response which might allow different strokes to be introduced
	4. Enjoys	Enjoyment shown by relaxation/smiling
Interactive massage	5. Responds cooperatively	Participates in some way, e.g. moving limbs to facilitate the massage. Less need for encouragement at this stage
	6. Leads	May offer a limb for massage once the previous one is finished. Follow the lead
	7. Imitates	Imitates the massage on the back of her own hand, with encouragement. Give verbal support and encouragement
	8. Imitates independently	Imitation occurs without verbal prompting, e.g. offering the oil for massage. Reciprocal massage between the learner and support worker may become possible

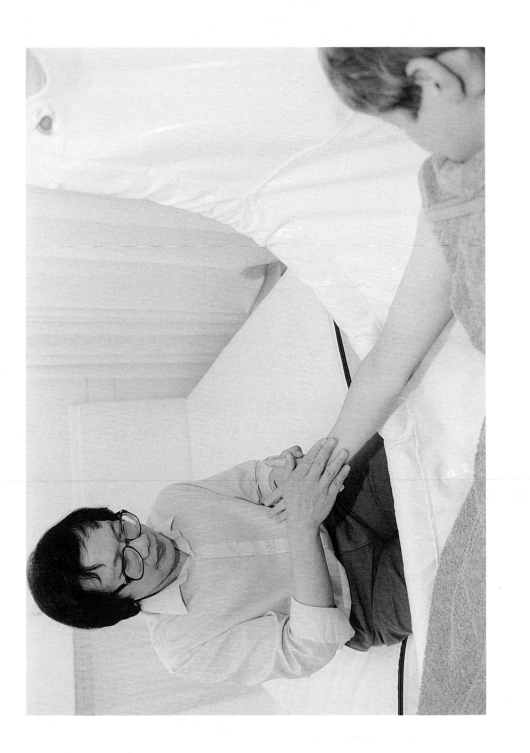

may show their distress by violent or erratic ('challenging') behaviour. This behaviour can be externally applied towards others or internally applied when it is termed self-injurious behaviour. Dosseter et al (1991) reported on the use of massage in the care of a 14-year-old girl with Cornelia de Lange syndrome and a 10-year history of self-injurious behaviour. The results were dramatic. She enjoyed twice-daily massage which soon developed into a form of reciprocal play over which the girl and care worker shared equal control. After 6 months of massage this girl no longer required medication, despite the fact that, before massage, she had had 100 bouts of self-injurious behaviour each day. This illustrates the creative ways in which massage can be shared with this client group.

Many people with severe developmental disabilities may be severely restricted physically, as well as intellectually, and may have disorders of muscle tone. Constipation can be a permanent problem in their nursing care and enemas are widely used to maintain bowel evacuation. Emly (1993) describes the use of abdominal massage in a 21-year-old man with profound disabilities. Massage (modified from the method first described by Prosser in 1938; Prosser (1941)) three times weekly reduced the enema requirement from twice weekly for 10 years to none for a whole month. The benefits of massage can be multifactorial in this group of patients and goals should be set accordingly.

Uses and Effects of Massage in People with Learning Disabilities

Massage can be used with this client group to:

- promote relaxation
- reduce anxiety
- stimulate
- calm challenging behaviour
- improve sleep patterns
- improve communication and interaction
- promote therapeutic rather than destructive sensory stimulus
- improve bowel function
- assist in the expression of emotional response
- promote pleasure and feelings of well-being.

The use of essential oils can be particularly beneficial in this client group (Harrison & Ruddle 1995). They provide useful sensory input and added enjoyment and their therapeutic effects can be chosen according to individual need. Clients may progress to choosing and communicating their preferred odours, which can also be applied in baths or burners. As with all client groups, it is essential that a full assessment is carried out before proceeding with massage. In particular, essential oils should be chosen with care with due regard to side-effects, especially in the presence of medical conditions such as epilepsy (when hyssop and rosemary should be avoided) and skin conditions. Weak blends and short treatment times should be used when treating young children.

KEY POINTS

♦ Ensure the client understands what you are doing.

♦ Take the steps very slowly; expect and acknowledge small amounts of progress.

♦ Remember the steps are not always linear: fluctuation between stages of achievement does not necessarily indicate regression.

♦ Respect individual moods and desires.

♦ When rejection of the massage occurs, switch immediately to another activity the individual enjoys.

♦ Take care in planning the environment – does this individual like music, privacy, require the presence of a trusted person or advocate?

♦ Choice of the massage position should be client led and should aspire towards facilitating absolute physical and emotional comfort.

♦ The massage should be learner led.

♦ Welcome and permit the interaction and leadership of the client.

♦ Persevere.

♦ Keep massage sessions short.

♦ Be exquisitely sensitive to responses.

♦ Keep input simple.

♦ Ensure that there is a clear start and finish to the activity.

ABDOMINAL MASSAGE

Individuals with altered muscle tone, reduced mobility or who are taking long-term medication may suffer from constipation, which is uncomfortable and increases feelings of being unwell. Although massage has long been advocated as being beneficial to those with constipation (Chin 1959), the results of studies have appeared contradictory. Klauser et al (1992) reported that colonic massage did not change parameters of colonic function in either healthy volunteers or constipated patients. They measured bowel function by transit time of swallowed radio-opaque markers and stool consistency, the latter being a subjective score which was averaged. They compared two 2-week control periods (before and after massage), separated by a 3-week massage period in the healthy volunteers, and compared a premassage period with a massage period in the constipated patients. It has been suggested that massage can have a delayed effect on constipated patients (Holey & Lawler 1995), so, in omitting a post-massage measurement period in the treatment group, the Klauser study missed what is possibly the most important time period.

In contrast, Resende et al (1993) found that massage and exercise improved bowel evacuation frequency and reduced the use of enemas and bouts of incontinence significantly. Unfortunately, the study was not well controlled as there was no control group, medication was stopped and exercise added. The results could be due to any one or a combination of these three interventions. Interestingly, bowel transit times were not increased, but frequency of bowel emptying *was* increased, demonstrating the dubious nature of the link between these two factors.

Emly (1993) advocates the use of abdominal massage in neurological patients, following success in her learning disability unit. She suggests that massage reduces spasticity in the abdominal wall, thereby promoting peristalsis. Evidence to support the widespread anecdotal evidence of massage-induced bowel emptying is clearly inconclusive but it may be a comfortable alternative to laxatives and enemas in individuals who are less mobile, on restricted diets or medication. Indeed, a pilot study conducted with subjects who were profoundly disabled and institutionalized found that massage was not more effective than laxative use. Colonic transit times, stool frequency, size and consistency, the requirement for enemas and client well-being were monitored (Emly et al 1998). It appears, then, that massage may be an alternative to laxative/enema use and a promising treatment for chronic constipation (Ernst 1999) but is not a superior intervention in terms of bowel function.

BABY MASSAGE

Massaging babies is a tradition in many countries and is becoming popular in the West. Babies spend their embryonic developing months in the cushioned enclosure of the womb, being massaged by the amniotic fluid, with additional sensory input from the mother's heartbeat. Tactile sense is developed at 7.5 months of gestation (Gottleib 1983). Once born, babies are comforted by cuddles, back patting, caresses and stroking, all of which are natural acts performed instinctively by most parents. A baby quickly comes to recognize the feel and smell of its primary carers and to enjoy the closeness involved in feeding and cuddling. This and the intimacy of personal hygiene maintenance (bathing and nappy changing) promotes a strong psychological bond between parents and child.

Babies, who are unable to reason, can learn some important things through sensation, for example danger (e.g. touching something hot) or self-esteem. Abusive touch can lead to confusion about touch, whereas positive and appropriate touch can lead to emotional security. If parents are stressed or depressed, or if they themselves have never learned the value of caring touch, their babies may become deprived of touch. Massage is one way in which bonding and caring touch can be facilitated and supported. There are various ways in which massage is being used with babies: in premature baby units, in baby massage classes which also function as postnatal health promotion sessions, and in private massage classes. Massage can also be used to increase mother–baby interaction where women have postnatal depression. Onozawa et al (2001) found that scores on the Edinburgh postnatal depression scale (EPDS) dropped in both the massage and support groups but only participation in the massage group improved mother–baby interaction. This study had a high drop-out rate but is worth repeating with a higher sample, to explore the validity of the results.

Much of the practice of baby massage is supported by research findings. Hartelius et al (1992) discuss their previous research in which they studied how premature babies responded to touch. The babies relaxed during *containment* (holding by their parents) but became restless and irritable when stroked. They preferred firm stroking on the back and arm to soft stroking on the back and arm. In a further study by the same workers, 11 preterm babies, born at 26–36 weeks' gestation, were videoed at weekly intervals while being touched in different ways (Hartelius et al 1992). Containment induced relaxation, and an initially reduced blood oxygen level, before restoring it to a higher level than before touch. The babies became alert and awake with fine controlled movements. Stroking appeared to trigger reflex activity, for example whole limb extension, clenched fists, legs fully flexed to the body, grimaces and crying, whimpering and grunting noises. They stared expressionlessly. When left alone, their movements and expressions changed. The touch also had a negative effect on breathing, resulting in reduced blood oxygen levels and occasionally apnoea. The conclusion drawn was that premature infants do not tolerate massage and this appeared to reinforce the widespread policy of minimal touch in special care baby units. This study was based on a small sample with no analysis of results to identify which age, condition or type of touching produced specific effects. Also, no oil was used, which could have influenced the babies' reaction. Field et al (1996d) found that massage with oil enhances the positive effects of massage on newborns.

Other studies have shown that massage does benefit preterm infants. Field et al (1986) monitored 20 premature babies, with a mean gestational age of 31 weeks, who were in transitional care. Following baby massage with oil and passive movements for three 15-minute periods daily for 10 days, the babies showed increased weight, activity, alertness and maturity, and required a hospital stay of 6 days less than the control group. Statistical significance was reached in this well-controlled study.

Adamson-Macedo (1990) discussed studies that have substantiated Macedo's (1984) TAC-TIC method of patterned tactile stimulation, finding that it produces better weight gain and better sucking and hand grasp reflexes. Acolet et al (1993) studied 11 stable premature babies with a median age of 29 weeks. Twenty minutes of massage with arachis (peanut) oil was applied to the back and limbs. No behavioural responses were monitored but eight infants had consistently reduced plasma cortisol levels. There were no consistent significant changes in adrenaline (epinephrine), noradrenaline (norepinephrine) or oxygen concentration, but skin temperature dropped.

Thus, it was shown that massage reduces the stress of intensive care but the need to maintain body temperature was demonstrated, although it must be acknowledged that the sample size was extremely small. In the same year, Wheeden et al (1993) conducted a randomized controlled study of 30 preterm neonates who had been exposed to cocaine. They were medically stable with a mean age of 30 weeks. Massage was given for 15 minutes, three times over 10 days, and the babies increased their weight, reduced stress behaviour and postnatal complications, and showed increased motor maturity above the control group. Similar positive effects were found in a subsequent study (Scafidi et al 1996) in cocaine-exposed newborns, who showed a 28% greater daily weight gain than controls, improved behavioural development and fewer complications. These results are transferable to babies born to HIV-positive mothers (Scafidi & Field 1997).

A variety of studies have been conducted in this subject which, on the whole, show positive beneficial effects of massage for normal preterm infants. The contradictory findings of the Hartelius studies perhaps show that the specific strokes are important and that oil should be used. The age, medical stability and reflex activity of the babies should be taken into account. Babies under 29 weeks' gestation may prefer holding and containment, and all babies should be stroked firmly, preferably through an oily medium which should not be peanut-based as it is thought that the increase in serious peanut allergies may be due to early exposure to peanuts in childhood. However, Vickers et al (2001), in one of the rigorous Cochrane Reviews, points out that the selective reporting of outcomes in a number of these studies weakens the assertion that massage is beneficial to preterm or low birth weight infants.

With older babies, massage can promote bonding. This is particularly important where there are social difficulties causing stress, postnatal depression, poor parenting skills, illness, disability or following a difficult birth. Massage can also help the mother who is apprehensive about handling her baby because, for example, it is a fragile baby. Mothers often want to do something extra for their baby beyond routine caring tasks and massage can provide an additional interest. Thus, massage has been utilized as a vehicle for health promotion, as it is attractive to a busy mother who would not necessarily find the time to seek health promotion advice for herself. Massage can be taught in a supportive class environment and the mother can be encouraged to continue massage at home. The principles therefore apply to both situations.

Baby massage classes can:

- promote bonding
- give the mother a chance to take 'time out' for relaxation
- create an opportunity to meet other parents and professionals and discuss feelings and problems
- provide an opportunity for health promotion: back care, postnatal exercises, prevention of incontinence
- offer support and monitoring of problems.

Principles of Baby Massage Classes

First, it is essential that the room is adequately warm, as babies lose heat quickly. Isherwood (1994) recommends the use of music and has found that slow rock music soothes restless babies while new age music is preferred by the mothers. The parent and class leader must be flexible and prepared to adapt to the reactions of individual babies and the needs of the mother. There should be an unhurried relaxed atmosphere and mothers should be encouraged to watch, listen to and cuddle their babies. The relaxation and rest offered to the mother is equally valid and there may be occasions where massage does not seem appropriate because the baby is asleep or upset or the mother is anxious. On these occasions, she can participate in other ways. Oil should always be used and it should be warmed in the hands first. Essential oils can be selected, but allergic reactions should be watched for and oil should not be used on broken or sore skin. Nut oils should be avoided. Mothers may develop an interest in massage for themselves and may then be advised to seek a preferred type such

BOX 14.1	*Baby massage routine*

The baby should be on the lap, looking at the mother. Eye contact is encouraged. Various routines can be taught, but the following is typical:

- Circle the crown of the head gently with the palm of the hand
- Stroke both hands from the crown of the head down the sides of the face
- Apply firm but gentle strokes across the shoulders
- Stroke down the arms
- Stroke down the chest, then the abdomen
- Stroke down the legs and feet
- If desired, these strokes can be followed by gentle 'squeezing' movements with the palm of the hand; this affects the tissues like a kneading technique
- Finish the front of the body by light strokes from the neck to the toes.

Turn the baby prone:

- Stroke down the back of the head and neck
- Continue long strokes down the back and buttocks
- Stroke down the legs and feet
- Follow with gentle 'squeezing' movements with the palms

The depth should be variable, depending on the tolerance of the individual baby, and should be appropriate to the age of the baby and its associated reflex activity.

as aromatherapy. For safety, the women in the group should be advised to keep fingernails short and to remove any jewellery that could scratch the baby. The maximum length of massage for a baby who is under 4 months old should be 10 minutes and this time can be increased gradually to suit individual babies. The baby should be allowed expression and comfort, so its wriggling or repositioning should be accommodated. A baby massage routine is shown in Box 14.1.

Specific Conditions

Massage is particularly useful in certain conditions. If a baby has a congenitally dislocated hip and must spend periods of time in immobilization, for example in a Paulik harness or plaster of Paris, then massage can facilitate bonding, self-esteem and comfort, especially between plaster changes. The so-called 'floppy' baby can be hyposensitive to stimulation and massage can be used as an extrasensory stimulus.

If the baby has difficulty weaning, massage can be followed by a bottle feed, stroking across the cheek to the mouth to stimulate the rooting reflex. When teething or constipated, massage can be soothing and is often applied naturally, although a particular routine may give the parent confidence in its application. A premature baby may be best massaged in side-lying and flexion, and a near foetal position can be encouraged if an upset baby begins arching its back.

MASSAGE IN OLDER CHILDREN

Children sometimes suffer from many of the same conditions which affect adults. It would be logical to assume, then, that massage could benefit children in terms of their mental and physical health. It can be carried out in much the same way, depending on the age of the child (short periods of massage and interactive massage, perhaps accompanied by some relaxing singing, may suit younger children). Research in this area is patchy but it has been conducted in the areas of attention deficit disorder, juvenile rheumatoid arthritis, burned children, diabetes mellitus and atopic eczema (Anderson et al 2000). Massage proved to be superior to relaxation in self-ratings of happiness and observed hyperactivity in a small group of hyperactive attention deficit adolescents (Field et al 1998b). Anxiety, stress and pain reduced in children with mild to moderate juvenile rheumatoid arthritis, compared with a relaxation therapy group. (Field et al 1997c). Massage was found to reduce distress during a painful change of dressings in children with burns (Hernandez-Reif et al 2001). The same research team used massage to lower blood glucose levels in children with diabetes mellitus (Field et al 1997d).

MASSAGE IN LABOUR AND PREGNANCY

Light superficial massage is safe to do in pregnancy. Gentle stroking and circular kneading can be done with oil over the abdomen to facilitate stretching of the skin. Massage with a partner can be done for support and closeness in pregnancy and labour. Circular stroking over the low back, or wherever the contractions are felt, can be soothing, and sensitive stroking over the lower abdomen can be helpful in early labour. Massage has been reported to be helpful in labour, but preferred non-pharmacological pain relieving methods vary from individual to individual (Brown et al 2001). It has also been found to improve psychological factors (such as anxiety and depressed mood) in labour (Field et al 1997e).

BREAST MASSAGE

This is often recommended for problems associated with breastfeeding. For example, hypoga lactia (insufficient milk, thought to be a mechanical problem) or stagnation mastitis. Breast massage is often done automatically by women who are suffering problems of tender breasts, reduced lactation and milk ejection. It can be taught and advised by midwives and physiotherapists postnatally. Yokoyama et al (1994) compared six women who suckled their babies with six who had Japanese breast massage, which involved stroking down and round the breast by both hands and squeezing the nipples. Blood samples taken every 2 and 10 minutes from 10 minutes before the start to the end of the experiment showed that oxytocin release was pulsatile during the suckling and steady, but higher, during the massage. Prolactin release was increased by suckling but not by massage. Unsurprisingly, suckling was found to be the best method to increase lactation. Prolactin is released by nipple stimulation and oxytocin stimulates milk ejection, so it would seem that massage is good for stagnation mastitis and as a precursor to breastfeeding, although the sample population in this study was extremely small. A further study on methods of expressing breast milk showed that simultaneous breast pumping is more effective than sequential pumping and that massage increased milk production even further in both pumping groups (Jones et al 2001).

MASSAGE IN GYNAECOLOGY

Massage has been used to try and reduce pain and anxiety in women undergoing genetic amniocentesis. Light effleurage of the leg was not found to be effective (Fischer et al 2000). Evidence suggests that massage may, however, produce short-term beneficial effects on mood, anxiety, pain and water retention over relaxation therapy in a small group of women with premenstrual dysphoric disorder (Hernandez-Reif et al 2000). Kuznetsov et al (1998) used intensive massage in 30 patients experiencing chronic salpingo-oophoritis. The results were remarkable – 78% of subjects are reported to have had a strong anaesthetic and anti-inflammatory effect with 33% recovering 'reproductive function'.

Summary

Massage can be used throughout the childbearing years to assist the well-being of the mother and can also provide benefit for the baby as an individual and within the family unit. It can be used as a means to educate women about their own and their babies' health; creative ways can be found to use massage to raise body awareness in children, enhance relationships between partners, children and parents, and between siblings, and assist psychological and physical growth and healthy family relationships.

KEY POINTS

- ◆ A baby's tactile sense is developed at 7.5 months of gestation.
- ◆ Touch is an important learning tool for a baby.
- ◆ A child's self-image and esteem are partly shaped through all forms of communication, including touch.
- ◆ Massage can be used to facilitate and support bonding and caring touch.
- ◆ Babies under 29 weeks of gestation may prefer holding and containment to massage.
- ◆ Ensure you understand the developmental sequence and reflex activity to inform your positioning and touching of babies.
- ◆ Oils, but not nut oils, should be used for baby massage.
- ◆ Breast massage can aid stagnation mastitis.
- ◆ Women may find massage supportive during labour.
- ◆ Massage can be used for creative health promotion sessions.
- ◆ Family relationships can be aided through massage.

REFERENCES

Acolet D, Modi N, Giannakoulopoulos X et al 1993 Changes in plasma cortisol and catecholamine concentrations in response to massage in preterm infants. Archives of Disease in Childhood 68: 29–31

Adamson-Macedo E N 1990 The effects of touch on preterm and fullterm neonates and young children. Journal of Reproductive and Infant Psychology 8: 267–273

Anderson C, Lis-Balchin M, Kirk-Smith M 2000 Evaluation of massage with essential oils on childhood ectopic eczema. Phytotherapy Research 14(6): 452–456

Aslan U B, Yüksel I, Yazici M 2001 A comparison of classical massage and mobilization techniques in the treatment in primary fibromyalgia. Fizyoterapi Rehabilitasyon 12(2): 50–54

Barnett K 1972 A theoretical construct of the concepts of touch as they relate to nursing. Nursing Research 21(2): 102–110

Beeken J E, Parks D, Cory J, Montopoli G 1998 The effectiveness of neuromuscular release in five individuals with chronic obstructive lung disease. Clinical Nursing Research 7(3): 309–325

Bodian M 1969 Use of massage following lid surgery. Eye Ear Nose and Throat Monthly 48: 542–545

Brouwer B, Sousa de Andrade V 1995 The effects of slow stroking on spasticity in patients with multiple sclerosis: a pilot study. Physiotherapy Theory and Practice 11: 13–21

Brown S T, Douglas C, Flood L P 2001 Women's evaluation of intrapartum nonpharmacological pain relief methods used during labor. Journal of Perinatal Education 10(3): 1–8

Chia S H 1995 Evaluating groups in learning disabilities. Nursing Standard 10(9): 25–27

Chin P C 1959 Experiences in 16 cases of intestinal obstruction cured by abdominal massage. Shandong Yikan 18: 15

Cohen-Mansfield J, Marx M S, Werner P 1989 Agitation and touch in the nursing home. Psychological Reports 64: 1019–1026

Cole E L 1992 Hands on hands: the effects of hand massage on mentally ill people on an acute admissions ward. Association of Chartered Physiotherapists in Mental Health student project housed at Queen Margaret College, University of Edinburgh, Edinburgh

De Wever M K 1977 Nursing home patients' perception of affective touching. Journal of Psychology 96: 163–171

Dennis M 1995 Pain stress and misdiagnosis. In: Everett T, Dennis M, Ricketts E (eds) Physiotherapy in mental health. Butterworth-Heinemann, London, pp. 127–142

Dosseter D R, Couryer S, Nicol A R 1991 Massage for severe self-injurious behaviour in a girl with Cornelia de Lange syndrome. Developmental Medicine and Child Neurology 33: 636–644

Emly M 1993 Abdominal massage. Nursing Times 89(3): 34–36

Emly M, Cooper S, Vail A 1998 Colonic motility in profoundly disabled people: a comparison of massage and laxative therapy in the management of constipation. Physiotherapy 84(4): 178–183

Ernst E 1998 Does post-exercise massage treatment reduce delayed onset muscle soreness? A systematic review. British Journal of Sports Medicine 32(3): 212–214

Ernst E 1999 Abdominal massage therapy for chronic constipation: a systematic review of controlled clinical trials. Forschende Komplementarmedizin 6(3): 149–151

Fakouri C, Jones P 1987 Relaxation treatment: slow stroke back rub. Journal of Gerontological Nursing 13(2): 32–35

Farber S D 1982 A multisensory approach in neurorehabilitation. In: Farber S D (ed) Neurorehabilitation – a multisensory approach. W B Saunders, Philadelphia, PA

Field D A, Miller S 1992 Cosmetic breast surgery. American Family Physician 45(2): 711–719

Field T M, Schanberg S M, Scafidi F et al 1986 Tactile/kinesthetic stimulation effects on preterm neonates. Pediatrics 77(5): 654–658

Field T, Ironson G, Scafidi F et al 1996a Massage therapy reduces anxiety and enhances EEG patterns of alertness and math computations. International Journal of Neuroscience 86: 197–205

Field T, Seligman S, Scafidi F, Schanberg S 1996b Alleviating post-traumatic stress in children following Hurricane Andrew. Journal of Applied Developmental Psychology 17: 37–50

Field T, Grizzle N, Scafidi F, Schanberg S 1996c Massage relaxation therapies: effects on depressed adolescent mothers. Adolescence 31(124): 903–911

Field T, Schanbergs S, Davales M et al 1996d Massage with oil has more positive effects on newborn infants. Pre and Perinatal Psychology Journal 11: 73–38

Field T, Quintino O, Henteleff T et al 1997a Job stress reduction therapies. Alternative Therapies in Health and Medicine 3(4): 54–56

Field T, Lasko D, Mundy P et al 1997b Brief report: autistic children's attentiveness and responsivity improve after touch therapy. Journal of Autism and Development Disorders 27(3): 333–338

Field T, Hernandez-Reif M, Seligman S et al 1997c Juvenile rheumatoid arthritis: benefits from massage therapy. Journal of Paediatric Psychology 22(5): 607–617

Field T, Hernandez-Reif M, Lagreca A et al 1997d Massage therapy lowers blood glucose levels in children with diabetes mellitus. Diabetes Spectrum 10: 237–239

Field T, Hernandez-Reif M, Taylor S et al 1997e Labor pain is reduced by massage therapy. Journal of Obstetrics and Gynaecology 18(4): 286–291

Field T, Henteleff T, Hernandez-Reif M et al 1998a Children with asthma have improved pulmonary functions after massage therapy. Journal of Paediatrics 132(5): 854–858

Field T, Quintino O, Hernandez-Reif M, Koslovsky G 1998b Adolescents with attention deficit hyperactivity disorder benefit from massage therapy. Adolescence 33(129): 103–108

Field T, Peck M, Hernandez-Reif M et al 2000 Postburn itching pain and psychological symptoms are reduced with massage therapy. Journal of Burn Care and Rehabilitation 21(3): 189–193

Fischer R L, Bianculli K W, Sehdev H, Hediger M L 2000 Does light pressure effleurage reduce pain and anxiety associated with genetic amniocentesis? A randomized controlled trial. Journal of Maternal–Fetal Medicine 9(5): 294–297

Fraser J, Kerr J R 1993 Psychophysiological effects of back massage on elderly institutionalized patients. Journal of Advanced Nursing 18: 238–245

Gottleib G 1983 The psychobiological approach to developmental issues In: Mussen P H (ed) Handbook of child psychology, 2. Infancy. Wiley, New York

Gurland B J, Toner J A 1982 Depression in the elderly: a review of recently published studies. In: Eisdorfer C (ed) Annual review of geriatrics and gerontology. Springer, New York

Harrison J, Ruddle J 1995 An introduction to aromatherapy for people with learning disabilities. British Journal of Learning Disabilities 23: 37–40

Hartelius I, Ramussen L, Sygehus O 1992 How little you are? Neonatal Network 11(8): 33–37

Hernandez-Reif M, Field T, Field T, Theakston H 1998 Multiple sclerosis patients benefit from massage therapy. Journal of Bodywork and Movement Therapies 2(3): 168–174

Hernandez-Reif M, Martinez A, Field T et al 2000 Premenstrual symptoms are relieved by massage therapy. Journal of Obstetrics and Gynaecology 21(1): 9–15

Hernandez-Reif M, Field T, Largie S et al 2001 Children's distress during burn treatment is reduced by massage therapy. Journal of Burn Care and Rehabilitation 22(2): 191–195

Holey E A, Lawler H 1995 The effects of classical massage and connective tissue manipulation on bowel function. British Journal of Therapy and Rehabilitation 2(11): 627–631

Hondras M A, Linde K, Jones A P 2001 Manual therapy for asthma. Cochrane Database of Systematic Reviews, Issue 4, Oxford

Hulme J, Waterman H, Hillier V F 1999 The effect of foot massage on patients' perception of care following laparoscopic sterilization as day case patients. Journal of Advanced Nursing 30(2): 460–468

Isherwood D 1994 Baby massage groups. Modern Midwife (February): 21–23

Jones E, Dimmock P W, Spencer S A 2001 A randomised controlled trial to compare methods of milk expression after preterm delivery. Archives of Disease in Childhood: Fetal and Neonatal Edition 85(2): F91–95

Katz J, Wowk A, Culp D, Wakeling H 1999 Pain and tension are reduced among hospital nurses after on-site massage treatments: a pilot study. Journal of Perianesthesia Nursing 14(3): 128–133

Klauser A G, Flaschentrager J, Gehrke A, Muller-Lissner S A 1992 Abdominal wall massage: effect on colonic function in healthy volunteers and in patients with chronic constipation. Zeitschrift für Gastroenterologie 30: 247–251

Kleinke C L 1977 Compliance to requests made by gazing and touching experimentors in field settings. Journal of Experimental and Social Biology 13: 218–223

Kuznetskov O F, Makarova M R, Markina L P 1998 The comparative effect of classic massage of different intensities on patients with chronic salpingo-oophoritis. Voprosy Kurortologii Fizioterapii I Lechebnoi Fizicheskoi Kultury 2: 20–23

Langland R M, Panicucci C L 1982 Effects of touch on communication with elderly confused clients. Journal of Gerontological Nursing 8(3): 152–155

Levoska S, Keinanen-Kiukaanniemi S 1993 Active or passive physiotherapy for occupational cervico-brachial disorders? A comparison of 2 treatment methods with a 1 year follow-up. Archives of Physical Medicine 74(4): 425–430

Lindsay W R, Picaithly D, Geelen N et al 1997 A comparison of the effects of four therapy procedures on concentration and responsiveness in people with profound learning disabilities. Journal of Intellectual Disability Research 41(3): 201–207

Macedo E N 1984 Effects of very early tactile stimulation on very low birth weight infants: a 2-year follow-up study. Doctoral thesis, University of London, London

Marin I, Lepresle C, Mechet M A, Debesse B 1991 Postoperative pain after thoracotomy: a study of 116 patients. Revue des Maladies Respiratoires 8(2): 213–218

McInnes J, Treffry J 1982 Deaf–blind infants and children – a developmental guide. Open University Press, Milton Keynes

O'Brien J 1987 A guide to lifestyle planning. In: Wilcox B, Bellamy G T (eds) A comprehensive guide to the activities catalogue: an alternative curriculum for youth and adults with severe disabilities. Paul H Brookes, Baltimore, MD

Onozawa K, Glover V, Adams D et al 2001 Infant massage improves mother–infant interaction for mothers with postnatal depression. Journal of Affective Disorders 63(1–3): 201–207

O'Sullivan S B 1988 Strategies to improve motor control. In: O'Sullivan S B, Schmitz T J (eds) Physical rehabilitation: assessment and treatment. F A Davis, Philadelphia, PA

Partridge C J, Johnstone M, Morris L 1991 Disability and health services: perceptions beliefs and experiences of elderly people. Centre for Physiotherapy Research, King's College, London. Cited in: Smyth L 1993 Positive ageing. Physiotherapy 79(12): 823–824

Pheasant S T 1992 Does RSI exist? Occupational Medicine 42: 167–168

Pheasant S T 1994 Musculoskeletal injury at work: natural history and risk factors. In: Richardson B, Eastlake A (eds) Physiotherapy in occupational health. Butterworth-Heinemann, Oxford, pp. 146–170

Poon K 1991 Hand massage and music: the effectiveness of each as forms of relaxation therapy with dementia sufferers. Association of Chartered Physiotherapists in Mental Health course project housed at Queen Margaret College, University of Edinburgh, Edinburgh

Prosser E M 1941 A manual of massage and movements, 2nd edn. Faber and Faber, London

Resende T L, Brocklehurst J C, O'Neill P A 1993 A pilot study on the effect of exercise and abdominal massage on bowel habit in continuing care patients. Clinical Rehabilitation 7: 204–209

Rose N 1995 Psychiatric illnesses. In: Everett T, Dennis M, Ricketts E (eds) Physiotherapy in mental health. Butterworth-Heinemann, London, pp. 3–17

Rosenberg M W, Moore E G 1995 Demography of aging and disability. In: Pickles B, Compton A, Cott C, Vandervoort A (eds) Physiotherapy with older people. W B Saunders, London, pp. 19–28

Sanderson H, Harrison J, Price S 1991 Aromatherapy and massage for people with learning difficulties. Hands on Publishing, Birmingham

Scafidi F, Field T 1997 Massage therapy improves behaviour in neonates born to HIV positive mothers. Journal of Pediatric Psychology 21: 889–897

Scafidi F, Field T, Wheeden A et al 1996 Cocaine-exposed preterm neonates show behavioural and hormonal differences. Pediatrics 97: 851–855

Sirotkina A V 1964 Materials for the study of massage influence on paresis and paralysis of different etiology. PhD thesis, USSR. Cited in: Wine Z K 1995 Massage Magazine 55: 101–102. Noah Publishing Company, Davis, California

Sunshine W, Field T, Schanbergs S et al 1996 Massage therapy as compared to TENS improved sleep patterns and decreased pain fatigue anxiety depression and cortisol levels. Journal of Clinical Rheumatology 2: 18–22

Valentine K E 1984 Massage in psychological medicine – modern use of an ancient art. New Zealand Journal of Physiotherapy (December): 15–16

Vickers A, Ohlsson A, Lacy J B, Horsley A 2001 Massage for promoting growth and development of preterm and/or low birth-weight infants. Cochrane Library, Issue 4, Oxford

Weinrich S P, Weinrich M C 1990 The effect of massage on pain in cancer patients. Applied Nursing Research 3(4): 140–145

Wheeden A, Scafidi F A, Field T et al 1993 Massage effects on cocaine-exposed neonates. Developmental and Behavioral Pediatrics 14(5): 318–322

Wolfsenberger W 1983 Social role valorisation: a proposed new term for the principle of normalisation. Mental Retardation 21(6): 234–239

Yokoyama Y, Ueda T, Irahara M, Aono T 1994 Releases of oxytocin and prolactin during breast massage and suckling in puerperal women. European Journal of Obstetrics Gynecology and Reproductive Biology 53: 17–20

Index